Recurrent Pregnancy Loss

Sumita Mehta • Bindiya Gupta
Editors

Recurrent Pregnancy Loss

Springer

Editors
Sumita Mehta
Department of Obstetrics & Gynecology
Babu Jagjivan Ram Memorial Hospital
New Delhi
India

Bindiya Gupta
Department of Obstetrics and Gynecology
UCMS & GTB Hospital
New Delhi
India

ISBN 978-981-10-7337-3   ISBN 978-981-10-7338-0 (eBook)
https://doi.org/10.1007/978-981-10-7338-0

Library of Congress Control Number: 2018930908

Printed on acid-free paper

This Springer imprint is published by Springer Nature
The registered company is Springer Nature Singapore Pte Ltd.
The registered company address is: 152 Beach Road, #21-01/04 Gateway East, Singapore 189721, Singapore

Preface

"Let me recognize the gift in my ability to conceive and carry life however briefly.

Let me take joy in my ability to love so deeply and desire to nurture a soul unbeknownst to me.

Let a part of this soul be reflected in the spirit of my future children, born or adopted, so that I may know it through them."

Stacey Dinner-Levin

Recurrent pregnancy loss (RPL) is one area of reproductive medicine that is filled with controversy and confusion. With much ongoing research, new concepts are evolving and new treatment strategies are developed every now and then. Not only is the controversy restricted to management principles, even the definition has been variably given by two different societies.

The book has been divided into four parts for the reader's convenience. Part I deals with the definitions, epidemiology, and physiologic basis of a normal pregnancy. Etiology of recurrent pregnancy loss is a topic of much debate, and many theories and conflicting data exist to explain its causation. Part II describes in detail each causative factor and their respective management supported by latest evidence and research. The last two chapters in this part have effectively summarized all the latest recommendations and practices. An RPL couple is emotionally wrecked, and stress further increases the risk of abortion. We have specially introduced chapters covering this aspect. Parts III and IV discuss the areas of controversy and address management options and latest research clarifying the role of immunological and genetic therapy.

All the authors of the chapter are experts in their respective fields and have contributed immensely by sharing their vast clinical experience, expertise, and research. Overall, it is our honest effort to bring to you a book which has all relevant and updated information on this topic to facilitate decision making and optimal treatment for a couple with RPL.

Sumita Mehta
Bindiya Gupta

Contents

About the Editors

Sumita Mehta, DGO, DNB, FICOG, MAMS is a specialist and head at the Department of Obstetrics and Gynecology at Babu Jagjivan Ram Memorial Hospital, Delhi, India. She is the secretary of the Indian Society of Colposcopy and Cervical Pathology and a national expert for the project ECHO (Extension for Community Healthcare Outcomes) at the National Institute of Cancer Prevention and Research. She is an executive member and has served as an editor for the Association of Obstetricians and Gynecologists of Delhi. She is on the editorial board of journals *Heliyon* and the *Journal of Gynecology and Obstetrics Forecast* and is a reviewer for many international journals. Her special area of interest is in the field of gynecologic oncology, especially cervical cancer. She has conducted several colposcopy workshops throughout India and has delivered numerous lectures at various academic forums. She is the editor of 8 books and has published over 75 articles in national and international journals of repute.

Bindiya Gupta, M.D., AIIMS is presently working as an assistant professor at the Department of Obstetrics and Gynecology, UCMS and GTB Hospital, Delhi. She has published over 50 articles in national and international journals and has edited 2 books. She is presently editor for the Association of Obstetricians and Gynecologists of Delhi and was an editorial board member of the Indian College of Obstetricians and Gynecologists. She was web editor of NARCHI 2014–2016 and was coeditor of AOGD 2011–2012. A reviewer for various international journals, she also serves on the editorial board of two international journals. Her work has been recognized with several awards, including the FIGO best prize paper award from a developing country and FOGSI Junior Corion award.

Contributors

Nutan Agarwal Department of Obstetrics and Gynecology, All India Institute of Medical Sciences, New Delhi, India

Pakhee Aggarwal Obstetrics and Gynecology, Fortis Healthcare, New Delhi, India

Fortis Memorial Hospital, Gurgaon, India

Flt Lt Rajan Dhall Hospital and Aashlok Hospital, New Delhi, India

Darukshan Anjum Obstetrics and Gynecology, Babu Jagjiwan Ram Memorial Hospital, New Delhi, India

Nidhi Arora Apollo Center of Fetal Medicine, Indraprastha Apollo Hospital, New Delhi, India

Anupama Bahadur Obstetrics and Gynecology, All India Institute of Medical Sciences, Rishikesh, Uttrakhand, India

Sanskriti Batra Obstetrics and Gynecology, Institute of Obstetrics and Gynecology, Sir Ganga Ram Hospital, New Delhi, India

Punita Bhardwaj Obstetrics and Gynecology, Institute of Obstetrics and Gynecology, Sir Ganga Ram Hospital,, New Delhi, India

Juhi Bharti Obstetrics and Gynecology, All India Institute of Medical Sciences, New Delhi, India

Sruthi Bhaskaran Obstetrics and Gynecology, University College of Medical Sciences and GTB Hospital, New Delhi, India

Jaya Chaturvedi Obstetrics and Gynecology, All India Institute of Medical Sciences, Rishikesh, Uttrakhand, India

Latika Chawla Department of Obstetrics and Gynecology, All India Institute of Medical Sciences, Rishikesh, Uttrakhand, India

Sonia Chawla Obstetrics and Gynecology, University College of Medical Sciences and GTB Hospital, New Delhi, India

Tarun Das Obstetrics and Gynecology, Institute of Obstetrics and Gynecology, Sir Ganga Ram Hospital, New Delhi, India

Deepika Obstetrics and Gynecology, ESI Post Graduate Institute of Medical Science and Research, New Delhi, India

Shivaji Dhopte Obstetrics and Gynecology, Institute of Obstetrics and Gynecology, Sir Ganga Ram Hospital, New Delhi, India

Priyanka Gogoi Department of Pathology, University College of Medical Sciences and GTB Hospital, New Delhi, India

Aparna Goyal Department of Psychiatry, University College of Medical Sciences and Guru Teg Bahadur Hospital, Dilshad Garden, New Delhi, India

Anshul Grover Obstetrics and Gynecology, Babu Jagjiwan Ram Memorial Hospital, New Delhi, India

Namita Grover Obstetrics and Gynecology, ESIC Model Hospital, Industrial Area II, Chandigarh, India

Bindiya Gupta Obstetrics and Gynecology, University College of Medical Sciences and GTB Hospital, New Delhi, India

Monika Gupta Obstetrics and Gynecology, VMMC and Safdarjung Hospital, New Delhi, India

Nupur Gupta ESI Post Graduate Institute of Medical Science and Research, New Delhi, India

Sangeeta Gupta ESI Post Graduate Institute of Medical Science and Research, New Delhi, India

Taru Gupta ESI Post Graduate Institute of Medical Science and Research, Basaidarapur, Delhi, India

Vasudha Gupta Obstetrics and Gynecology, University College of Medical Sciences and GTB Hospital, New Delhi, India

Sandhya Jain Obstetrics and Gynecology, University College of Medical Sciences and GTB Hospital, New Delhi, India

Ritu Khatuja Obstetrics and Gynecology, Baba Sahib Ambedkar College of Medical Sciences, New Delhi, India

Kavita Khoiwal Obstetrics and Gynecology, All India Institute of Medical Sciences, New Delhi, India

Vidushi Kulshrestha Obstetrics and Gynecology, All India Institute of Medical Sciences, New Delhi, India

Sumita Mehta Obstetrics and Gynecology, Babu Jagjiwan Ram Memorial Hospital, New Delhi, India

Divya Pandey Obstetrics and Gynecology, Vardhman Mahavir Medical College and Safdarjung Hospital, New Delhi, India

Shalini Rajaram Obstetrics and Gynecology, University College of Medical Sciences and GTB Hospital, New Delhi, India

Rashmi Obstetrics and Gynecology, University College of Medical Sciences and GTB Hospital, New Delhi, India

Komal Rastogi Obstetrics and Gynecology, Maulana Azad Medical College and Lok Nayak Hospital, New Delhi, India

K. Aparna Sharma Obstetrics and Gynecology, All India Institute of Medical Sciences, New Delhi, India

Pooja Sikka Obstetrics and Gynecology, Postgraduate Institute of Medical Education and Research, Chandigarh, India

Alpana Singh Obstetrics and Gynecology, UCMS and GTB Hospital, New Delhi, India

Manpreet Singh Department of Anaesthesia and Intensive care, Government Medical College and Hospital, Chandigarh, India

Nilanchali Singh Obstetrics and Gynecology, Maulana Azad Medical College and LokNayak Hospital, New Delhi, India

Nisha Singh Obstetrics and Gynecology, King George Medical University, Lucknow, India

Pooja Singh Obstetrics and Gynecology, University College of Medical Sciences and GTB Hospital, New Delhi, India

Shweta Singh ESI Post Graduate Institute of Medical Science and Research, New Delhi, India

Seema Singhal Obstetrics and Gynecology, All India Institute of Medical Sciences, New Delhi, India

Anshuja Singla Obstetrics and Gynecology, University College of Medical Sciences and GTB Hospital, New Delhi, India

Sumeet Singla Department of Medicine, Maulana Azad Medical College and Lok Nayak Hospital, New Delhi, India

Ankita Srivastava Lok Nayak Jai Prakash Hospita, New Delhi, India

Mala Srivastava Institute of Obstetrics and Gynecology, Sir Ganga Ram Hospital, New Delhi, India

Shruti Srivastava University College of Medical Sciences and GTB Hospital, New Delhi, India

Amita Suneja Obstetrics and Gynecology, University College of Medical Sciences and GTB Hospital, New Delhi, India

Vaishali Upadhyaya Department of Radiodiagnosis, Vivekananda Polyclinic and Institute of Medical Sciences, Ramkrishna Mission Sewashram, Lucknow, India

Garima Vats Obstetrics and Gynecology, University College of Medical Sciences and GTB Hospital, New Delhi, India

Menka Verma Obstetrics and Gynecology, BSA Hospital, New Delhi, India

Swati Verma Obstetrics and Gynecology, ESIC Model Hospital, Industrial Area II, Chandigarh, India

Leena Wadhwa Obstetrics and Gynecology, ESI Post Graduate Institute of Medical Science and Research, New Delhi, India

Part I

Overview

Background, Epidemiology and Definition of Recurrent Pregnancy Loss

1

Alpana Singh, Ritu Khatuja, and Menka Verma

1.1 Background

Spontaneous pregnancy loss is often a common occurrence. Miscarriage is a spontaneous loss of pregnancy before the fetus reaches viability, i.e., gestation age up to 20 weeks or a weight of 500 g. The World Health Organization considers birth weight of 500 g to be used to define viability in developing countries, where gestational age is not certain [1]. Large numbers of pregnancies are lost before clinical confirmation, whereas around 15% of all clinically diagnosed pregnancies result in spontaneous abortion, and live births are seen in about 30% of all conceptions [2]. Spontaneous miscarriage is a physical and emotional trauma for the woman as well as for the family, especially when faced with recurrent losses. RPL is traditionally referred to as three or more consecutive pregnancy losses before 20 weeks of gestation. (Ectopic, molar, and biochemical pregnancies are excluded.)

1.2 Definitions and Terminology

Stirrat defined recurrent miscarriage as three or more pregnancy losses on the basis of epidemiological evidence [3]. Till date, the available data suggests that the risk of abortion is 30% and 33% after two miscarriages and three miscarriages, respectively. This strongly supports the role of evaluation after two miscarriages in women with history of no previous live birth [4]. Also the latest guidelines by the

A. Singh (✉)
Obstetrics and Gynecology, UCMS and GTB Hospital, Delhi, India
e-mail: dralpanasingh@gmail.com

R. Khatuja • M. Verma
Obstetrics and Gynecology, BSA Hospital, Delhi, India
e-mail: drritu.kj@gmail.com

S. Mehta, B. Gupta (eds.), *Recurrent Pregnancy Loss*,
https://doi.org/10.1007/978-981-10-7338-0_1

American Society for Reproductive Medicine define RPL as two or more pregnancy losses, which have been confirmed by either sonography or histopathological examination [5].

Studies also consider RPL as primary or secondary. Primary RPL miscarriages have never been carried to viability, whereas in the secondary type, live birth has occurred at some time [6, 7]. However, there is no specific terminology given to multiple spontaneous miscarriage interspersed with normal pregnancy. It is important to do an early evaluation in cases where fetal cardiac activity had been documented prior to the loss, in women who are older than 35 years and/or in couples with history of infertility. The timing of fetal demise provides etiologic clue, and its documentation is important in investigating the causes and treatment for RPL.

The European Society for Human Reproduction Special Interest Group for Early Pregnancy has revised terms for use in early pregnancy loss to confirm consistency for usage [8]. Pertinent recommendations are summarized in Table 1.1.

The European Society for Human Reproduction Special Interest Group for Early Pregnancy has defined recurrent miscarriage as three early consecutive losses or two late pregnancy losses.

Miscarriages can be divided into various types as follows:

Threatened miscarriage**:** There is uterine bleeding in early pregnancy which is associated with lower backache and cramping, but cervical os remains closed. This bleeding is usually due to implantation of embryo in the uterus. In this condition the process of abortion has been initiated, but further progression can be averted and pregnancy can be continued.

Inevitable miscarriage**:** In this condition uterine bleeding is associated with abdominal or lower back pain with an opening, dilatation, and effacement of the cervix. In this type of abortion, continuation of pregnancy is impossible as the changes have reached to advanced state.

Incomplete miscarriage**:** Type of abortion where some products are expelled, while some products are still inside the uterine cavity.

Complete miscarriage**:** In this type of abortion, the products of conception have been expelled from the uterus completely, and so subsequently bleeding, cramps, or pain also subside. The ultrasound confirms the diagnosis of complete abortion.

Table 1.1 Revised nomenclature in early pregnancy loss

Term	Definition
Biochemical pregnancy loss	Pregnancy not found by ultrasound
Empty sac	Ultrasound showing sac without any structure or minimal structures
Fetal loss	Previous CRL measurement with subsequent absence of fetal cardiac activity (FCA)
Early pregnancy loss	Scan showing empty sac or sac with fetus but no FCA (less than 12 weeks of gestation)
Late pregnancy loss	Loss of FCA in more than 12 weeks of gestation
Pregnancy of unknown location (PUL)	Pregnancy not identified on scan with positive hCG

***Missed miscarriage*:** Women can experience a miscarriage without knowing it. In this type of abortion, embryonic death has occurred without any expulsion of the embryo. There is loss of symptoms of pregnancy, and on ultrasound cardiac activity is absent.

***Blighted ovum*:** This is an anembryonic pregnancy. The fertilized egg implants into the uterine cavity, but the development of the fetus never begins. Usually gestational sac is there, but yolk sac may or may not be present, and the fetal pole is also absent.

***Septic abortion*:** Any type of abortion when accompanied by clinical evidence of pelvic infection.

1.3 Epidemiology

1.3.1 Incidence

RPL affects 0.4–1% of couples [9]. The risk of losing the pregnancy is more in early gestations, mostly in the first trimester. There is 22–57% of risk of miscarriage with pregnancy less than 6 weeks [10].

1.3.2 Prevalence

Prevalence of RPL is very uncertain since there is no nationwide registration of miscarriages or RPL in most of the places and many early miscarriages will not be treated in hospitals and are thus not registered. However, from various studies the prevalence of RPL is found to be between 0.6% and 2.3% [11, 12].

1.3.3 Risk Factors and Etiology

The couple with RPL has main concern for cause and risk of recurrence. Etiologies for RPL include genetic abnormalities, endocrine diseases, uterine anomaly, antiphospholipid syndrome (APS), thrombophilias (heritable or acquired), infections, immunologic abnormalities, and environmental factors. Also increased number of previous miscarriages, maternal age, lifestyle factors, and familiar factors are risk factors for RPL.

1.3.3.1 Number of Previous Miscarriages

The risk of future pregnancy losses can be predicted by the obstetric history of women. It has been reported that with every miscarriage, the risk of subsequent pregnancy loss increases (Table 1.2) [3].

Recurrent miscarriages occur generally at same gestation age in each pregnancy. In epidemiological studies three or more pregnancy losses are being considered for RPL, but clinical evaluation should be considered after two early pregnancies losses [5].

Table 1.2 Risk of miscarriage with consecutive pregnancies

Consecutive pregnancy	Risk of miscarriage (%)
First pregnancy	5–13
After first pregnancy loss	14–21
After second pregnancy loss	24–29
After third pregnancy loss	31–45

1.3.3.2 Maternal Age

Change in social and lifestyle leads to a trend of delay in child birth. Varies studies show that increasing maternal age is associated with the incidence of miscarriage [13, 14]. The miscarriage rates in women with RPL were almost identical in women of age 31–35 years and 36–39 years (38–40%) but increased to 70% in women of age 40–44 years [14]. It shows that the impact of age after 40 years is the strongest prognostic factor in RPL. The age of women with RPL has a role in the findings of studies of endocrinological and nongenetic immunological biomarkers. With progressing age the ovarian reserve as well as secretion of ovarian steroid hormones will be reduced. Immune parameters such as production of autoantibodies and T helper 2 cytokines are affected both directly by increased maternal age and diminished secretion of ovarian steroids [15].

1.3.3.3 Lifestyle Factors

It has been observed from different epidemiological studies that RPL is associated with obesity, high intake of caffeine or alcohol daily, use of nonsteroidal anti-inflammatory drugs, and excessive high impact physical exercise. The rate of pregnancy loss is also affected by social class and occupation. These women are at high risk of physical or psychical stress. It is also seen that women with PCOS exhibit an increased rate of miscarriage and RPL, but studies also showed the miscarriage rate in PCOS is not dependent on polycystic ovarian pathology if obesity is adjusted. Previous history of infertility also has an increased risk of miscarriage [16–22].

1.3.3.4 Family History

There are studies suggesting that RPL is increased in first-degree relatives [23, 24], and Christiansen et al. found the RPL frequency significantly increased in sisters of RPL [25]. Kolte et al. [26] found in their study a clinical miscarriage rate of 25.3% per pregnancy in siblings of RPL women, which is significantly higher ($p < 0.001$) than the rate of 13.1% in the background population.

It is also suggested that most RPL cases are probably caused by several genetic polymorphisms, each contributing only modestly to the total RPL risk, i.e., multifactorial inheritance [26].

1.4 Etiopathogenesis

Etiologies for RPL is summarized in Table 1.3 [27]. Despite a thorough evaluation for these causes, around 50% still remain unexplained.

1.4.1 Genetic Causes

Genetic factors comprise approximately 3.5–5% of RPL etiologies. These include structural chromosomal abnormalities like translocations, insertions, inversions, and mosaicism of which parental balanced and Robertsonian translocations have been reported as common causes of RPL. Monogenic disorders have also been reported as rare causes of repeated pregnancy losses. It is important to evaluate the karyotype of both partners as well as the abortus. Genetic counselling is imperative in such cases by a geneticist or a genetic counsellor, and preimplantation genetic diagnosis or donor gametes can be given as an option [27].

1.4.2 Anatomical Causes

Twelve to sixteen percent of RPL cases are associated with anatomic abnormalities. These include congenital uterine anomalies (incomplete mullerian fusion or septum, uterine artery anomalies, DES exposure, and cervical insufficiency) and acquired anomalies (intrauterine adhesions and uterine fibroids or polyps). Defective vascularization of endometrium leads to improper placentation and finally pregnancy loss. Congenital uterine anomalies are usually also linked with second trimester pregnancy losses. Septate uterus accounts for 76% risk of spontaneous abortion in affected women and it is the commonest uterine anomaly associated with RPL. Other uterine anomalies, like bicornuate, unicornuate, and didelphous uterus, have very low risk for RPL. Intrauterine adhesions result in early pregnancy losses due to its impact on placentation. It is found that RPL results if there is submucosal fibroid or intramural fibroids more than 5 cm size [28–30].

1.4.3 Endocrine Causes

Endocrinological causes are implicated for approximately 17–20% of RPL. These include luteal phase insufficiency, androgen disorder, thyroid disorders, and increased serum levels of prolactin. Also metabolic diseases such as polycystic ovarian syndrome (PCOS) and diabetes mellitus are included here.

Luteal phase defect, characterized by insufficient progesterone production resulting in retarded endometrial development, is thought to be associated with RPL. But there is no accurate test to evaluate the exact effect of LPD on RPL. In women with PCOS, there may be increase in level of luteinizing hormone or androgens or both leading to premature oocytes aging and defect in endometrium maturation [22, 31, 32]. There is correlation between insulin resistance and the resultant hyperinsulinemia in PCOS and diabetes mellitus with RPL, as there is the decreased in spontaneous pregnancy loss after getting treatment with the insulin sensitizing oral hypoglycemic agents [33]. Untreated hypothyroidism is clearly related with spontaneous miscarriage and RPL, but the association between antithyroid antibodies and RPL in euthyroid patients is not established [34–36]. The study by Hirahara F. et al.

Table 1.3 Proposed etiologies for RPL

Etiology	Incidence
Genetic factors	*3.5–5%*
(a) Chromosomal (b) Single gene defect (c) Multifactorial	
Anatomic factors	*12–16%*
(a) Congenital • Exposure to diethylstilbestrol • Uterine malformations • Cervical incompetence	
(b) Acquired • Cervical insufficiency • Synechiae • Leiomyomas • Adenomyosis	
Endocrine factor	*17–20%*
(a) Luteal phase defect (Lpd) (b) Polycystic ovarian syndrome (PCOS) (c) Other androgen abnormalities (d) Diabetes, thyroid disorders, hyperprolactinemia	
Infectious factors	*0.5–5%*
(a) Bacteria (b) Viruses (c) Parasites (d) Zarasites (e) Fungal	
Immunologic factors	*20–50%*
(a) Cellular mechanism • Suppressor cell or factor deficiency • Alteration in major histocomptibility antigen expression • Alteration in cellular immune regulation – TH1 immune responses to reproductive antigens (embryo or trophoblast) – TH2 cytokine or growth factor deficiency – Hormonal—progesterone, estrogen, prolactin, and androgen alterations – Tryptophan metabolism (b) Humoral mechanism • Antiphospholipid antibodies • Antithyroid antibodies • Antisperm antibodies • Antitrophoblast antibodies • Blocking antibodies deficiency	
Thrombotic factors	Not known
(a) Heritable thrombophilias • Single gene defect (FVL, MTHFR factors deficiency) • Antibody-mediated thrombosis (APS, anti-β-2 G1) (b) Acquired thrombophilias: Antiphospholipid antibody syndrome	
Other factors	*10%*

Table 1.3 (continued)

Etiology	Incidence
(a) Altered uterine receptivity (integrins, adhesion molecules) (b) Environmental • Toxins • Illicit drugs • Cigarettes and caffeines (c) Placental abnormalities (circumvallete and marginate) (d) Maternal medical illnesses (cardiac, renal, and hematological) (e) Male factors (f) Exercise (g) Dysynchronous fertilization	

suggested that a normal level of prolactin has an important role in maintaining early pregnancy [37].

1.4.4 Infections

The relation between infection and recurrent pregnancy losses is not established. But infections like *Listeria monocytogenes*, herpes simplex virus, measles, toxoplasmosis, rubella, and cytomegalovirus are associated with sporadic spontaneous abortion. The mechanism of miscarriage can be due to infection of the uterus, fetus, or placenta, placental insufficiency, or infected intrauterine device [27].

1.4.5 Immunologic Causes

Immunologic causes account for 20–50% of all RPL cases [38]. The autoimmune and alloimmune mechanisms are associated with this. The role of aberrant immunologic factors in pregnancy losses is not clear as the mechanism of the mother to accept semi-allogenic zygote is not well understood.

Several autoimmune diseases have been linked to RPL, but the most common autoimmune disorder, Anti phospholipid antibody syndrome (APS), is associated with poor obstetric outcomes, including RPL. Despite incompletely understood mechanism of recurrent miscarriage due to autoimmune factors, anticardiolipin antibodies and lupus anticoagulant should be included in RPL evaluation.

Other immunological factors, i.e., alloimmune factors, may cause RPL by the same principle of graft rejection in transplant recipients. It has been found in cases of RPL that there is deficiency of essential constituents of the immunological pathways which provide protection to the embryos, such as appropriate expression of complement regulatory proteins (e.g., mannan-binding lectin, apoptosis-inducing TNF superfamily members, macrophage inhibitory cytokine 1, Th1/Th2/Th3-type cytokines, and HLA-DR, HLA-G or HLA-E) [27, 39].

1.4.6 Thrombotic Causes

Factor V Leiden mutation and mutations in the gene encoding methylene tetrahydrofolate reductase (MTHFR) and prothrombin gene are the most common thrombotic etiology. The heritable thrombophilias associated with RPL are increased levels of serum homocysteine, prothrombin promoter mutations, protein C and protein S deficiencies, and antithrombin mutations. Hyperhomocysteinemia and activated protein C resistance are linked with acquired thrombophilias .The proposed mechanism is thought to be thrombosis of spiral arteries, and the intervillous space on the maternal side of the placenta can impair adequate placental perfusion. The resulting abnormalities of the uteroplacental circulation may cause late fetal loss, intrauterine growth restriction, placental abruption, or preeclampsia [27, 40].

1.4.7 Other Causes

Environmental and occupational exposures to organic solvents, toxins, ionizing radiation, and medications can affect uterine receptivity which may have a role in causation of RPL. However, no strong co-relation has been found between RPL and occupational factors, stress, or chemicals factors as most evidence in this respect is retrospective [27].

Smoking, alcohol, and caffeine addiction are associated with RPL in a dose-dependent manner, or they also may act synergistically to increase sporadic miscarriages.

Key Points

- Miscarriage is defined as the spontaneous loss of pregnancy before the fetus reaches viability, i.e., until 20 weeks of gestation. The World Health Organization considers a birth weight of 500 g to define viability in developing countries, when gestation age is not certain.
- Recurrent miscarriage is defined as the loss of three or more consecutive pregnancies, but clinical evaluation should be started following two first trimester pregnancy losses.
- Studies suggest that the effect of maternal age, lifestyle, and parental factors and risk of miscarriage with each subsequent pregnancy loss have a strong correlation with RPL.
- RPL is multifactorial, and the causes include genetic abnormality, uterine anatomic abnormalities, endocrinal disorder, immunological factors, and thrombotic factors. Although infections and environmental factors are also included in the list, their association to RPL is not clear.
- In spite of a large list of etiology, approximately half of all cases will remain unexplained.
- Assessment and counselling of couple with recurrent pregnancy losses should be done in a committed clinic. They should be given psychological support and reassurance, and detailed information should be documented so that decision for future pregnancies is optimal.

References

1. WHO recommended definitions, terminology and format for statistical tables related to the perinatal period. Acta Obstet Gynecol Scand. 1977;56:247–53.
2. Macklon NS, Geraedts JPM, Fauser BCJM. Conception to ongoing pregnancy: the "black box" of early pregnancy loss. Hum Reprod Update. 2002;8:333–43.
3. Stirrat GM. Recurrent miscarriage: definition and epidemiology. Lancet. 1990;336:673–5.
4. The American College of Obstetricians and Gynecologists. Management of recurrent early pregnancy loss. Washington, DC: The American College of Obstetricians and Gynecologists; 2001. ACOG Practice Bulletin No. 24.
5. Practice Committee of the American Society for Reproductive Medicine. Definitions of infertility and recurrent pregnancy loss. Fertil Steril. 2008;89:1603.
6. Ansari AH, Kirkpatrick B. Recurrent pregnancy loss: an update. J Reprod Med. 1998;43:806.
7. Paukku M, Tulppala M, Puolakkainen M, et al. Lack of association between serum antibodies to Chlamydia trachomatis and a history of recurrent pregnancy loss. Fertil Steril. 1999;72:427.
8. Farquharson RG, Jauniaux E, Exalto N, ESHRE Special Interest Group for Early Pregnancy (SIGEP). Updated and revised nomenclature for description of early pregnancy events. Hum Reprod. 2005;20:3008–11.
9. Salat-Baroux J. Recurrent spontaneous abortions. Reprod Nutr Dev. 1988;28:1555–68.
10. Wilcox AJ, Weinberg CR, O'Connor JF, et al. Incidence of early loss of pregnancy. N Engl J Med. 1988;319(4):189–94.
11. Warburton D, Strobino B. Recurrent spontaneous abortion. In: Bennet MJ, Edmonds DK, editors. Spontaneous and recurrent abortion. Oxford: Blackwell Scientific; 1987. p. 193–213.
12. Fertility and Employment 1979. The Danish Data Archives no. 0363, Odense University.
13. Lund M, Kamper-Jørgensen M, Nielsen HS, Lidegaard Ø, Andersen AM, Christiansen OB. Prognosis for live birth in women with recurrent miscarriage. What is the best measure of success? Obstet Gynecol. 2012;119:37–43.
14. Nybo Andersen AM, Wohlfahrt J, Christens P, Olsen J, Melbye M. Maternal age and fetal loss: population based register study. BMJ. 2000;320:1708–12.
15. Raghupathy J, Al-Mutawa E, Al-Azemi M, Makhseed M, Azizieh H, Szekeres-Bartho J. Progesterone-induced blocking factor (PIBF) modulates cytokine production by lymphocytes from women with recurrent miscarriage or preterm birth. J Reprod Immunol. 2009;80:91–9.
16. Rasch V. Cigarette, alcohol, and caffeine consumption: risk factors for spontaneous abortion. Acta Obstet Gynecol Scand. 2003;82:182–8.
17. Fedorcsak P, Storeng R, Dale PO, Tanbo T, Abyholm T. Obesity is a risk factor for early pregnancy loss after IVF or ICSI. Acta Obstet Gynecol Scand. 2000;79:43–8.
18. Li DK, Liu L, Odouli R. Exposure to non-steroidal anti-inflammatory drugs during pregnancy and risk of miscarriage: population based cohort study. BMJ. 2003;327:368–72.
19. Brandt LP, Nielsen CV. Job stress and adverse outcome of pregnancy: a causal link or recall bias? Am J Epidemiol. 1992;35:302–11.
20. Madsen M, Jørgensen T, Jensen ML, Juhl M, Olsen J, Andersen PK, et al. Leisure time physical exercise during pregnancy and the risk of miscarriage: a study within the Danish National Birth Cohort. BJOG. 2007;114:1419–26.
21. Wang JX, Norman RJ, Wilcox AJ. Incidence of spontaneous abortion among pregnancies produced by assisted reproductive technology. Hum Reprod. 2004;19:272–7.
22. Wang JX, Davies MJ, Norman RJ. Polycystic ovarian syndrome and the risk of spontaneous abortion following assisted reproductive technology treatment. Hum Reprod. 2001;16:2606–9.
23. Alexander SA, Latinne D, Debruyere M, Dupont E, Gottlieb W, Thomas K. Belgian experience with repeat immunization in recurrent spontaneous abortion. In: Beard RW, Sharp F, editors. Early pregnancy loss: mechanisms and treatment. London: Springer; 1988. p. 355–63.
24. Ho H, Gill TJ, Hsieh C, Yang YS, Le TY. The prevalence of recurrent spontaneous abortion, cancer, and congenital anomalies in the families of couples with recurrent spontaneous abortions or gestational trophoblastic tumors. Am J Obstet Gynecol. 1991;165:461–6.
25. Christiansen OB, Mathiesen O, Lauritsen JG, Grunnet N. Idiopathic recurrent spontaneous abortion. Evidence of a familial predisposition. Acta Obstet Gynecol Scand. 1990;69:597–601.

26. Kolte AM, Nielsen HS, Moltke I, Degn B, Pedersen B, Sunde L, et al. A genome-wide scan in affected sibling pairs with idiopathic recurrent miscarriage suggests genetic linkage. Mol Hum Reprod. 2011;17:279–85.
27. Fox-Lee L, Schust DJ. Recurrent pregnancy loss. In: Berek JS, editor. Berek and Novak's gynecology. Philadelphia: Lippincott Williams & Wilkins; 2012. p. 1190–232.
28. Lin PC. Reproductive outcomes in women with uterine anomalies. J Womens Health. 2004;13:33–9.
29. Bajekal N, Li TC. Fibroids, infertility and pregnancy wastage. Hum Reprod Update. 2000;6:614–20.
30. Raga F, Bauset C, Remohi J, et al. Reproductive impact of congenital Müllerian anomalies. Hum Reprod. 1997;12:2277–81.
31. Bussen S, Sutterlin M, Steck T. Endocrine abnormalities during the follicular phase in women with recurrent spontaneous abortion. Hum Reprod. 1999;14:18–20.
32. Watson H, Kiddy DS, Hamilton-Fairley D, et al. Hypersecretion of luteinizing hormone and ovarian steroids in women with recurrent early miscarriages. Hum Reprod. 1993;8:829–33.
33. Glueck CJ, Wang P, Goldenberg N, Sieve-Smith L. Pregnancy outcomes among women with polycystic ovary syndrome treated with metformin. Hum Reprod. 2002;17:2858–64.
34. Vaquero E, Lazzarin N, De Carolis H, et al. Mild thyroid abnormalities and recurrent spontaneous abortion: diagnostic and therapeutical approach. Am J Reprod Immunol. 2000;43:204–8.
35. Kutteh WH, Yetman DL, Carr AC, et al. Increased prevalence of antithyroid antibodies identified in women with recurrent pregnancy loss but not in women undergoing assisted reproduction. Fertil Steril. 1999;71:843–8.
36. Rushworth FH, Backos M, Rai R, et al. Prospective pregnancy outcome in untreated recurrent miscarriers with thyroid autoantibodies. Hum Reprod. 2000;15:1637–9.
37. Hirahara F, Andoh N, Sawai K, et al. Hyperprolactinemic recurrent miscarriage and result of randomized bromocriptine treatment trials. Fertil Steril. 1998;70:246.
38. Thellin O, Coumans B, Zorzi W, et al. Tolerance of the foeto-placental "graft": ten ways to support a child for nine months. Curr Opin Immunol. 2000;12:731–7.
39. Porter TF, LaCoursiere Y, Scott JR. Immunotherapy for recurrent miscarriage. Cochrane Database Syst Rev. 2006;(2):CD000112.
40. Kruse C, Steffensen R, Varming K, Christiansen OB. A study of HLA-DR and -DQ alleles in 588 patients and 562 controls confirms that HLA-DRB1*03 is associated with recurrent miscarriage. Hum Reprod. 2004;19:1215.

Normal Implantation, Placentation, and Fetal Development

2

Taru Gupta, Shweta Singh, Sangeeta Gupta, and Nupur Gupta

2.1 Introduction

Implantation is defined as a process of attachment and invasion of the uterine endometrium by the blastocyst [1]. A healthy female will have predictable, regular, cyclical, and spontaneous ovulation which is regulated by complex interaction of the HPO axis, ovaries, and genital tract. With ovulation, secondary oocyte and cumulus oocyte complex is released in the peritoneal cavity and is picked up by the fimbrial end of the fallopian tube. This oocyte is transported to the ampullary end of the fallopian tube by its ciliary action where fertilization takes place. Fertilization window is narrow, and almost all pregnancies are reported when successful intercourse occurs 2 days preceding or on the day of ovulation.

After fertilization, a diploid cell with 46 chromosomes is formed called as zygote. The zygote undergoes cleavage, and further cleaved cells are called blastomeres. As the cleavage proceeds, after 3 days of fertilization, the ovum comes to a 16-cell stage. It looks like a mulberry and is called as morula. And at this stage, it enters in the uterine cavity. Morula is surrounded by zona pellucida and consists of inner cell mass and outer cell layer called as trophectoderm. The inner cell mass later on gives rise to embryo proper, and trophoblast provides nutrition to the inner cell mass. Once morula enters the uterine cavity, there is gradual accumulation of fluid which partially separates inner cell mass from trophectoderm and is now called as the blastocyst [2]. The cavity of the blastocyst is called as blastocele as shown in Fig. 2.1. Zona pellucida prevents the embryo from sticking to the fallopian tube and upper uterine cavity as it travels down and hence prevents implantation of embryo at abnormal site. Once blastocyst is formed and reaches the uterine cavity, the zona pellucida disappears under the influence of specific proteases which are released from the endometrium during the secretory phase.

T. Gupta (✉) • S. Singh • S. Gupta • N. Gupta
ESI Post Graduate Institute of Medical Science and Research, Basaidarapur, Delhi, India
e-mail: tarugupta1971@yahoo.com

S. Mehta, B. Gupta (eds.), *Recurrent Pregnancy Loss*,
https://doi.org/10.1007/978-981-10-7338-0_2

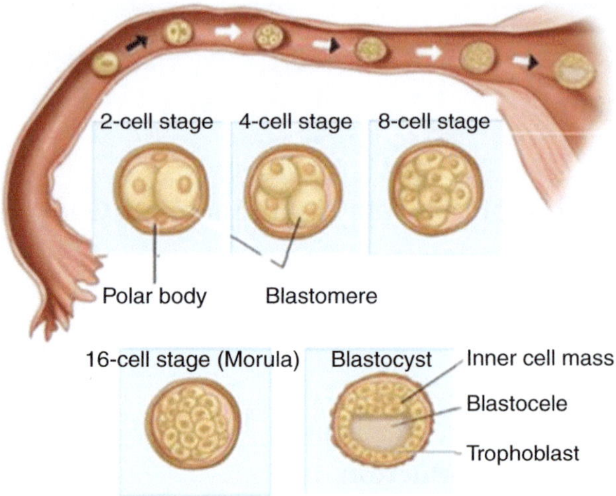

Fig. 2.1 Zygote cleavage, morula, and blastocyst formation [3]

2.2 The Decidua

The endometrium of pregnancy is highly modified and specialized for proper hemochorial implantation, that is, one in which maternal blood comes in contact with trophoblast. This specialized endometrium is known as decidua, and decidualization is the transformation of secretory endometrium in which the stromal cells of secretory endometrium enlarge, become vacuolated, and store glycogen and lipids. This change in stromal cells is called decidual reaction, which is completed only after blastocyst implantation. The attachment of trophoblast is enhanced by the pericellular matrix which is secreted by the decidual cells (Fig. 2.2).

Decidualization depends on estrogen, progesterone, cytokines, and hormones secreted from the blastocyst, once it gets hatched from the zona pellucida. Blastocyst secretes IL-1 and IL-2 cytokines and hCG hormone which influence the endometrium receptivity, and it secretes leukemia inhibitory factor (LIF) and colony-stimulating factor-1 (CSF-1). These increase the trophoblast protease which by degradation of extracellular matrix helps in "hatching" leading to trophoblast invasion. Bone morphogenic protein 2 (BMP 2) which is a nonactive precursor protein is cleaved by proprotein convertase 5/6 (PC6) to produce active form, which helps in decidualization [4]. If there is deletion of BMP2 or PC6, it leads to inhibition of decidualization and implantation, thereby causing infertility [3].

The decidua is classified into three parts based on anatomical location as shown in Fig. 2.3.

Decidua basalis: this is the decidua directly beneath the blastocyst implantation site, where the placenta will be formed. It is invaded by trophoblasts and is also referred as decidual plate.

Decidua capsularis: this is the part of the decidua which overlies the enlarging blastocyst and separates the conceptus from the uterine lumen. This is more prominent during the second month of pregnancy and contains flattened single layer of decidual cells.

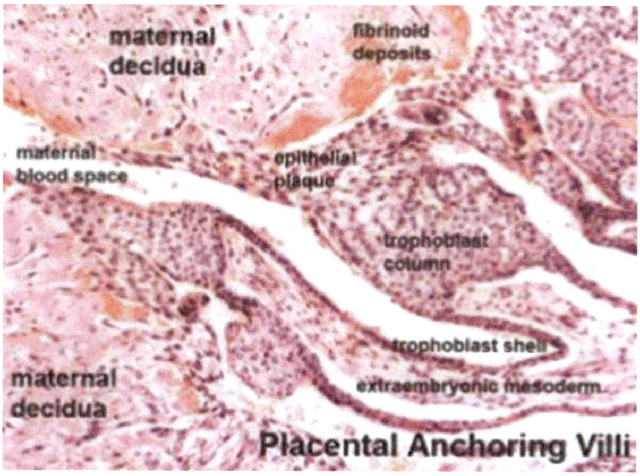

Fig. 2.2 Decidual reaction with placental anchoring villi

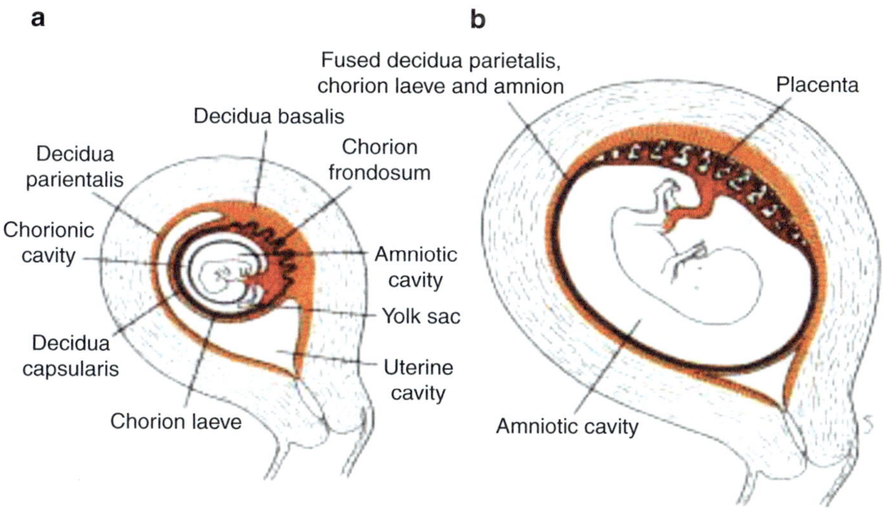

Fig. 2.3 The decidua and fetal membranes. (**a**) Second month of pregnancy, (**b**) third month [2]

Decidua parietalis: the remainder of uterine cavity is lined by the decidua parietalis.

Initially, there is a space between the decidua capsularis and decidua parietalis; after 14–16 weeks, this space is obliterated by the growing sac, which results in apposition of the decidua capsularis and parietalis and forms the decidua vera functionally obliterating the uterine cavity.

Decidua consists of three zones: the outer most compact layer is called as zona compacta, middle spongy layer called zona spongiosa, and a basal layer with glands and small blood vessels known as zona basalis. Zona compacta and zona spongiosa together form zona functionalis. In the initial stages, glands of the decidua serve as a source of essential nutrients for the embryo till these are supplied by the maternal blood. The decidua also contributes to the protection of the embryo from immunologic rejection and the uterine wall from excessive invasion by the embryo. During delivery, decidua sheds off, along with the placenta and membranes, and the basal zone remains and helps in regeneration of endometrium.

2.3 Blastocyst Implantation

After 6 days of fertilization, the blastocyst implants in the decidua. The process of implantation is divided into three steps: apposition, adhesion, and invasion [1, 2] (Fig. 2.8).

Apposition: Initially, a blastocyst comes in contact with the endometrium, and the process is called as apposition or adplantation. This process requires the adhesion interaction of newly hatched blastocyst with endometrium during the "receptive window." If implantation has not proceeded sufficiently during this receptive window of menstrual cycle, then there is loss of conceptus.

When the blastocyst initially implants, the endometrium is 5 mm thick making the cavity of the uterus only slit like which helps in apposition of blastocyst with endometrium.

Adhesion: It is defined as increased physical contact between the blastocyst and decidua. The process of adhesion of the blastocyst starts at the site of apposition. For successful adhesion formation, expression of certain local cytokines, trophinin, and galectin-9 and cellular adhesion molecules (CAM) are required. The integrins—one of four families of CAMs—are cell-surface receptors that mediate cell adhesion to extracellular matrix proteins.

Leukemia inhibitory factor (LIF): leukemia inhibitory factor (LIF) is also associated with successful implantation [5] (Figs. 2.4 and 2.5). LIF upregulates endometrial expression of heparin-binding epidermal growth factor (HB-EGF), which causes growth of the trophoblast and hatching of the blastocyst. hCG from the blastocyst further stimulates the production of LIF.

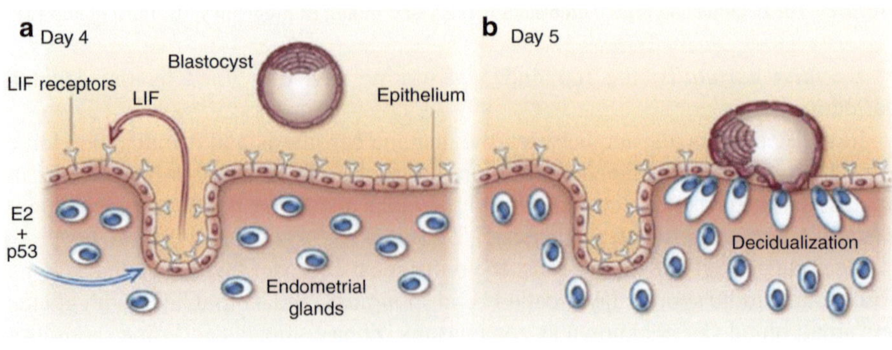

Fig. 2.4 (**a**) Day 4 of pregnancy, estrogen (E2) induces LIF expression in the endometrial glands, and LIF is secreted into the uterine lumen [5]. (**b**) Implantation by day 5 of pregnancy [5]

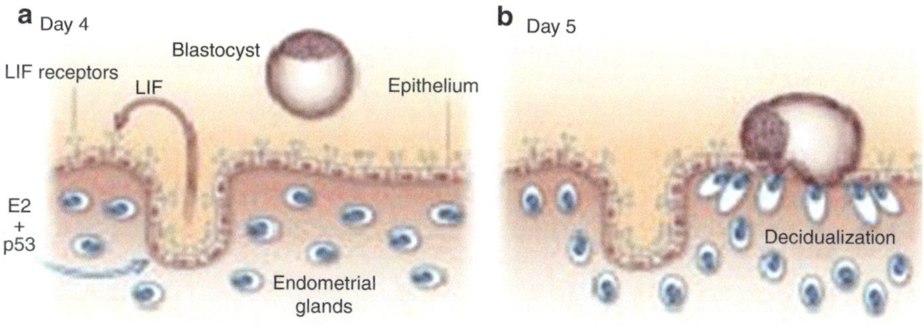

Fig. 2.5 LIF expression

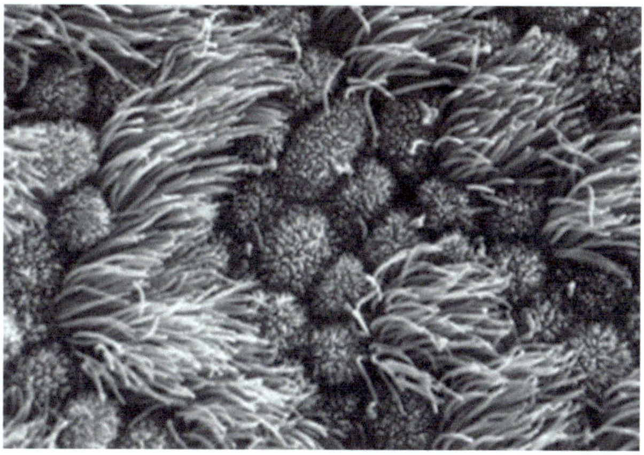

Fig. 2.6 Human uterine tube ciliated epithelium on electron microscopy

MUC-1: The luminal cells of the endometrium have a mucus-coated microvillous border. Mucin forms major component and MUC-1 a trans-membrane protein which acts as antimicrobial, anti-adhesive, and anti-infective. Expression of MUC-1 varies over the menstrual cycle and is upregulated by progesterone. Decreased MUC-1 expression is associated with receptivity, and hence, high levels of mucin are inhibitory to implantation, while later on this mucin is expressed on placental amnion where it acts as antibacterial and has antimicrobial roles.

Trophinin: Trophinin are expressed on blastocyst trophectoderm cells and on uterine epithelial cells. Adhesion occurs through this trophinin-trophinin binding, and it also triggers trophectoderm cells for invasion and proliferation and induces programmed cell death (apoptosis) in maternal endometrial epithelial cells.

Uterine epithelium and uterodomes: Uterine epithelial cilia (Fig. 2.6) help in initial movement of oocyte and conceptus, while epithelial microvilli help in the implantation process. Both are hormone regulated but have different physical properties as shown in Table 2.1

Table 2.1 Properties of endometrial cilia and microvilli

Cilia	Microvilli
• Have long processes	• Have short processes
• Epithelial cells have apical membrane specialization	• Epithelial cells have apical membrane specialization
• Microtubules are filled with motile structure	• Microfilament is filled with non-motile structure
• Ciliated cell numbers are under control of estrogen	• Microvilli length is hormonally controlled. While progesterone has control over short microvilli, estrogen controls long and thin microvilli

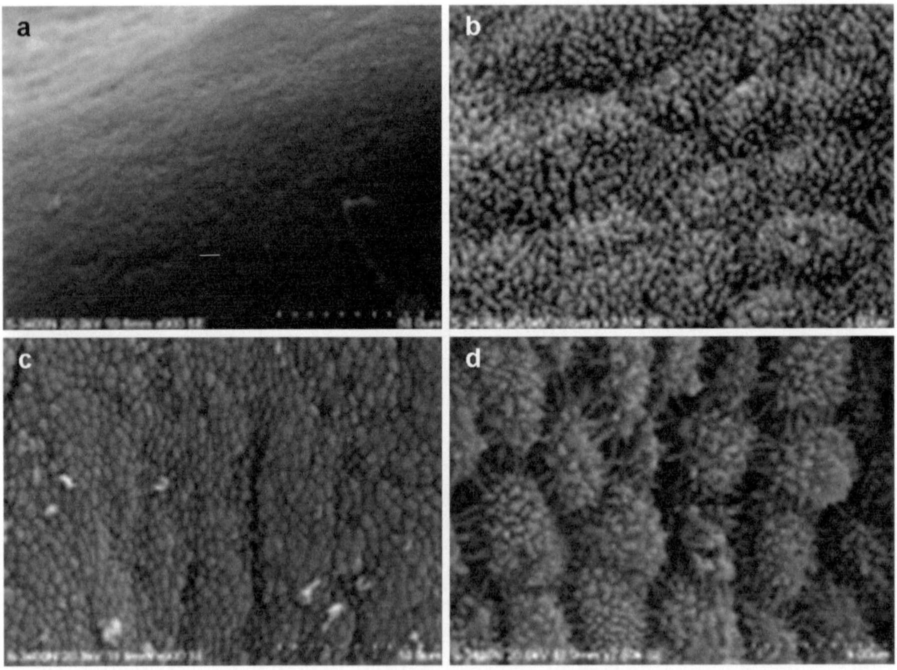

Fig. 2.7 Electron microscopic view of uterodomes

Changes in the cytoskeleton of endometrial epithelial lining cells also occur during the receptive phase; apex of microvilli fuse to form pinopods, which facilitates adhesion between the syncytiotrophoblast and endometrial epithelial cell membranes. Since their role is not only limited to pinocyte activity, hence, an alternative name is given as "uterodomes" depending upon their appearance in electron microscope [6] (EM) (Fig. 2.7). For the process of apposition and adhesion, it is important that the blastocyst is not rejected. This is achieved by HLA-G which inhibits cytotoxic T cells. In addition the populations of both T and B cells are reduced at the site of invasion.

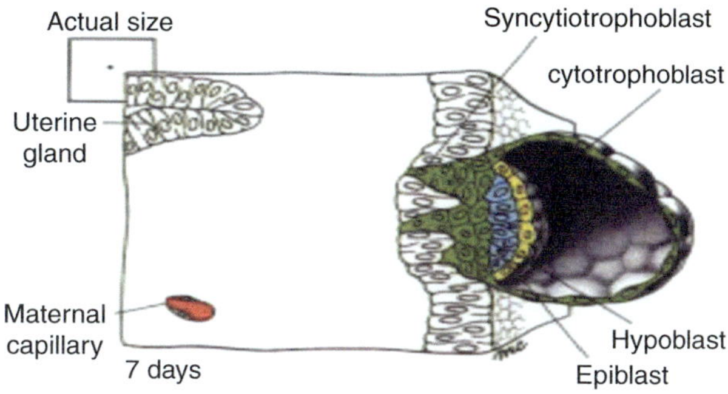

Fig. 2.8 Day 8: Syncytiotrophoblast invades the uterine epithelium

Galectin-9: Galectin-9 is a protein that binds galactosides and is a maker for mid- and late secretory phase of human endometrium and decidua [7]. It is also expressed at uterodomes during implantation which suggests that it may also help in endometrial receptivity.

Invasion: It is defined as penetration and invasion of syncytiotrophoblast and cytotrophoblasts into the endometrium, inner third of myometrium, and uterine vasculature. Implantation is completed by day 9, and a coagulation plug is formed where the blastocyst has entered the uterine wall by day 12 (Fig. 2.8). As the blastocyst invades the endometrium, the syncytiotrophoblast cells form junctional complexes with the endometrial epithelial cells, and the trophoblast insinuates between the epithelial cells and into the basal laminae. The decidual cells themselves may contribute to the breakdown of the basal lamina. Also, syncytiotrophoblast cells also secrete agents that induce apoptosis in local endometrial cells, which they phagocytize. There are specific set of integrins which are involved in implantation. Specifically, Vβ3 and α4β1 integrins are expressed on endometrial epithelium and considered as receptive marker for blastocyst attachment. Aberrant expression of Vβ3 is associated with infertility.

Nitabuch's layer: Also called as fibrinoid layer, it is formed at the maternal/fetal interface during placental development and helps in prevention of deeper implantation of conceptus.

2.4 Factors Preventing Immune Rejection of Implanting Conceptus

The embryo being implanted is actually foreign to maternal immune system, so to prevent it from rejection, there are various maternal and embryonic mechanisms which act simultaneously.

Decidual cells

1. *Decidual macrophages*: play a regulatory role at fetal-maternal interface by helping in tissue remodeling and inhibiting inflammation.

2. *Decidual T cell*: these are activated by fetal HLA-C expressed in extravillous trophoblast cells. They are specific to immune tolerance to fetal alloantigens.
3. *Uterine natural killer cells*: HLA-C activates killer inhibitory receptors and hence prevents immune rejection.

Chemokine gene silencing: it prevents the attraction of maternal immune cells by epigenetic silencing of chemokine expression in the decidual stromal cells [8].

Corticotropin-releasing hormone: CRH which is secreted by both mother and conceptus kills the maternal immune cells. CRH is secreted by both maternal and implanting conceptus at the site of implantation. It binds to the receptors on the surface of trophoblast cells and activates an extrinsic cell death pathway on local maternal immune cells [9].

2.5 Placental Development

The blastocyst consists of flattened trophoblastic cells and inner cell mass which is eccentrically attached to trophoblast. Inner cell mass differentiates into endoderm, ectoderm, and mesoderm. The human placenta originates from the trophectoderm, which originates from trophoblast.

2.5.1 Role of Trophoblast

It helps in formation of all components of placenta. Its invasiveness promotes implantation, it provides nutrition to the early embryo, and it secretes some hormones which are essential for maternal physiological adaptation and maintenance of pregnancy [10].

2.5.2 Trophoblast Differentiation

After implantation, the trophoblast differentiates into outer multinucleated syncytium, primitive syncytioblast, and inner layer of primitive mononuclear cells called as cytotrophoblasts. Cytotrophoblasts retain their cell wall and have ability to undergo DNA synthesis and mitosis and lie deep to syncytium and rest on extra-embryonic mesoderm. Syncytiotrophoblast which remain nearest to decidua lose their cell boundaries and have continuous sheet of cytoplasm containing multiple nuclei form a loose amorphous syncytium and it helps in transport.

After implantation is complete, cytotrophoblast further differentiates into **villous trophoblast and extravillous trophoblast** [11]. The villous trophoblast gives rise to chorionic villi, which primarily help in transport of oxygen and nutrients and exchange of compounds between fetus and mother. Extravillous trophoblast migrates into decidua and myometrium and maternal vasculature and helps in penetration. They are further divided into two types, **interstitial trophoblast and**

endovascular trophoblast. Interstitial trophoblast invades the decidua and myometrium and forms placental bed, while endovascular trophoblast invades the spiral artery lumina and helps in transformation of high-resistance blood flow to low-resistance blood flow.

2.5.3 Chorionic Villous Formation

Syncytiotrophoblast has property of invasion and hence invades maternal deciduas basalis and thickens. By 12th day of fertilization, small cavities appear in this layer and form lacunae (Fig. 2.9). Lacunae are radially arranged around the blastocyst and separated by portions of syncytium which are called as trabeculae. Eventually, these small lacunae join to form large lacunar spaces which surround each trabecula. By the 12th postfertilization day, extravillous cytotrophoblasts line the trabeculae which were formed initially by syncytiotrophoblast, and now trabeculae are called as primary villous, and lacunar space is called as inter villous space. The extraembryonic mesoderm invades the primary villous and forms secondary villous. Later on a blood vessel arises in the core of the mesoderm, and now it is called as tertiary villous (Fig. 2.10). By the 17th postfertilization day, the fetal blood vessels are functional, and feto-placental circulation is established in villi (Fig. 2.11) [2].

Villi thus formed are covered by outer layer of syncytium and an inner layer of cytotrophoblasts (Langerhans cells). Villous tips are proliferated by cytotrophoblasts and form trophoblastic cell column that are called as anchoring villi which are not invaded by fetal mesenchyme and anchored to decidua at basal plate. Hence, the basal plate consists of cytotrophoblasts from cell column, the covering shell of syncytiotrophoblast, and maternal decidua. The base of intervillous space faces the maternal side. The chorionic plate consists of two layers of trophoblast externally and fibrous mesoderm internally. The base of chorionic plate forms the roof of intervillous space. By 8–10 weeks definitive chorionic plate is formed, and amniotic and

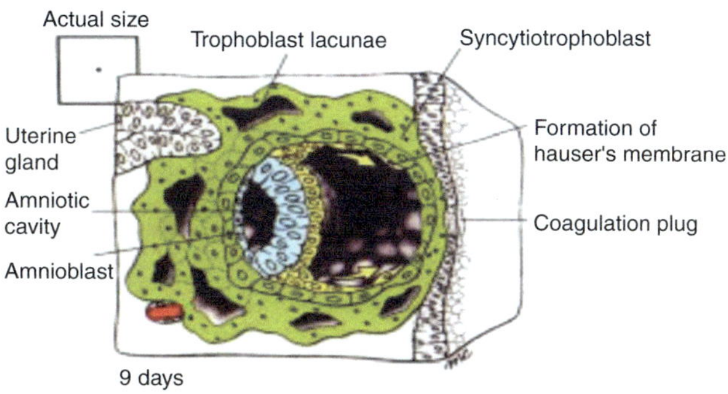

Fig. 2.9 By 9 days the embryo is completely implanted [2]

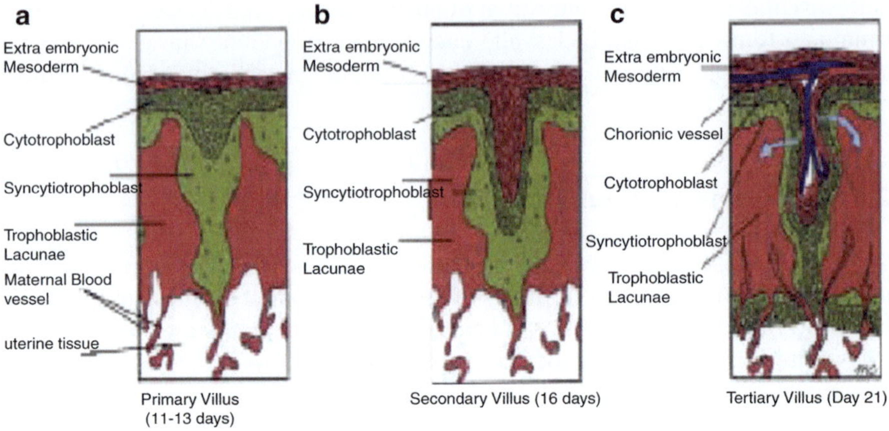

Fig. 2.10 Formation of the chorionic villi. (**a**) Primary stem is seen as cytotrophoblastic proliferation bud into the overlying syncytiotrophoblast. (**b**) Secondary villi are formed by day 16. (**c**) Tertiary villi are formed by day 21

Fig. 2.11 Embryonic blood vessels exchange nutrients with maternal plasma in intervillous space [2]

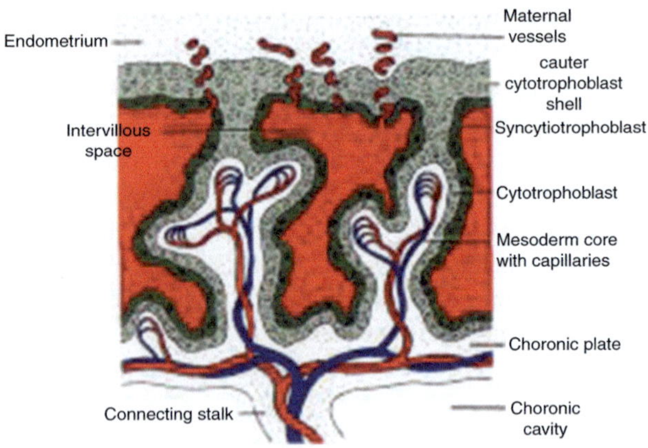

chorionic mesenchyme fuses together (Fig. 2.12). Simultaneously, amniotic sac expands, surrounds the connective stalk and the allantois, and joins to form the umbilical cord.

Chorionic villi are distributed all over the blastocyst. The villi facing the decidua capsularis are called as chorionic leave. Villous beneath the decidua basalis proliferates and forms the fetal component of the placenta and is called as chorionic frondosum. As the embryo grows, the chorionic villi beneath the decidua capsularis degenerate. As the amniotic cavity obliterates, the extracelomic cavity, amnion, and chorion come in close contact. Chorion leave is generally more translucent and rarely exceeds 1 mm in thickness.

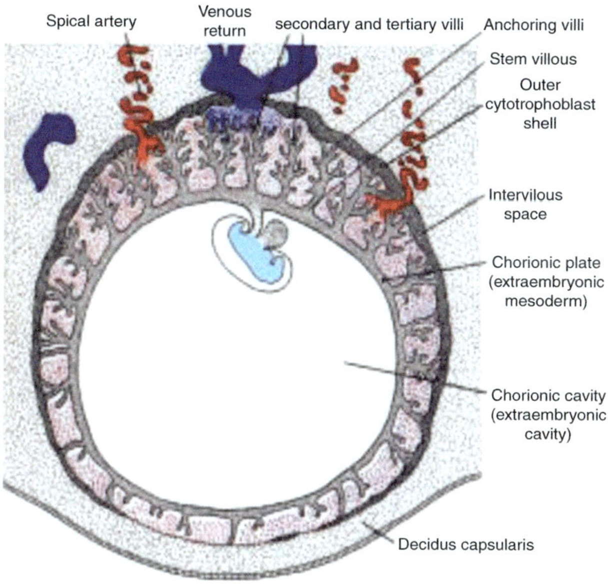

Fig. 2.12 By 8 weeks, embryo surrounded by amnion is attached to the chorionic plate by connecting stalk [2]

2.5.4 Formation of Amnion, Chorion, Amniotic Cavity

By the tenth day, the blastocyst is completely encased and invades the decidua. The lining of cells of the blastocyst facing the uterine cavity is called anembryonic pole and is lined by single layer of flattened cells. The other pole of blastocyst adjoining decidua called as embryonic pole/embryonic disc contains inner cell mass. Some cells differentiate into flattened cells forming the first germ layer called as endoderm; the remaining inner cell mass becomes columnar and forms the ectoderm.

Small flattened cells arising from the trophoblast called as amniogenic cells derived from trophoblast appear between the ectoderm below and trophoblast above and form a cavity filled with fluid called as amniotic cavity. A flattened layer of cells arising from endoderm line the blastocystic cavity and forms primitive yolk sac.

The cells of trophoblast gives rise to mass of cells called as extraembryonic mesoderm or primary mesoderm, which lies between the trophoblast and yolk sac. This also separates the wall of amniotic cavity from the trophoblast. Later on, a cavity appears in the extraembryonic mesoderm which is known as extraembryonic coelom or chorionic cavity. This chorionic cavity splits the extraembryonic mesoderm into inner parietal/somatopleuric extraembryonic mesoderm and outer layer called visceral/splanchnopleuric extraembryonic mesoderm. Hence, chorion is formed by the parietal extraembryonic mesoderm and the overlying trophoblast, and amnion is formed by amniogenic cells forming the wall of the amniotic cavity. Some mesenchymal cells eventually will condense to form body stalk. This stalk joins the embryo and later develops into the umbilical cord [2].

Eventually the amniotic sac distends and obliterates the extraembryonic coelom and leads to apposition of chorion and amnion. Placental amnion covers the placenta and chorionic vessels, and umbilical amnion covers the umbilical cord.

2.6 Formation of Amniotic Fluid, Its Properties and Its Functioning

2.6.1 Production and Circulation

Amniotic fluid (AF) is produced by:

1. Transudation of maternal serum across the placental membranes, from fetal circulation across the umbilical cord and from fetal skin before keratinization takes place at 20 weeks.
2. Excretion of fetal urine and fetal lung fluid also contributes to the amniotic fluid production [11].

Amniotic fluid is removed by fetal swallowing and intramembrane absorption. It is usually replaced every 3 h.

Volume: according to period of gestation, the amount varies as shown in Table 2.2.

2.6.2 Physical Features and Composition

AF is usually colorless to pale straw colored, and it is highly hypotonic compared to maternal serum. It is alkaline with a low specific gravity of 1.010 and osmolarity of 250 mOsmol/L at term which indicates fetal lung maturity.

It is usually composed of water 98–99% and 1–2% of solid components which constitute protein, glucose, urea, uric acid, creatinine, lipids, and electrolytes. It also contains suspended particles like lanugo, vernix caseosa, and exfoliated squamous epithelial cell from the fetal skin, respiratory tract, and urinary bladder.

Table 2.2 Approximate amount of liquor in mL corresponding to period of gestation (weeks)

Period of gestation (weeks)	Volume (approx.) (mL)
12	50
20	400
36–38	1000
40	600–800
42	200

2.6.3 Function

AF functions as a cushion and protects the fetus.

During pregnancy:

1. It acts as cushion and protects fetus from extraneous injury.
2. Maintains even temperature.
3. Helps growth and development of fetus and prevents any adhesion formation between fetal parts and allows free movement of fetus.

During labor:

1. AF helps in dilatation of cervix by acting as a hydrostatic wedge.
2. It prevents the interference with placental circulation till the membranes remain intact.
3. It acts as an antiseptic and bactericidal and flushes the birth canal and prevents ascending infection to the fetus and uterine cavity.

2.7 Trophoblastic Invasion and Spiral Artery Remodeling

Extravillous trophoblast invades the endometrium and inner third of myometrium via some regulatory factors. They secrete proteolytic enzymes which digest extracellular matrix and activate proteinase, which is already present in the endometrium. They also activate matrix metalloproteinases which digest matrix proteins. The autocrine and paracrine activity of trophoblasts controls the ability of invasion into maternal tissue. Trophoblasts secrete insulin-like growth factor II, which promotes invasion, while decidual cells produce insulin-like growth factor-binding protein type 4, which blocks the invasion of trophoblasts.

Estriol levels also play a critical role in invasion and remodeling of spiral arteries. While low levels of early pregnancy promote invasion, as the pregnancy advances and levels escalate, it downregulates VEGF and integrin receptors and hence controls the invasion.

Maternal vasculature undergoes extensive modification in the first half of pregnancy to convert a high-resistance blood flow to low-resistance blood flow. If uteroplacental blood flow remodeling is impaired, it can lead to pathological conditions like preeclampsia, fetal growth restriction, and preterm birth. There are two types of extravillous trophoblast performing different roles in spiral artery modification. Interstitial trophoblast penetrates the decidua and adjacent myometrium. They are aggregated around spiral arteries and prepare the vessels for endovascular trophoblastic invasion. Endovascular trophoblast penetrates the spiral artery lumen and forms cellular plugs which destroy the vascular endothelium and allow only maternal blood plasma to flow into the intervillous space. This helps in keeping the oxygen levels low. During this time, anaerobic glycolysis provides the energy requirements for the early stages in organogenesis, thereby minimizing the risk of

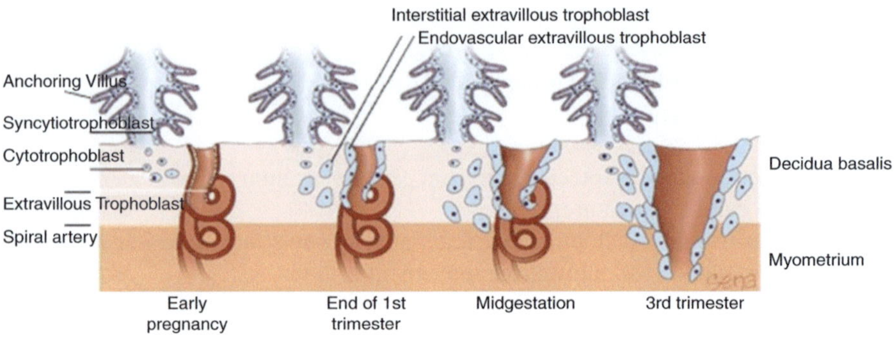

Fig. 2.13 Spiral artery modification

damage to DNA by reactive oxygen species generated during aerobic metabolism. Low oxygen levels also lead to proliferation of cytotrophoblasts helping in their invasion and anchoring to decidua. By 10–12 weeks of gestation, these plugs break down the placenta and further invade and modify the vasa media of the vessel and replace the smooth muscle of vasa previa to fibrinoid material, and later on the endothelium regenerates and maternal whole blood then flows into the intervillous space. As the walls of the spiral arteries do not contain maternal endothelium, they do not respond to hormonal and neural signals from the mother, and blood is delivered steadily to the placenta. This spiral artery modification occurs in decidua basalis only and does not involve the decidua parietalis, and only spiral arteries undergo modification while decidual veins are spared (Fig. 2.13).

Ramsay and Donner described the vessel modification in two waves or stages. During the first wave which occurs before 12 weeks, there is invasion and modification of spiral arteries up to the border between decidua and myometrium. The second wave occurs between 12 and 16 weeks and involves some invasion of intramyometrial segments of spiral arteries. These processes convert narrow lumen high-resistance muscular arteries into dilated low-resistance vessels. This conversion event plays crucial role in pathogenesis of preeclampsia and fetal growth restriction.

2.8 Mature Placenta at Term and Villous Branching

A fully formed human placenta is discoidal in shape. Grossly, it is around 15–20 cm in diameter and 3 cm in thickness at center and thins out toward the ends. It feels spongy and weighs around 500 g and occupies approximately 30% of uterine wall.

It has two surfaces, fetal and maternal surfaces, as shown in Fig. 2.14.

Fetal surface: it is smooth and lined by glistening amnion and the umbilical cord is attached to the center of the placenta mostly. Beneath the amnion, the radiating branches of umbilical vessels can be seen. Fourth/fifth of the placenta is fetal origin formed from chorionic villous.

Maternal surface: it is somewhat rough and spongy and covered by remnants of decidua basalis which gives it a thin grayish color and maternal blood which gives

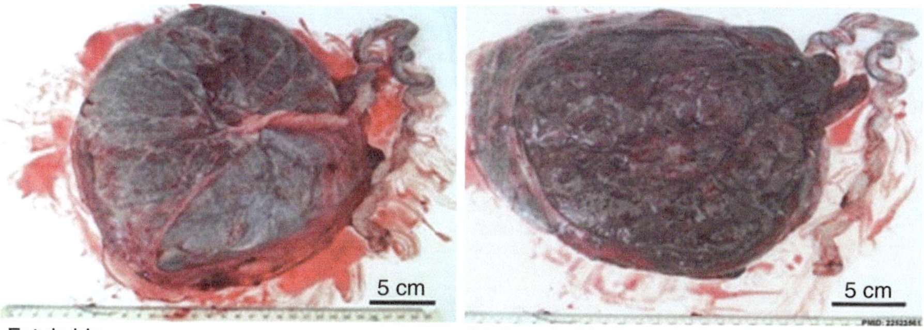

Fig. 2.14 Fetal and maternal side of term placenta

it a dull red color. Maternal surface is divided into 15–20 convex polygonal areas known as lobes or cotyledons. Lobes are incompletely separated by grooves of variable depth that arise from folding of basal plate. The total number of lobes remains constant, and each lobe grows individually. Lobules are functional units supplied by each main stem villous. As placenta grows, the early thick stem villi progressively form finer subdivision, and there is increase in number of smaller villi. Each of truncal or main stem villi and its ramification constitute a placental lobule. Each lobule is supplied with single truncal branch of chorionic artery and drained by single chorionic vein. At margins the basal and chorionic plates fuse and chorionic leave and amnion are in close contact. Attachment of placenta is firm and effective due to anchoring villi which connect the chorionic plate and basal plate.

2.9 Placental Circulation

Placental circulation constitutes two systems: uteroplacental circulation or maternal circulation and feto-placental circulation or fetal circulation (Fig. 2.15).

2.9.1 Uteroplacental Circulation/Maternal Circulation

Maternal arterial blood enters through the basal plate to reach the chorionic plate. Once blood comes in contact with the microvillous surface of chorionic villi, it drains back through venous orifices in the basal plate and enters the uterine veins.

Mixing of arterial and venous blood is prevented by the increased pressure of endometrial arteries with which they release the blood toward chorionic plate. As explained earlier, due to spiral artery modification, low-resistance vessels are formed, and it helps to increase the uterine perfusion as the gestation advances.

Blood flow is constantly maintained during uterine contraction also, due to the special arrangement of spiral arteries and veins. Spiral arteries are perpendicular to

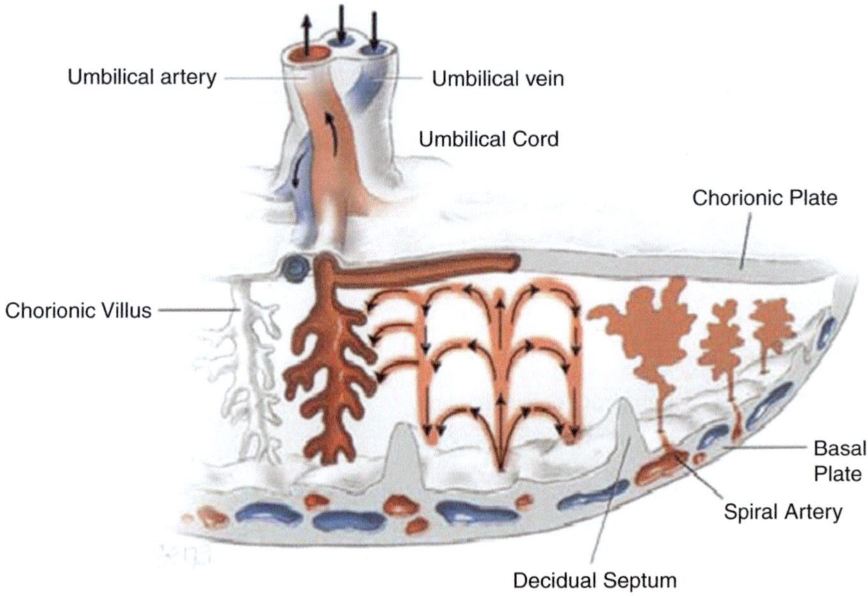

Fig. 2.15 Section through a full term placenta [3]

the uterine walls, while veins are parallel to the uterine wall. Hence, during contraction veins are occluded, but the arterial blood flow is maintained in the intervillous space, and during relaxation venous flow is facilitated. With this arrangement large volume of blood is available for exchange in spite of decreased rate of blood flow. This concept was also supported by Bleker and associates who used serial sonography during normal labor and found that placental length, thickness, and surface area increased during contraction. Due to occluded venous flow as compared to arterial inflow, there is distention of intervillous space. Hence, larger volume of blood is available for exchange.

2.9.2 Feto-Placental Circulation/Fetal Circulation

The fetus has two umbilical arteries, and as the cord joins the placenta, these umbilical arteries branch beneath the amnion and form villi. These villi form capillary network in terminal villous branches for adequate exchange. Deoxygenated blood is carried out from the fetus to placenta via umbilical arteries, and oxygenated blood returns from the placenta to fetus via a single umbilical vein. The chorionic vessels are branches of umbilical vessels that traverse along the fetal surface of placenta in chorionic plate. Chorionic arteries always cross over chorionic veins and are responsive to vasoactive substances. These arteries further break into smaller branches and enter the stem of chorionic villi, which further divide into primary, secondary, and tertiary vessels of corresponding villi.

The perforating branches of surface arteries are called truncal arteries, which pass through the chorionic plate. Each truncal artery supplies one main stem villous and thus one cotyledon. As these arteries branch, their caliber increases, and amount of smooth muscle decreases, and hence end diastolic flow is maintained throughout the normal pregnancy, which is usually established by 10 weeks of pregnancy.

2.10 Placental Barrier

The placenta does not make a perfect barrier as fetal cells are usually found in maternal circulation and vice versa. The two are separated by placental membranes in the following order which consists of syncytiotrophoblast, cytotrophoblasts, basement membrane, stromal tissue, and endothelium of fetal capillary wall with basement membrane (Fig. 2.16).

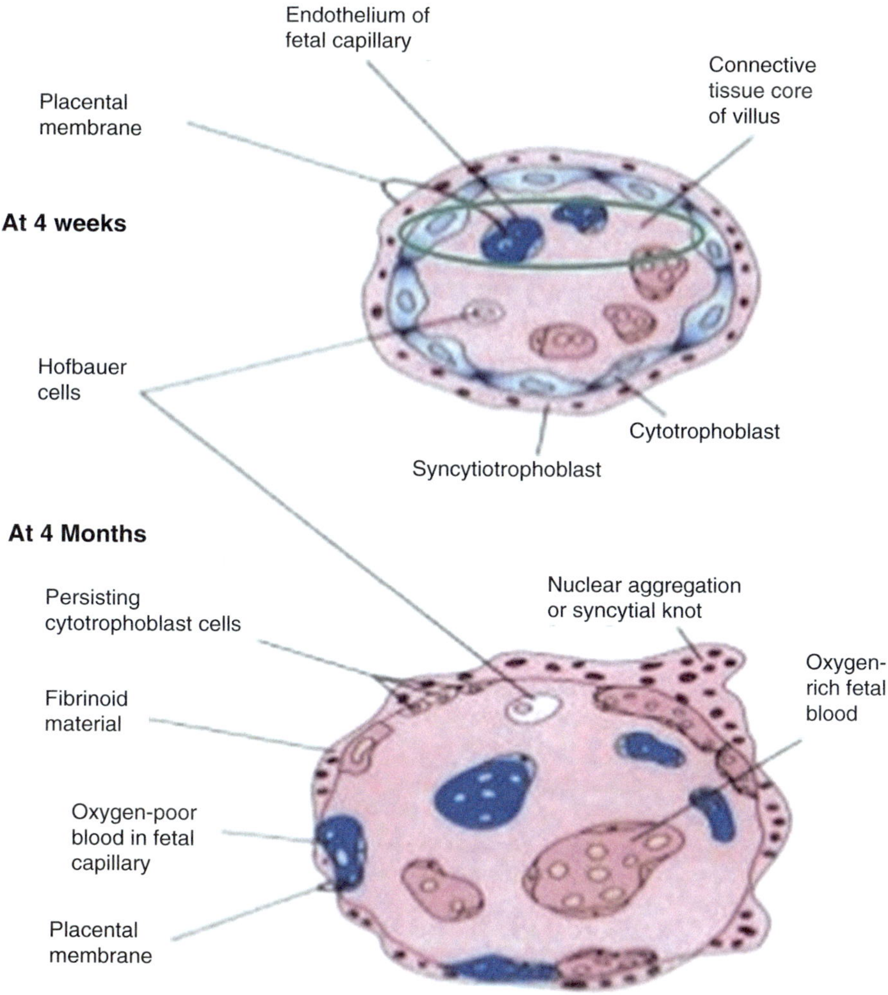

Fig. 2.16 (**a**) Placental barrier at 4 weeks; (**b**) at 4 months

2.11 Placental Aging

As the gestation age increases, there is degeneration of some villi, piling up of fibrin-like material between villi, and, at times, heaping up of syncytial cells to form syncytial knots. However, a functional proportion of the placenta continues to proliferate and grows as pregnancy advances.

2.12 Umbilical Cord

2.12.1 Development

During early pregnancy yolk sac and umbilical vesicle develop. Initially the embryonic disc is interposed between the amnion and yolk sac. Later on with differential growth of embryonic disc, the dorsal surface of the embryo grows faster than the ventral surface, in association with elongation of its neural tube. With this type of differential growth, the embryo eventually bulges into the amniotic sac, and the dorsal part of yolk sac incorporates into the embryo body to form the gut. Anterior wall of hind gut is formed by the allantois which projects into base of body stalk from the caudal wall of yolk sac.

With further growth, the yolk sac decreases in size and its pedicle becomes relatively longer. The amnion expands and obliterates the extraceolomic cavity and fuses with chorionic leave and covers the bulging placental disc and lateral surface of body stalk which is now called as the umbilical cord or funis.

2.12.2 Content

Initially the umbilical cord consists of two umbilical veins and two umbilical arteries. During fetal development, the right umbilical vein usually disappears and only the "left umbilical vein is left." Umbilical arteries do not have internal elastic lamina. They have well-developed muscular coat which helps in effective closure of arteries due to reflex spasm as soon as the baby is delivered. Both arteries and veins do not have vasa vasorum. Content of the umbilical cord is shown in Fig. 2.17.

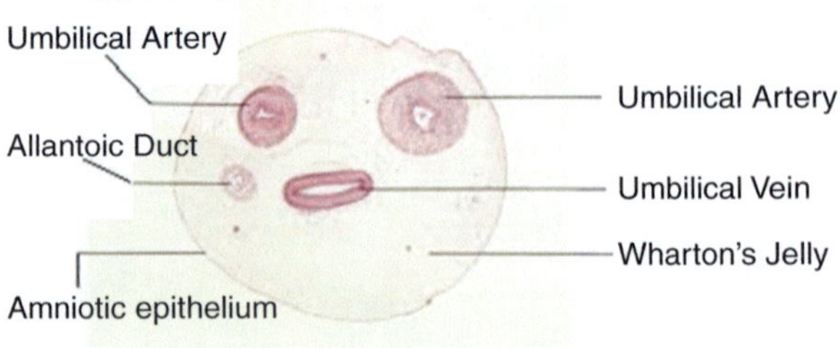

Fig. 2.17 Cut section of the umbilical cord

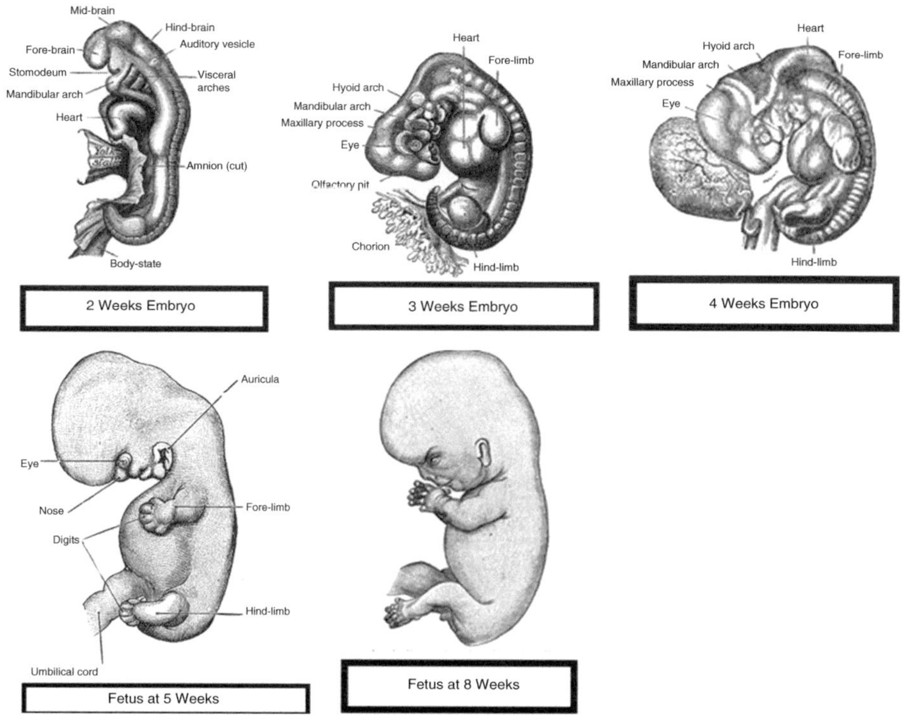

Fig. 2.18 Stages of fetal development

Near its insertion to the placenta, the cord contains a small duct of umbilical vesicle which is lined by flattened or cuboidal epithelium. Intra-abdominal portion of umbilical vesicle which extends from the umbilicus to intestine usually atrophies, but if it remains patent, then it is called as Meckel's diverticulum.

The umbilical cord is covered by single layer of amniotic epithelium. Umbilical vessels are supported by gelatinous fluid which is formed by mucoid degeneration of extraembryonic mesodermal cells which are rich in mucopolysaccharides called as Wharton's jelly.

The umbilical cord is usually 40 cm in length but may vary from 30 to 100 cm, and its average diameter is 1.5 cm. Thickness of the cord is not uniform, and few areas have local collection of Wharton's jelly which are called as false knots.

Initially, the cord is attached to ventral surface of the embryo close to the caudal extremity, but as the coelom closes and yolk sac atrophies, the point of attachment is shifted permanently to the center of the abdomen at the fourth month. The placental attachment of the cord may be central which is more common.

2.13 Fetal Development

Fetal growth and development has been calculated from the first day of the last menstrual period up to 280 days or 40 weeks. The whole prenatal development is divided into three periods:

1. Ovular period—this is the period of ovulation till fertilization of ovum. It corresponds to 2 weeks following ovulation.
2. Embryonic period—it corresponds to the development of the embryo. This begins from third week following ovulation till 10 weeks (8 weeks postconception).
3. Fetal period—it begins with 8 weeks postconception or 10 weeks from LMP and ends with delivery. The embryo is approximately 4 cm long.

Gestational age can be calculated from the first day of the last menstrual period. It is 2 weeks greater than the postconception age. The period of gestation can also be divided into three units, each 13–14 weeks long. These three trimesters are important obstetrical milestones for fetal growth and development. The fetal development has been explained in Table 2.3, according to weeks.

2.14 Fetal Nutrition

The fetus absorbs nutrients in different ways depending upon the stage of the fetus:

1. *Absorption*: during early postfertilization period, the fetus attains nutrition via absorption. It absorbs nutrients stored in cytoplasm and from tubal and uterine secretions.
2. *Histotrophic transfer*: once the embryo undergoes implantation before establishment of uteroplacental circulation, the nutrition is derived from diffusion and later on via stagnant maternal blood in trophoblastic lacunae.
3. *Hematotrophic transfer:* as the feto-maternal circulation is established, the transfer of nutrients via active and passive transfer occurs after 3 weeks onward.

2/3 of total calcium, 3/4 of total proteins, and 4/5 of total iron are deposited during the last trimester.

2.15 Fetal Hemopoiesis

Hemopoiesis occurs first in the yolk sac from the 14th day of embryonic period. By the 10th week, the liver takes over, and finally this function is replaced by the bone marrow near term. In the early period, erythropoiesis is megaloblastic, and near term it becomes normoblastic. The type of hemoglobin depends on its globin chain. The hemoglobin produced from the yolk sac is, namely, Grower-1 (ξ-ε chain), Grower-2(α-ε chain), and Portland (ξ-γ chain). When the liver produces red cells, it produces fetal hemoglobin F ($\alpha 2$-$\gamma 2$). From 24 weeks onward, the bone marrow synthesizes adult-type hemoglobin A ($\alpha 2$-$\beta 2$). At term 3/4 of total hemoglobin is Hb F; during 6–12 months of life, the proportion of Hb F decreases and is replaced by adult type of hemoglobin Hb A.

Erythropoiesis is controlled by fetal erythropoietin, which primarily is secreted from the fetal liver initially, and later renal secretion begins. Fetal hemoglobin has higher affinity to oxygen due to lower binding of 2,3-diphosphoglycerate compared to adult hemoglobin. It is alkali resistant. Life span of fetal RBC is 2/3 of adult RBC, i.e., 80 days. The total feto-placental blood volume at term is 125 kg per body weight of the fetus. Cord blood levels of iron, ferritin, vitamin B 12, and folic acid are higher than maternal blood.

2.16 Coagulation Factors

Fetal fibrinogen appears as early as 5 weeks. The fetus produces normal, adult-type procoagulant, fibrinolysis and anticoagulant protein by 12 weeks. Serum levels of factors II, VII, IX, X, and XI, pre-kallikrein, protein S, protein C, antithrombin, and plasminogen are 50% of adult levels. Factors V, VIII, and XIII and fibrinogen levels are closer to adult value [12]. Vitamin K-dependent coagulation factors usually decrease during the first few days of birth.

2.17 Plasma Proteins

The fetus does not depend on mother as the fetal liver produces enzymes and plasma protein for its own requirement. At birth, total plasma protein and albumin concentration is equivalent to adult levels.

2.18 Leukocyte and Fetal Immunology

The thymus and spleen develop early in fetus. B lymphocytes are formed by 9 weeks in the fetal liver and the 12th week in the spleen. T lymphocytes are formed in the thymus by the 14th week. Maternal immunoglobulin Ig G crosses the placenta from 12 weeks onward and provides passive immunity. At term, fetal Ig G levels are 10% higher than maternal levels. Ig M, if found, is mainly of fetal origin and denotes some intrauterine infection. Colostrum contains Ig A which provides mucosal protection against enteric infection; if newborn encounters enteric infection, it produces Ig A antibody in response to antigen [13].

2.19 Urinary System

The fetal kidney is formed from metanephros by 9–12 weeks. Earlier to that, pronephros and mesonephros generate urine. The kidney and ureter develop from intermediate mesoderm. The bladder and urethra develop from urogenital sinus.

Table 2.3 Fetal development according to weeks of pregnancy (Fig. 2.18)

Embryo-fetal growth	
First 2 weeks	• Zygote develops to blastocyst stage • Implantation after 6–7 days following fertilization • Notochord develops • Ectoderm thickens to form neural plate and neural folds
3rd week	• Fetal blood vessels appear in chorionic villi • Neural folds fuse to form neural tube
4th week	• Cardiovascular system starts developing • Partition of primitive heart begins • Complete neural tube closure • Arm and leg buds are formed • Umbilical cord is formed
6th week	• Synapses of spinal cord develop • Heart is completely formed • Upper lip is completely formed • External ear appears as elevation
12th week	• Center of ossification of fetal bones and fingers and toes appear • Skin and nails form • Rudimentary hair appears • External genitalia is formed
16th week	• CRL 12 cm, wt. 110 g • External genitalia well formed • Eye movement begins • Midbrain maturation develops
20th week	• Fetal movement present • Skin is less transparent and lanugo develops • Scalp hair develops
22th week	• Cochlear function develops
24th week	• Fat deposition begins • Head larger than the body • Lung development starts
26th week	• Pain receptors develop
28th week	• Skin red, covered with vernix caseosa • Isolated eye blinking present • Testes descend to internal inguinal ring
32th week	• Wt. 1800 g • Skin is shiny, wrinkled, and red
36th week	• Wt. 2500 g • Body becomes more round • One testes descends into the scrotum • Lanugo disappears
40th week	• Wt. 3400 g • Fetus is well formed • Both testes descend to scrotum • Posterior fontanelle closes

Allantois also contributes to bladder formation. By 14 weeks, nephrons develop and become active to produce urine. Near term 650 mL of urine is produced per day. However, the fetal kidney is not essential for fetal survival in utero but is important for formation of amniotic fluid. Any urinary tract obstruction or renal aplasia or hypoplasia may lead to oligoamnios.

2.20 Lung Development

The lungs are more like glands and have pseudo-glandular pattern with intersegmental bronchial tree between 6 and 16 weeks. By 16–26 weeks, bronchial cartilage plates extend peripherally. Terminal bronchioles are formed and divided into several respiratory bronchioles, which later form multiple saccular ducts. At 26 weeks, primitive pulmonary alveoli are formed from respiratory bronchioles, and the alveoli formation begins by 32 weeks. Extensive capillary network is formed, lymphatic system develops, and type II pneumocytes start producing surfactant. Surfactant lowers the surface tension of lung fluid so that alveoli expand easily following delivery. Lecithin-sphingomyelin (L/S) ratio of 2:1 in amniotic fluid signifies fetal lung maturity. Fetal cortisol is a natural trigger for augmentation of lung surfactant production. At birth 15% of adult type of alveoli are present, and the lung continues to grow till the age of 8 years.

Breathing movement is established by 11 weeks [14], and by 20 weeks these movements become regular at an interval of 30–70 per minute and help in circulation of amniotic fluid in the respiratory system.

2.21 Gastrointestinal Tract

By the 12th week swallowing begins, and simultaneously the small intestine undergoes peristalsis and transports glucose actively. Much of water is absorbed, and unabsorbed material appears in the colon called as meconium by the 20th week. If swallowing is inhibited because of any obstructive pathology, it leads to polyhydramnios. Term fetus swallows around 200–750 mL of fluid per day.

Meconium: the fetal bowel content is mainly composed of secretions from the lung, liver, desquamated fetal cells, lanugo, scalp hair, and vernix. It is usually the undigested, unabsorbed debris of amniotic fluid which was swallowed by the fetus. Biliverdin from the liver gives it a greenish black color. Intrauterine hypoxia causes vagal stimulation which leads to anal sphincter relaxation and meconium-stained liquor.

Liver: enzyme production in the liver increases with gestational age. However, the fetal liver is not capable of converting free unconjugated bilirubin to conjugated bilirubin completely. The small amount which gets converted into conjugated bilirubin oxidizes to form biliverdin, and majority of unconjugated bilirubin is excreted in amniotic fluid after 12 weeks and is transferred across the placenta.

2.22 Endocrinology

Fetal pituitary secretes growth hormone, ACTH, prolactin, TSH, and gonadotrophic hormones by the 10th week. By the 12th week, posterior pituitary secretes vasopressin and oxytocin. Fetal adrenal undergoes hypertrophy of reticular zone and synthesizes estriol precursor, cortisol, and dehydroepiandrosterone. Adrenal medulla secretes small amounts of catecholamines. Thyroxine production is started from the fetal thyroid by the 11th week. The pancreas secretes insulin by the 12th week and glucagon by the 8th week of gestation.

2.23 Skin

Lanugo (thin colorless hairs) appears by the 16th week and disappears at term. Sebaceous glands are formed by the 20th week. Vernix caseosa which is secretions of sebaceous glands smears the skin. Horny layer of epidermis is formed after the 20th week and prevents transudation from fetal capillaries into amniotic fluid.

2.24 The Fetal Circulation

Fetal circulation differs from adult circulation as deoxygenated blood from the fetus is carried via umbilical arteries toward the placenta, where oxygen transport occurs. Then oxygenated blood via the umbilical vein is carried back to the fetus. Fetal blood does not enter the pulmonary vasculature for oxygenation, and most of the blood bypasses the lung. Schematic representation is shown in Fig. 2.19.

Oxygenated blood along with required nutrients is carried toward the fetus via a single umbilical vein. The umbilical vein divides into the ductus venosus and portal sinus in the liver. Most of the oxygenated blood shunts to the IVC via the ductus venosus. Small amounts of blood from portal sinuses drain into hepatic vein and supply oxygenated and nutrient-rich blood to the liver, and after that relatively deoxygenated blood enters into the IVC via the hepatic vein. Hence, blood in the IVC contains less oxygen content than which was present in the umbilical vein. Blood from the IVC drains into the right atrium. From right atrium, due to configuration of upper inter-atrial septum (Crista Dividens) maximum amount of blood (75%) shunts toward left atrium via foramen ovale. The left atrium pumps oxygenated blood toward the left ventricle and supplies the heart and brain.

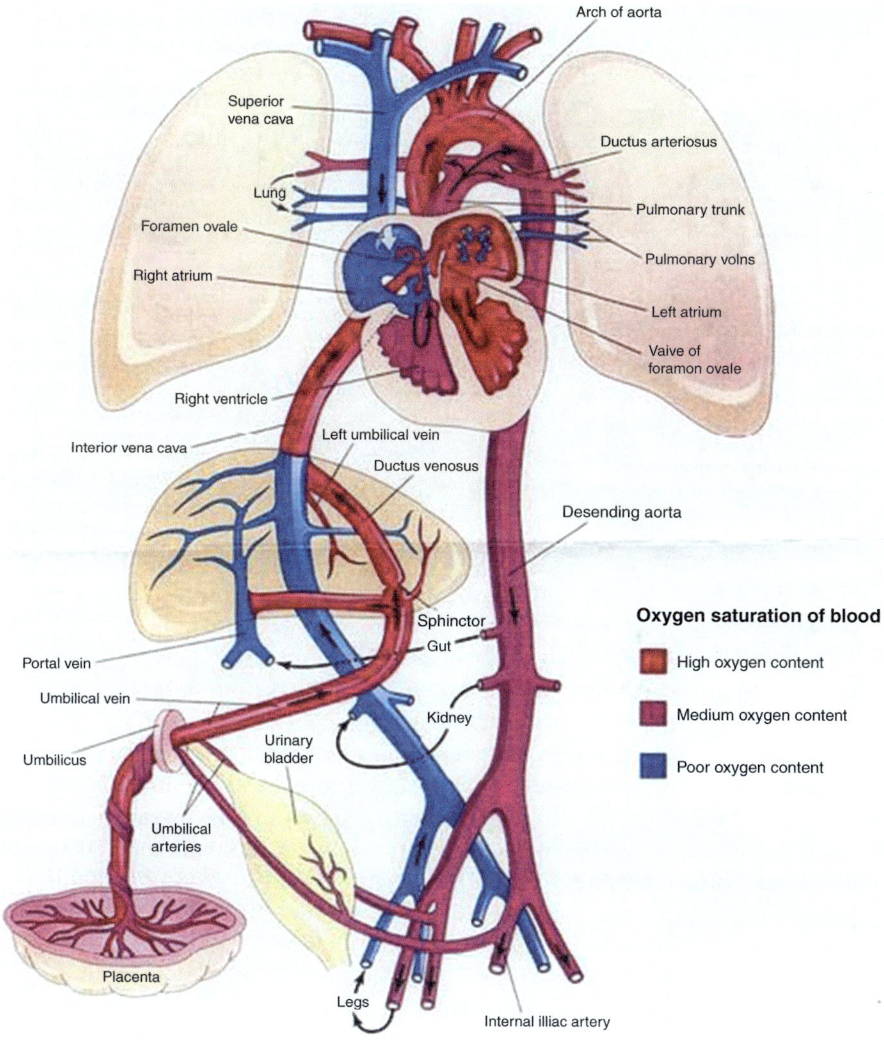

Fig. 2.19 The fetal circulation

The deoxygenated blood from the SVC enters the right atrium, and blood is shunted to the right ventricle. While entering into the right atrium, the SVC courses along the inferior and anterior aspect of the atrium, and hence most of the deoxygenated blood returning from the brain and upper body enters directly to the right ventricle. The ostium of coronary sinus also lies superior to the tricuspid valve, and hence deoxygenated blood from the heart also drains directly to the right ventricle. Because of this shunting, blood in the right ventricle is 15–20% less oxygenated than in the left ventricle. Due to high resistance of pulmonary arteries, the right ventricular blood with low oxygen content which is discharged

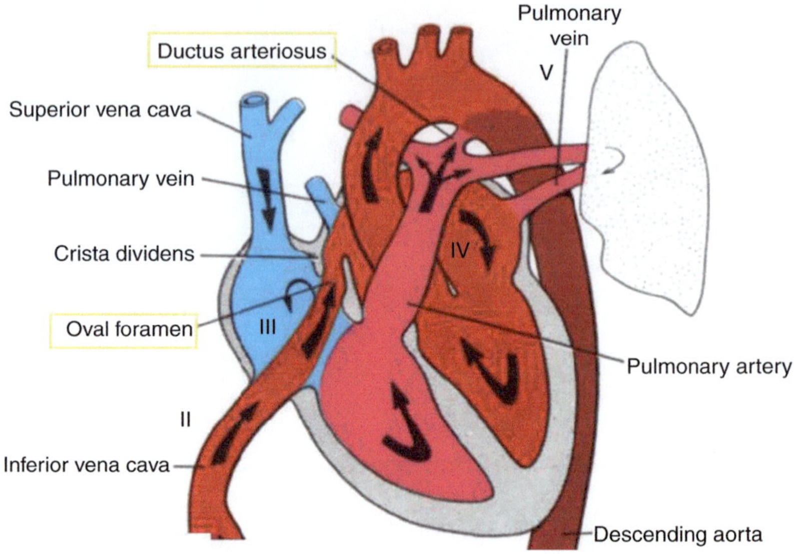

Fig. 2.20 Blood flow in the fetal heart

into the pulmonary trunk shunts to the descending aorta via the ductus arteriosus and, hence, bypasses the lung and mixes with the blood from the proximal aorta (shown in Fig. 2.20). Seventy percent of cardiac output (60% from right and 10% from left ventricle) is carried by ductus arteriosus to the descending aorta. Forty percent of combined output goes to the placenta through the umbilical arteries. The deoxygenated blood leaves the body by way of two umbilical arteries to reach the placenta where it is oxygenated and gets ready for recirculation. The mean cardiac output is comparatively high in the fetus and is estimated to be 350 mL per kg per minute.

2.25 Changes in Fetal Circulation at Birth

Soon after birth, there are hemodynamic changes in circulation as the oxygenation of blood has to be carried out via the lungs and there is cessation of placental flow. With initiation of respiration, the pulmonary vascular resistance decreases and leads to the following changes:

1. *Closure of umbilical arteries*: initially there is immediate functional closure of umbilical vessel, and actual obliteration occurs after 2–3 months. The distal parts form the lateral umbilical ligaments and the proximal parts remain open as superior vesicle arteries.
2. *Closure of umbilical vein*: the umbilical vein gets obliterated after closure of umbilical arteries and hence allows extra amount of blood to be received by the fetus via the placenta. As the ductus venosus collapses, the pressure of the IVC

and right atrium falls. After obliteration, the umbilical vein forms the ligamentum teres, and ductus venosus becomes ligamentum venosum.

3. *Closure of ductus arteriosus*: once respiration is attained after a few hours, the muscular wall of ductus arteriosus contracts due to rising oxygen content of blood which is flowing from the duct. Functional closure occurs soon after the establishment of pulmonary circulation; the anatomical obliteration takes 1–3 months. After closure it becomes ligamentum arteriosum.
4. *Closure of foramen ovale*: with increase in pressure of the left atrium and fall in pressure of the right atrium, there occurs functional closure of the foramen ovale soon after birth, and anatomical closure occurs after 1 year.

Within 1–2 h following birth, the cardiac output is estimated to be about 500 mL per minute, and heart rate varies from 120 to 140 beats per minute.

Key Points

- Implantation is defined as a process of attachment and invasion of uterine endometrium by the blastocyst.
- The endometrium of pregnancy known as Decidua is highly modified and specialized for proper hemochorial implantation.
- After 6 days of fertilization, the blastocyst implants in the decidua, and the process of implantation is divided into three steps: apposition, adhesion, and invasion.
- The human placenta originates from the trophectoderm, which originates from the trophoblast.
- After implantation, the trophoblast differentiates into primitive syncytioblast and cytotrophoblast, which later on helps in formation of chorionic villi, which form the placenta.
- By 8–10 weeks definitive chorionic plate is formed, and amniotic and chorionic mesenchyme fuses together.
- Extravillous trophoblast invades the endometrium and inner third of myometrium and converts spiral arteries from high-resistance vessels to low-resistance vessels for adequate flow of blood to the fetus.
- Fetal growth and development has been calculated from the first day of the last menstrual period up to 280 days or 40 weeks.

References

1. Cha J, Sun X, Dey SK. Mechanisms of implantation: strategies for successful pregnancy. Nat Med. 2012;18(12):1754–67.
2. Sadler TW. Langman's medical embryology. 8th ed. Philadelphia: Lippincott Williams & Wilkins; 2000.
3. Cunningham FG, et al. Implantation and placental development. In: Cunningham FG, Lenevo KJ, et al., editors. Williams obstetrics. New York: McGraw-Hill; 2014. p. 80–110.

4. Sood R, Zehnder JL, Druzin ML, Brown PO. Gene expression patterns in human placenta. Proc Natl Acad Sci U S A. 2006;103(14):5478–83.
5. Hu W, Feng Z, Teresky AK, Levine AJ. p53 regulates maternal reproduction through LIF. Nature. 2007;450(7170):721–4.
6. Ren Q, Guan S, Fu J, Wang A. Temporal and spatial expression of MUC1 during implantation in sows. Int J Mol Sci. 2010;11(6):2322–35.
7. Shimizu Y, Kabir-Salmani M, Azadbakht M, Sugihara K, Sakai K, Iwashita M. Expression and localization of galectin-9 in the human uterodome. Endocr J. 2008;55(5):879–87.
8. Nancy P, Tagliani E, Tay C-S, Asp P, Levy DE, Erlebacher A. Chemokine gene silencing in decidual stromal cells limits T cell access to the maternal-fetal interface. Science. 2012;336(6086):1317–21.
9. Makrigiannakis A, Zoumakis E, Kalantaridou S, Coutifaris C, Margioris AN, Coukos G, Rice KC, Gravanis A, Chrousos GP. Corticotropin-releasing hormone promotes blastocyst implantation and early maternal tolerance. Nat Immunol. 2001;2(11):1018–24.
10. Arnholdt H, Meisel F, Fandrey K, et al. Proliferation of villous trophoblast of the human placenta in normal and abnormal pregnancies. Virchows Arch B Cell Pathol Incl Mol Pathol. 1991;60:365.
11. Adzick NS, Harrison MR, Glick PL, et al. Experimental pulmonary hypoplasia and oligohydramnios: relative contributions of lung fluid and fetal breathing movements. J Pediatr Surg. 1984;19:658.
12. Corrigan JJ Jr. Norma hemostasis in the fetus and newborn: coagulation. In: Polin RA, Fox WW, editors. Fetal and neonatal physiology. Philadelphia: Saunders; 1992. p. 1368.
13. Bloch EM, Reed WF, Lee TH, et al. Male microchimerism in peripheral blood leukocytes from women with multiple sclerosis. Chimerism. 2011;2(1):6.
14. Boddy K, Dawes GS. Fetal breathing. Br Med Bull. 1975;31:3.

3 Normal Immune Function: Journey of the Fetus

Vidushi Kulshrestha

3.1 Introduction

Pregnancy is a unique immunological challenge. Fetus carrying both maternal and paternal genes is a semi-allogenic graft to maternal immune system, yet it escapes immune rejection and is tolerated throughout pregnancy [1]. This immunological relationship between the pregnant mother and her antigenically foreign fetus was first described as a "paradox of pregnancy" by Medawar in 1953 which led to the origin of reproductive immunology [2]. He later won the Nobel Prize for his pioneering work in laws of transplantation immunology.

This immunological paradox exists because of the maternal immune tolerance seen toward the fetus which inherits paternal polymorphic genes [2]. Surrogate mothers have a bigger alloantigen challenge and this paradox holds true for them also [3].

Medawar originally proposed three mechanisms to explain maternal tolerance of the fetus. The antigenic immaturity of the fetus and physical separation between the fetus and mother were later proven incorrect. Though the fetus itself is not in direct contact, the fetal-derived trophoblasts are in contact with the mother's immune system which present antigens to the maternal immune system.

Then came the concept of placenta being a neutral shield between mother and fetus which lacks the major histocompatibility complex (MHC) antigens. However, this was also refuted, as class I MHC antigens do exist on the trophoblast and uterus has antigen-presenting capacity. Another view thought the uterus as an immunologically privileged site [4] where fetal tissue directs the maternal immune response toward a protective one. But the occurrence of ectopic pregnancies demonstrates that the uterus is not the only unique immune-privileged site.

V. Kulshrestha
Department of Obstetrics and Gynaecology, AIIMS, New Delhi, India
e-mail: drvidushi.kul@gmail.com

S. Mehta, B. Gupta (eds.), *Recurrent Pregnancy Loss*,
https://doi.org/10.1007/978-981-10-7338-0_3

The focus of reproductive immunology research has therefore been based on Medawar's third hypothesis, i.e., deviation of maternal immune system toward the immunological inertness. During pregnancy, maternal immune system has to be modulated in such a way so as to avoid rejection of the semi-allogenic fetus and also allowing for placental invasion and preserving maternal defense against infections.

3.2 Initiating Signal for Developing Maternal Tolerance to the Developing Embryo

The immune processes occurring at maternal fetal interface are highly dynamic with both maternal and fetal contributions. The embryo expresses its genome as early as the two-cell stage and signals its presence to the mother. Development of maternal tolerance depends on unique embryo-derived signaling between the embryo and mother, and this signaling must take place prior to embryo-maternal contact, i.e., implantation, and prior to the activation of embryo genome [5]. The fertilized egg is surrounded by semipermeable zona pellucida and cumulus oophorus which protects it against access to maternal immune cells. Further, cytokines secreted by cumulus may serve as the embryo-derived signaling [5]. Both in natural conception and in embryo transfer following assisted reproductive techniques (ART), there is a lag of 5–7 days between embryo presence and implantation, which is required for priming the endometrium and to make maternal system receptive to the embryo. The maternal system of recognition is not confined only to the uterus; rather it is systemic, as is evident by occurrence of ectopic pregnancy [6].

3.3 Factors and Mechanisms for Maternal Immune Tolerance

Pregnancy success depends on embryo-driven autocrine signaling followed by appropriate maternal response [6]. Various factors and their mechanisms are involved in endometrial priming and development of maternal immune tolerance after the signaling has been initiated by the developing embryo. These dynamic changes leading to successful development of semi-allogenic fetus are as follows.

3.3.1 Altered HLA Expression (HLA-G, HLA-C)

The major histocompatibility complex (MHC), referred to as the human leukocyte antigen (HLA) complex, is a tightly linked cluster of genes, which helps in T cell immune recognition and reaction. The HLA genes are located within the short arm of chromosome 6 and are grouped into Class I, II, and III regions. The class I genes are subdivided into:

Class Ia: This includes HLA-A, HLA-B, and HLA-C.

Class Ib: This includes HLA-E, HLA-F, and HLA-G.

Placental trophoblast cells are unique as they only express one class Ia molecule (HLA-C) and all three class Ib (HLA-E, HLA-F, and HLA-G) molecules [7]. HLA-G shows less polymorphism, and so paternal HLA-G is very similar to maternal one, thereby decreasing the risk of immune rejection.

HLA-G antigen expression is restricted to extravillous cytotrophoblasts, i.e., uNK cells. They help in increasing maternal immune tolerance by suppression of cytotoxic activity of decidual killer cells and by preventing apoptosis of cytotoxic CD8+ T cells by Fas ligand pathway [8].

Embryos used for in vitro fertilization do not implant if they do not express HLA-G [8]. Hence, HLA-G testing has been used to select embryo to be transferred after IVF [9]. But HLA-G is not essential as pregnancy can occur in its absence as well, though there is higher pregnancy rate if HLA-G is present.

3.3.2 Role of Preimplantation Factor (PIF)

PIF is a peptide secreted by viable embryos which has multiple effects and prepares the mother for successful implantation by promoting embryo development, uterine priming, trophoblast invasion, and systemic immunoregulation [6]. PIF is secreted only by viable embryos and is measurable since 2-cell stage; hence, it is being evaluated as a possible biomarker for embryo tolerance and viable pregnancy [6], with an advantage over βhCG, as it is not positive in chemical pregnancies and unviable pregnancies unlike βhCG. Detection of PIF has been associated with good pregnancy outcome [10]. Immunoregulatory effects of PIF are both systemic and local. The last phase in embryo-maternal interaction is trophoblast adherence and invasion, through matrix metalloproteinases (MMP), which actually decides the fate of pregnancy; PIF also reduces natural killer (NK) cell toxicity [6].

3.3.3 Role of Progesterone

Progesterone is essential for maintenance of pregnancy. Progesterone is produced by corpus luteum in early pregnancy till placenta takes over at 12 weeks. Progesterone can affect immune response by various cellular and molecular mechanisms such as inhibition of monocyte-dependent T cell activation, stimulation of MMP and adhesion molecules, inhibition of antibody production, suppression of T cell activation and cytotoxicity, modification of NK cell activity, and secretion of protective asymmetric antibodies [11].

Maternal lymphocytes especially peripherally produced CD8+ lymphocytes are extremely sensitive to progesterone during pregnancy which exert a receptor-mediated action and release a 34 kDa protein, called the progesterone-induced blocking factor (PIBF). This PIBF mediates the biological effects of progesterone and facilitates immune tolerance [12]. The level of progesterone receptor-positive lymphocytes increases throughout gestation, and in turn, the PIBF concentration also increases until 37th gestational week, followed by a slow decrease until term. PIBF signals through the JAK/STAT pathway and through cytokines; it results in a preferential Th2-type production of cytokines and inhibition of NK cell activity [12]. Progesterone may also stimulate Treg cells even in physiological doses [13] though further evidence is needed to evaluate this role.

3.3.4 Altered Th1-Th2 Ratio with Th2 Dominance

T cells are defined as helper T lymphocytes and cytotoxic T lymphocytes. Helper T lymphocytes are particularly important in pregnancy as they affect the function of other immune cells by producing cytokines. Helper T lymphocytes are further classified into T helper type 1 (Th1) and type 2 (Th2) based on their cytokine secretion through which they mediate their effects. A correctly regulated cytokine environment is essential for survival of the feto-placental unit.

- Cytokines secreted by Th1 are tumor necrosis factor (TNF)-α, interferon, and interleukin (IL)-2.
- These promote cellular immune responses and have deleterious effects on fetal growth [14].
- Cytokines secreted by Th2 are IL-4, IL-5, IL-9, IL-10 and IL-13, granulocyte-macrophage colony-stimulating factor, and IL-3.
- These promote humoral responses and enhance fetal survival. Also, Th2 cytokines inhibit Th1 responses, improving fetal survival [14].

Th1/Th2 paradigm: This hypothesis was proposed by Wegmann which stated that "successful pregnancy is a Th2 phenomenon i.e. the maternal immune response during pregnancy is biased towards a preferential production of Th2 humoral response and away from cell-mediated immunity' [15]. This hypothesis was in reference to the post-implantation period till labor rather than for implantation and conception; however, the adjusted uterine immune response with Th1/Th2 homeostasis may play a role in creating an optimal environment for implantation also. The balance between levels of Th1 and Th2 depends on serum progesterone levels, PIBF, TGF-α, and βand IL-10 [16].

Th1/Th2/Th17/Treg paradigm: Recently, the paradigm has been expanded into the Th1/Th2/Th17/Treg paradigm [14]. The Th1 and Th17 cells are mediators of inflammation and are found in high levels in spontaneous abortion. Treg cells which suppress inflammation play an important role in the induction of antigen-specific tolerance by inhibiting NK cell destruction of trophoblast cells. In pregnancy, there is a shift from a Th1/Th17 toward a Th2/Treg cell response to prevent rejection.

3.3.5 Synthesis of Immunosuppressive Molecules

Synthesis of immunosuppressive molecules by placental exosomes, such as FasL, PDL1, IDO, and MHC molecules, may modulate the immune response. Transforming growth factor α (TGF-α) generates Treg cells from CD4+CD25− precursors. Treg cells maintain transplantation tolerance through a TGF-α-dependent FOXP3 induction. Thus, TGF-α is a key regulator of the signaling pathways which initiate and maintain FOXP3 expression and suppressive function among CD4+CD25− precursors. The suppressive effects of TGF-α and IL-10 on lymphocytes and antigen-presenting cells are synergic [17].

3.3.6 Regulatory T Cells (Tregs)

Tregs are the most potent suppressive cells in the immune system and are required to prevent autoimmunity and help in tolerating allogeneic organ grafts. These unique properties of T cells help in maternal immune tolerance during pregnancy. The three main subsets of Treg cells are, viz., type 1 regulatory T cells (Tr1), T-helper 3 cells, and CD4+ CD25+ Treg cells [18].

The factors which help in promoting increase in number of Treg cells are found mainly in seminal fluid. They increase before implantation of the embryo especially CD4+ and CD25+. A trigger for their release is also through embryo signaling which is independent of semen's presence as this is also present in IVF pregnancy [6].

Decrease in Treg cells is associated with pregnancy complications like spontaneous abortions, unexplained infertility, and preeclampsia. CD4+CD25+ Treg cells in these women are lower in peripheral blood and decidual tissue compared to normal pregnant women [19].

3.3.7 Complement System

The complement system leads to lysis of cell membrane by causing aggregation of inflammatory cells and formation of membrane attack complexes. The complement cascade, in turn, is regulated by complement regulatory proteins (CRP) that are critical for protecting tissues from inflammation. The complement cascade when activated leads to cleavage of C3 component into C3a and C3b fragments. MAC which activates cell lysis is released by binding of C5b which in turn is activated by C3a and C3b fragments. The MAC is a pore-forming lipophilic complex that increases cell membrane permeability and ultimately causes cell death [20].

Appropriate complement inhibition is required for successful outcome of a pregnancy [21]. The complement system is inhibited by decay-accelerating factor (DAF), membrane cofactor protein (MCP), and CD59 which are expressed by the placenta.

3.3.8 Uterine Natural Killer Cells (uNK Cells) or Decidual NK Cells

These distinctive lymphocytes originate in bone marrow and belong to the natural killer cell lineage and are different from mature circulating NK cells. NK cell function is regulated by an array of inhibitory receptors, including killer immunoglobulin-like receptors (KIR) and activating receptors (KAR). Uterine NK cells gradually increase in midluteal phase at the expected time of implantation and are crucial for normal implantation. These uNKs have a distinct phenotype characterized by a high surface density of CD56 or neural cell adhesion molecule. Their proliferation is increased by progesterone, by production of IL-15 by stromal cell and placental macrophages and by decidual prolactin; and activity is increased by increased expression of IL-15 receptor on CD56+ uNK cells and embryonic signals such as hCG [22]. These CD56+ NK cells accumulate at the decidua parietalis in close proximity to extravillous trophoblast and facilitate deep invasion of cytotrophoblasts into myometrial segments, thereby promoting spiral artery remodeling and angiogenesis. These processes are controlled by NK cell receptors that recognize MHC class I molecules as their ligands. These cells can damage trophoblast and secrete Th1 products causing fetal death unless suppressed by HLA-G interaction with KIR.

Near the end of the luteal phase of nonfertile ovulatory cycles, uterine NK cell nuclei begin to disintegrate. But if implantation proceeds, they persist in large numbers in the decidua during early pregnancy.

3.3.9 Phosphocholination

Phosphocholination is the posttranslational addition of phosphocholine to certain secretory glycoproteins, which has inhibitory effects on T and B lymphocytes. Lowry suggested that the presence of phosphocholine moieties in placental secreted peptides and proteins plays an important role in maternal immune tolerance during pregnancy [11].

3.3.10 Programmed Death Ligand 1 (PDL1)

Maternal immune response is altered by programmed death 1 (PD1) receptor and its ligands, PDL1 and PDL2. Expression of PDL1 which is found on all trophoblast cells increases throughout pregnancy; PDL2 is found mainly on syncytiotrophoblast of the early placenta and decreases throughout gestation. PD1 levels increase in response to fetal antigen-specific lymphocytes, and in its absence lymphocytes accumulate in the maternal uterine draining lymph nodes due to lack of their deletion [23].

3.3.11 Tryptophan Catabolism Mediated by Indoleamine 2,3-Dioxygenase (IDO)

L-tryptophan which is required for protein biosynthesis is catabolized by the enzyme IDO. Infection in an area leads to IFN secretion by the leukocytes which, in turn, triggers IDO production and tryptophan catabolism and subsequent inhibition of unwanted T cells and infection. Links between the IDO pathway with T-regulatory

(Treg) cell biology are also emerging [24]. Placental catabolization of tryptophan suppresses T cell activity and protects against fetal rejection.

On the other hand, many studies have shown that IDO is not essential for continuation of pregnancy as IDO expression has not been found to be significantly different between proven fertile women and women with a history of miscarriages.

3.3.12 Corticotropin-Releasing Hormone (CRH) and Its Regulation of FasL Expression

CRH is a peptide hormone that controls the stress response through adrenocorticotropic hormone (ACTH). It has a role in placental growth and remodeling, prostaglandin generation, gestation length, and the onset of labor.

Though hypothalamic CRH has been considered to act indirectly as an anti-inflammatory hormone, CRH produced at peripheral inflammatory sites has been shown to possess potent pro-inflammatory properties. Intrauterine CRH helps in embryo implantation by causing an aseptic inflammatory response, and in the ovary it has important interactions with the proapoptotic cytokine, Fas ligand [25].

3.3.12.1 Fas Ligand (FasL)

FasL is a member of TNF family and its release is controlled by CRH. It is expressed in activated T and B lymphocytes, NK cells, and macrophages. The Fas-FasL system is involved in apoptosis, lymphopoiesis and immunopoiesis, and cytolytic pathways of NK cells and regulates responses to viruses, elimination of tumor cells, cellular turnover, and deletion of autoimmune cells in lymphoid organs. FasL is expressed on the trophoblast and decidual cells during pregnancy and helps in implantation and maternal immune tolerance [25]. But other mechanisms controlling the maternal immune responses in absence of FasL have been reported.

3.4 Local Immune Tolerance

Immune tolerance at the local interface in the decidua is attained by downregulating T cell activity by various mechanisms:

- *Induction of anergy*: NK cells activate T cells and monocytes and also induce trophoblast apoptosis at the invasion front. Afterward, macrophages present peptides from phagocytosed apoptotic trophoblast cells to Th1 cells. This induces anergy of the T cells.
- *Fas ligand system-induced apoptosis*: Increased FasR expression leads to increased susceptibility of the T cells for induction of apoptosis, called activation-induced cell death (AICD). Consequently the precise balance between cytotoxic

T cell activity, controlling the amount of trophoblast invasion, and AICD or anergy induction of T cells is necessary for an implantation process.

- *Haptoglobins as immunomodulators*: Maternal proteins like haptoglobins are taken up and accumulated within the blastocyst fluid. Its secretion increases during the midluteal phase and peaks at the implantation window. They act on maternal immune cells: reduce NK activity by competitive binding and also reduce NK cell adhesion/invasion to extracellular matrices. Prostaglandin E in blastocyst fluid may also decrease cytotoxic NK cell activity.

The uterus is tailored to tolerate the fetal allograft and to allow controlled invasiveness of trophoblast only during the window of implantation. However, none of the compounds are pregnancy-specific and therefore cannot be the prime signal for tolerance. Abnormal embryo may fail to create necessary signaling [6].

Recently, three models of immune tolerance have been described in context of pregnancy [20]. The first is classic "self-nonself model" of immunity according to which recognition of nonself initiates T cell activation. A harmful immune response that is mediated by cytotoxic T cells is suppressed by shifting of immune response to one that produces noncytotoxic antibody. This is achieved by limiting trafficking or function of T cells via highly complex underlying mechanisms described above. The second is "danger model" which states that T cell, and therefore immune system activation, depends on recognition of "danger," rather than on recognition of nonself. This danger is expressed in fetal tissues and decidua through dysregulation of critical metabolic processes, necrosis etc. which produces a signal that alters the processing of locally expressed antigens. This may explain a shift toward Th2-type immune responses in decidua or the systemic circulation during pregnancy. The third is the "evolutionary nonself model" according to which activation of the innate immune response is the critical mechanism for overall immune response.

Conclusion

There are many mechanisms involved in maternal immune tolerance of the semi-allogenic fetus in a normal pregnancy. Failures in any of these assumed essential systems may cause recurrent pregnancy losses. A common difficulty lies in distinguishing between cause and effect when identifying immunological changes in such patients. Association of RPL with HLA typing, embryotoxic factors, HLA-G polymorphisms, anti-paternal antibodies, decidual cytokine profiles, and natural killer cells has been inconsistent and non-reproducible [26]. Immunomodulation treatments have not proven to be effective in management of RPL [26]. Treatments such as lymphocyte immunization therapy with paternal or third-party leukocytes to develop immune tolerance [27] and intravenous immunoglobulins for maternal immunosuppression are not found effective as treatment of RPL. Further research may lead to a greater understanding of the process and can contribute to developing new therapeutic strategies.

Key Points

- The immune processes occurring at maternal fetal interface are highly dynamic with both maternal and fetal contributions.
- Development of maternal tolerance depends on unique embryo-derived signaling between the embryo and mother.
- Preimplantation factor is being evaluated as a possible biomarker for embryo tolerance and viable pregnancy, as it is not positive in chemical pregnancies and unviable pregnancies unlike βhCG.
- HLA-G promotes maternal tolerance by immunosuppression of cytotoxic activity of the decidual/uterine NK cells.
- Progesterone-induced blocking factor mediates the biological effects of progesterone and facilitates immune tolerance.
- In pregnancy, there is a shift from a Th1/Th17 immune response which promotes rejection toward a Th2/Treg cell response that promotes tolerance as it inhibits uterine NK cell cytotoxicity against trophoblast cells.
- Synthesis of immunosuppressive molecules by placental exosomes such as FasL, PDL1, and IDO may modulate the immune response.
- CD4+ CD25+ Treg cells are the most potent suppressive cell lineage in the immune system.
- Appropriate complement inhibition is required for successful pregnancy.
- Uterine NK cells facilitate deep invasion of cytotrophoblasts into myometrial segments, thereby promoting spiral artery remodeling and angiogenesis.

References

1. Rao KA. In: Rao KA, editor. Principles & practice of assisted reproductive technology. 1st ed. New Delhi: Jaypee Brothers Medical Publishers; 2013. p. 116.
2. Medawar PB. Some immunological and endocrinological problems raised by the evolution of viviparity in vertebrates. Symp Soc Exp Biol. 1953;44:320–38.
3. Billingham RE. Transplantation immunity and the maternal-fetal relation. N Engl J Med. 1964;2(270):720–5.
4. Billington WD. The immunological problem of pregnancy: 50 years with the hope of progress. A tribute to Peter Medawar. J Reprod Immunol. 2003;60(1):1–11.
5. Piccinni MP, Scaletti C, Mavilia C, Lazzeri E, Romagnani P, Natali I, Pellegrini S, Livi C, Romagnani S, Maggi E. Production of IL-4 and leukemia inhibitory factor by T cells of the cumulus oophorus: a favorable microenvironment for pre-implantation embryo development. Eur J Immunol. 2001;31(8):2431–7.
6. Barnea ER. Chapter 2: Signalling between and mother in early pregnancy: basis for development of tolerance. In: Carp HJA, editor. Recurrent pregnancy loss: causes, controversies and treatment. 2nd ed. Boca Raton: CRC Press, Taylor and Francis Group; 2015. p. 17–28.
7. Hunt JS. Stranger in a strange land. Immunol Rev. 2006;213:36–47.
8. Fuzzi B, Rizzo R, Criscuoli L, Noci I, Melchiorri L, Scarselli B, et al. HLA-G expression in early embryos is a fundamental prerequisite for the obtainment of pregnancy. Eur J Immunol. 2002;32(2):311–5.

9. Criscuoli L, Rizzo R, Fuzzi B, Melchiorri L, Menicucci A, Cozzi C, et al. Lack of Histocompatibility Leukocyte Antigen-G expression in early embryos is not related to germinal defects or impairment of interleukin-10 production by embryos. Gynecol Endocrinol. 2005;20(5):264–9.
10. Ramu S, Stamatkin C, Timms L, Ruble M, Roussev RG, Barnea ER. PreImplantation factor (PIF) detection in maternal circulation in early pregnancy correlates with live birth (bovine model). Reprod Biol Endocrinol. 2013;11:105.
11. Schjenken JE, Tolosa JM, Paul JW, Clifton VL, Smith R. Mechanisms of maternal immune tolerance during pregnancy. In Recent advances in research on the human placenta, J Zheng (ed). Croatia, InTech, 2012, pp 211–242. Available at http://www.intechopen.com/books/recentadvances-in-research-on-the-humanplacenta/mechanisms-of-maternal-immune-tolerance-during-pregnancy.
12. Szekeres-Bartho J. Immunological relationship between the mother and the fetus. Int Rev Immunol. 2002;21(6):471–95.
13. Lee JH, Ulrich B, Cho J, Park J, Kim CH. Progesterone promotes differentiation of human cord blood fetal T cells into T regulatory cells but suppresses their differentiation into Th17 cells. J Immunol. 2011;187(4):1778–87.
14. Chaouat G, Ledee-Bataille N, Dubanchet S, Zourbas S, Sandra O, Martal J. Reproductive immunology 2003: reassessing the Th1/Th2 paradigm? Immunol Lett. 2004;92(3):207–14.
15. Wegmann TG, Lin H, Guilbert L, Mosmann TR. Bidirectional cytokine interactions in the maternal-fetal relationship: is successful pregnancy a TH2 phenomenon? Immunol Today. 1993;14(7):353–6.
16. Druckmann R, Druckmann MA. Progesterone and the immunology of pregnancy. J Steroid Biochem Mol Biol. 2005;97(5):389–96.
17. Gregori S, Goudy KS, Roncarolo MG. The cellular and molecular mechanisms of immunosuppression by human type 1 regulatory T cells. Front Immunol. 2012;3:30.
18. Guerin LR, Prins JR, Robertson SA. Regulatory T-cells and immune tolerance in pregnancy: a new target for infertility treatment? Hum Reprod Update. 2009;15(5):517–35.
19. Jasper MJ, Tremellen KP, Robertson SA. Primary unexplained infertility is associated with reduced expression of the T-regulatory cell transcription factor Foxp3 in endometrial tissue. Mol Hum Reprod. 2006;12(5):301–8.
20. Bonney EA. Immune regulation in pregnancy: a matter of perspective? Obstet Gynecol Clin North Am. 2016;43(4):679–98.
21. Girardi G. Complement inhibition keeps mothers calm and avoids fetal rejection. Immunol Invest. 2008;37(5):645–59.
22. Gubbay O, Critchley HO, Bowen JM, King A, Jabbour HN. Prolactin induces ERK phosphorylation in epithelial and CD56(+) natural killer cells of the human endometrium. J Clin Endocrinol Metab. 2002;87(5):2329–35.
23. Taglauer ES, Yankee TM, Petroff MG. Maternal PD-1 regulates accumulation of fetal antigen-specific CD8+ T cells in pregnancy. J Reprod Immunol. 2009;80(1–2):12–21.
24. Lippens C, Duraes FV, Dubrot J, Brighouse D, Lacroix M, Irla M, et al. IDO-orchestrated crosstalk between pDCs and Tregs inhibits autoimmunity. J Autoimmun. 2016;75:39–49.
25. Kalantaridou SN, Zoumakis E, Makrigiannakis A, Godoy H, Chrousos GP. The role of corticotropin-releasing hormone in blastocyst implantation and early fetal immunotolerance. Horm Metab Res. 2007;39(6):474–7.
26. Practice Committee Opinion of the American Society of Reproductive Medicine. Evaluation and treatment of recurrent pregnancy loss: a committee opinion. Fertil Steril. 2012;98:1103–11.
27. Wong LF, Porter TF, Scott JR. Immunotherapy for recurrent miscarriage. Cochrane Database Syst Rev. 2014;(10):CD000112.

Part II

Etiology and Management of RPL

Immunology and Pregnancy Loss

4

Monika Gupta

4.1 Introduction

Recurrent pregnancy loss (RPL) is typically defined as two or three or more consecutive pregnancy losses. Genetic, hormonal, metabolic, uterine anatomical, infectious, environmental, occupational and personal habits, thrombophilia, or immune disorders have been reported as possible etiologies. However, a majority of women with recurrent miscarriage have no discernible cause.

The immune system of pregnant women is tightly controlled to defend against microbial infections and to accept an embryo or the fetus, and inflammation-like processes are crucial for tissue growth, remodeling, and differentiation of the decidua during pregnancy.

Immunologic aberrations may lead to reproductive failure, such as implantation failure, recurrent pregnancy loss (RPL), preterm birth, intrauterine fetal growth restriction, and preeclampsia.

4.2 Mechanism of Fetal Tolerance

The key concepts of reproductive (allo)immunology have been described:

1. The embryo-fetus is a semi-allograft as it bears paternal immunogenetic traits inherently foreign to the mother.
2. The semi-allogeneic fetal tissues live in intimate contact with maternal tissues.

M. Gupta
Department of Obstetrics and Gynaecology, VMMC and Safdarjung Hospital, New Delhi, India
e-mail: drmonikagupta@hotmail.com

S. Mehta, B. Gupta (eds.), *Recurrent Pregnancy Loss*,
https://doi.org/10.1007/978-981-10-7338-0_4

3. The inclination toward an adverse immunologic interaction between the conceptus and the mother must be very highly regulated, to allow for successful pregnancy.

The mechanism for fetal tolerance suggests that in allogeneic reactions such as transplant and pregnancy, the immune response can be either harmful or favorable to the target cells expressing alloantigens. The harmful effect or rejection as observed in transplantation is characterized by cytotoxic antibodies and cells that damage the antigenic target. The enhancing effect or facilitation reaction is characterized by a predominance of humoral responses, which may counteract the rejection reaction and have a beneficial effect on the antigenic target. In normal pregnancy there is predominance of this facilitation reaction over the rejection reaction, and this occurs because of the local adaptation of the maternal immune system which allows for successful coexistence between the mother and fetus/placenta expressing both maternal (self) and paternal (nonself) genes [1–3].

If the coexisting but suppressed rejection reaction is upregulated, the embryo is rejected. The suggestion that the facilitation reaction prevails over the rejection reaction and results in fetal tolerance has been followed by a plethora of studies that have focused on the mechanisms mediating this specific response.

The normal reproductive immunology is now considered that of a unique immunologic interplay of various factors at the maternal-fetal interface and an appropriate balance in immunoregulatory factors so as to favor, and even promote, implantation and embryo-fetal survival. Cytotoxic adaptive immune responses are diminished, bypassed, or even abrogated, while regulatory adaptive immunity is enhanced. By contrast, innate (natural) immunity remains intact, serving two purposes: one, to continue to provide host defense against infection and, two, to interact with fetal tissues to promote successful placentation and pregnancy [4, 5].

4.2.1 Local Immune Adaptation

Various changes taking place in the uterus during pregnancy that contribute in the immune acceptance of the fetus or placenta have been described below. The interplay of these factors has a bearing in order to promote a successful pregnancy, and their alterations have been proposed to result in RPL.

4.2.1.1 Differences in Lymphocyte Populations

The first histologically apparent maternal immunologic adjustment to the embryo is a dramatic change in the relative proportions of leukocyte subpopulations in the uterus.

Natural Killer (NK) Cells

They are part of the innate immune system, and in contrast to T lymphocytes, they can recognize and react against target antigens typically on cells affected by intracellular infection or malignancy without prior sensitization. Natural killer cells are the most abundant cell population in endometrium and constitute 50–90% of lymphocytes in human uterine decidua in early pregnancy. These cells have a different phenotypic expression (CD16−/CD56bright) than peripheral blood NK cells (CD16+/CD56dim). In term placentas higher percentages of CD56dim/CD16+ NK cells are found in decidua basalis, whereas the percentage of CD56bright/CD16− uterine NK cells is significantly higher in decidua parietalis.

These findings suggest functional differences may occur even in different tissues during implantation and growth of the maternal-fetal unit. Due to their increased presence and direct contact with invading trophoblast, decidual NK (dNK) cells have been considered as important for the establishment of normal pregnancy. There is evidence that, coincident with blastocyst implantation and decidualization, when uterine NK cells become activated, they produce IFN-γ, perforin, and other molecules, including angiogenetic factors.

Invading fetal trophoblasts become admixed with decidual NK cells, macrophages, and dendritic cells. The major roles of decidual NK cells are unique to pregnancy in trophoblast attraction and invasion, decidual and placental angiogenesis and possibly fetal vasculogenesis, and vascular modifications in the uterus [6].

Alterations in decidual NK cell numbers and activation status may play a role in pregnancy complications, such as immunologic infertility, recurrent spontaneous abortion, and preeclampsia [7]. Flow cytometric analysis of decidual lymphocytes from normal pregnancy demonstrated that the relative proportion of decidual NK cells was increased to approximately the same extent in normal, anembryonic pregnancies, and recurrent pregnancy losses. Nonetheless, higher decidual NK activity has been found in tissue from women with anembryonic pregnancy and recurrent spontaneous abortion than in normal pregnancies. Thus increased decidual NK cell activity or numbers have been correlated with pregnancy losses.

Regulatory T Cells and Th17 Inflammatory Cells

Regulatory T Cells (Treg cells) are a subset of immunoregulatory T lymphocytes (CD4+CD25+Foxp3+), which derive either from the thymus or by activation of CD4+ T-cells following antigen stimulation under the influence of TGF-β. CD4+CD25+ regulatory T cells (Treg) are triggered in both alloantigen-dependent and alloantigen-independent manners [8]. Mechanisms of action of Tregs include cell contact-dependent and cytokine-dependent mechanisms for maintaining peripheral immunological self-tolerance. After being activated by antigen-presenting cells (APC's), decidual Treg cells can suppress the generation and the effector function of type 1 T-cell-mediated immune responses, which are considered harmful to pregnancy. By secretion of inhibitory cytokines (TGF-β, IL-10, and IL-35), and consumption of γc-family cytokines (IL-2, IL-4, IL-7, IL-15), decidual Treg cells may suppress activation and expansion of conventional T lymphocytes, inhibit the release of proinflammatory cytokine, increase T-cell apoptotic rates, and modulate the functions of decidual dendritic cells.

Forkhead box P3 (FoxP3) expression in Treg cells is a critical factor in the maintenance of Treg cell suppressive function. Upregulation of the transcription factor Foxp3 allows decidual Treg cells to begin their suppressive effect on decidual immune cells and transfer suppressive capabilities and the ability to inhibit downstream steps in the maternal anti-fetal immune cascade. However, the mechanism is not well defined. These fetal-specific Tregs persist after delivery and rapidly reaccumulate during subsequent pregnancies [9].

A recent study regarding the role of dendritic cells and Tregs in RPL has shown that the percentage of Tregs was significantly lower in women with miscarriage than in controls. In the risk evaluation of the factors such as age; BMI; percentage of mDCs, pDCs, and Tregs; and mDC/pDC ratio affecting the occurrence of miscarriage, the percentage of Tregs was the best predictive factor, with a cutoff point of 1.50, and the sensitivity and specificity of this test were 70% and 75%, respectively. The area under the curve was 0.74 for the Tregs [10].

A subpopulation of CD4+ interleukin (IL)-17-producing T cells (Th17) have also been recently described in pregnancy. Th17 cells have recently been described as a key effector T-cell subset, which has changed our understanding of immune regulation, immune pathogenesis, and host defense. They represent the third member of the T-cell trilogy having probably evolved to enhance host clearance of a range of pathogens distinct from those targeted by Th1 and Th2. Th17 are differentiated from naïve T-cells in response to a combination of cytokine signals distinct from, and antagonized by, cytokines of the Th1 and Th2 lineages (TGF-β, IL-1β, and IL-23) [11]. Their numbers are also expanded in the pregnant uterus, although not as much as CD4+CD25+ Tregs. In the absence of IL-6, TGF-β suppress the conversion of naïve T-cells to Th17 cells, while in the presence of IL-6, naïve T-cells are converted to Th17 cells, and existing Treg cells can function as inducers of Th17 cells and themselves convert to Th17 cells. Apart from TGF-β and IL-6, other factors can also influence the antagonism between Treg cells and Th-17 cells. IL-1 can induce Th17 cells as opposed to Treg cells; Th17 cells may play a role in protecting the maternal-fetal interface from microbes. The mutual antagonism and plasticity between Treg cells and Th17 cells illustrates the fine balance between a suppressive or pro-inflammatory immune outcome at the fetomaternal interface and the major importance of the cytokine environment for the success of pregnancy.
Increased Th17 cells and Th17 cytokines (e.g., IL-17 and IL-23) have been shown in unexplained RPL patients [12]. In addition, altered numbers of Th17 and/or ratio of Th17 to Tregs are associated with pregnancy complications, such a spontaneous abortion, preeclampsia, and preterm birth [13].

4.2.1.2 Soluble Immunomodulatory Agents

Uterine immune regulation is also provided by the induction of immune-modulatory molecules like cytokines, progesterone, and prostaglandins that permeate the uterine environment.

Cytokines

Cytokines are the signaling molecules secreted from immune cells and bind to receptors on other immune cells causing stimulation or inhibition of their function. Cytokines promoting the T-lymphocyte cytotoxicity and inflammation are called T helper type 1 cytokines, namely, IL-2 and interferon γ [IFN-γ]). Cytokines promoting antibody production and anti-inflammation are called T helper type 2 cytokines, namely, IL-4, IL-5, and IL-10. Normal human pregnancy is considered to be a Th2 anti-inflammatory condition and that a shift toward Th1 cytokines will lead to abortion or pregnancy complications. The appropriate balance of cytokine and chemokine expression at the maternal-fetal interface can govern the immune cell profile and function within the decidua.

Different cell populations are potentially involved in the production of Th2 cytokines and Th1 cytokines as well as other cytokines (i.e., IL-12, -15, -18), chemokines, and growth factors that control the differentiation and the activation of immune cells locally. A cytokine that controls the shift to Th1 response is IL-12 that coexists with one enhancing the Th2 response (IL-10).

In response to the conceptus or other antigens, decidual lymphocytes secrete proinflammatory Th1-type cytokines which adversely affect the development of the embryo. Fetal rejection occurs through immune-induced inflammation (delayed-type hypersensitivity reactions which result in lymphocyte infiltration of the trophoblast) and tissue degradation (cytotoxic reactions which result in damage of the trophoblast by NK cells and cytotoxic antibodies produced by specific subpopulations of B lymphocytes).

The cytokine balance is determined by maternal genes, which regulate the response to stress, LPS, and paternally inherited trophoblastic antigens. Also, cytokine gene polymorphisms (i.e., TNF, IFN-γ) have been associated with recurrent miscarriage in women with Th1 immunity to the trophoblast. However, several studies investigating the relationship between cytokines, angiogenic mediators, hormones, gene polymorphisms, and RPL have produced contradictory results [14].

Progesterone

Progesterone is proven to be vital in creating a healthy intrauterine environment during pregnancy and vital for its continuation too. At high concentrations, progesterone is a potent inducer of Th2-type cytokines as well as of LIF and M-CSF production by T-cells. A protein called progesterone-induced blocking factor (PIBF), by inducing a Th2-dominant cytokine production, mediates the immunological effects of progesterone. PIBF binds to a novel type of the IL-4 receptor and signals via the Jak/STAT pathway, to induce a number of genes, that not only affect the immune response. It might also play a role in trophoblast invasiveness [15]. It also inhibits production of tumor necrosis factor-alpha (TNF-alpha) in macrophages. Thus the maternal immune response is suppressed by altering the T helper 1 (Th1)/T helper 2 (Th2) balance.

Prostaglandin E2

Prostaglandin E2 (PGE2) is produced by resident macrophages and decidual cells. Lymphocytes proliferate poorly in the presence of this compound.

4.3 Maternal Systemic Immune Responses

Circulating immune cells in pregnant women generally have a higher capacity for cytokine production than those from nonpregnant women. However, selective suppression or modulation may occur. There are at least two mechanisms for overcoming most immune reactions: One is active suppression, and the other is enhanced tolerance. Enhanced tolerance has been clearly demonstrated in normal pregnancy.

4.3.1 Altered Human Leukocyte Antigen Expression

The primary cellular immune response that develops against transplanted tissue is directed against the major histocompatibility complex (MHC) proteins called human leukocyte antigens (HLAs). HLA molecules play an important role in both the adaptive and innate immunity. Although multiparous women are excellent sources of antibodies to paternal HLAs, maternal B lymphocytes specific for paternal HLA are partially deleted during pregnancy. In addition, T lymphocytes specific for paternal HLA are difficult to demonstrate.

HLA class 1A antigens like HLA-A and HLA-B are primary stimulatory antigens for graft rejection, whereas other nonclassical HLA 1B antigens are HLA-E/F/G. Unlike the invading trophoblasts, syncytiotrophoblast forming the outermost layer of the placental villi that is exposed to maternal blood lacks HLA class IA mRNA (HLA-A, HLA-B, and HLA-C) and membrane-bound protein but has HLA class IB (HLA-E, HLA-F, and HLA-G) HLA-G5 mRNA and antigens both early and late in pregnancy [16]. Soluble HLA-G in maternal serum, now termed HLA-G5, is biochemically unique among the HLA-G isoforms and is associated with desirable immune suppression in both pregnancy and graft transplantation.

NK cells have receptors that can be activated (Th1 response) or inhibited (Th2 response) by HLA-C/G/E ligands depending on polymorphism of HLA molecule. Some of the receptors recognizing HLA-G and HLA-C epitopes are selectively expressed on dNK cell. The specific interaction of the NK cell receptors with trophoblastic antigens led to the concept of an embryo recognition model through an "NK cell allorecognition system."

HLA-G and HLA-E dampen an immune response by interacting with leukocyte inhibitory receptors (LIRs) on uterine natural killer (NK) cells and macrophages and with the T-cell receptor on CD8+ cells. These inhibitory dNK receptors are expected to inhibit dNK activation for trophoblast damage; otherwise dNK are allowed to develop anti-trophoblast activity [17].

Most studies that have investigated the effect of dNK receptors in the maintenance of pregnancy have specifically focused on the interactions involving HLA-G molecules, because of their restricted distribution to placental tissues. Expression of some HLA-G isoforms has been shown to protect trophoblastic cells from lysis by activated cytotoxic cell clones [18].

Among the different NK cell receptor interactions with their specific counterparts on the trophoblast, the interactions between inhibitory receptors of the KIR family (inhKIR) and their ligands HLA-C molecules appear to be those mainly involved in the function of an NK-cell-mediated allorecognition system in pregnancy [19].

As regards studies on HLA in RPL, the three major issues, viz., HLA allele incompatibility (sharing) between partners with RPL, HLA allele prevalence, and HLA-C, HLA-G, and HLA-E alleles in couples with RPL have been addressed in the recent meta-analysis of 41 studies by Meuleman et al. [20]. The allele sharing in HLA-B, HLA-DR, and HLA-DQ loci has been found with significantly higher frequency in RPL than control couples. There was an increased risk of RPL in mothers carrying a HLA-DRB1*4 (OR 1.41, 95% CI 1.05–1.90), HLA-DRB1*15 (OR 1.57, 95% CI 1.15–2.14), or HLA-E*01:01 allele (OR 1.47, 95% CI 0.20–1.81) and a decreased risk with HLA-DRB1*13 (OR 0.63, 95% CI 0.45–0.89) or HLA-DRB1*14 (OR 0.54, 95% CI 0.31–0.94) [20].

4.3.2 TNF Superfamily

Apoptosis-inducing members of the tumor necrosis factor (TNF) supergene family may also have important roles in protecting the placenta and its membranes by inducing apoptosis in potentially cytotoxic T cells. The ligands identified in and/or on human trophoblasts include TNF-alpha, Fas L, and TNF-related apoptosis-inducing ligand (TRAIL).

All of these molecules, which are expressed as both membrane and soluble forms, can kill activated immune cells targeting the trophoblast via specific receptors on activated leukocytes.

Placental-derived microparticles, such as microvesicles and exosomes containing an array of placental proteins, mRNA, and microRNAs, also play a role in regulating the maternal immune system during pregnancy. The release and content of these microparticles is increased and/or altered under certain pathologic conditions, and, as such, they may be involved in the pathogenesis of pregnancy complications such as preeclampsia [21].

4.4 T Cells in Peripheral Blood

4.4.1 NK Cells

In peripheral blood, 90% of NK cells carry the CD56dimCD16 markers, which are associated with high toxicity and low cytokine production. Majority of studies have found that percentage of CD56+ cells in peripheral blood taken prior to pregnancy in RPL women is significantly higher than in controls [22].

4.4.2 Regulatory T Cells (Tregs)

Tregs produce interleukin-10 (IL-10), which appears to play a role in maintaining pregnancy, though their exact role in RPL is still not very clear due to sparsity of relevant studies. Lee et al. reported that the percent of Tregs in peripheral blood at the time of pregnancy loss was significantly lower in first trimester loss [23]. The levels of IL-17(+) T cells and the IL-17(+) T/CD4(+)Foxp3(+) Treg cell ratio were significantly increased.

A population of IL-10 producing CD19+CD24hi CD27+ regulatory B cells also expands during normal pregnancy, and their role may be to suppress undesired immune responses from maternal T cells.

4.4.3 T Helper Cells

T helper cells can be characterized by their patterns of cytokine production into T helper 1 and 2 cells. Percentages of peripheral blood Th1 (CD3+/CD4+/TNF-alpha+, CD3+/CD4+/IFN-gamma+) and Th2 cells (CD3+/CD4+/IL-10+, CD3+/CD4+/IL-4+) in women with histories of recurrent pregnancy losses and normal fertile women are comparable. However, when the ratios of these cells (Th1/Th2) were compared in these two groups, women with recurrent pregnancy losses had significantly elevated Th1:Th2 ratios compared to that of normal fertile controls [24].

4.4.4 T Suppressor Cell

T suppressor cell (CD3+/CD8+) cytokine production pattern of CD3+/CD8+ cells has been observed to be parallel to that of CD3+/CD4+ cells. The ratio of CD3+/CD8+/TNF-α to CD3+/CD8+/IL-10 cells is significantly elevated in women with RPL as compared to those of normal controls. Thus there are significantly elevated Th1 immune responses in peripheral blood lymphocytes of women with recurrent pregnancy losses or multiple implantation failures, which may reflect the systemic contribution of Th1 cytokines.

4.4.5 GM-CSF

Granulocyte-macrophage colony-stimulating factor (GM-CSF) plays an important role in Th1/Th2 balance as it stimulates the production of prostaglandins, tumor necrosis factor (TNF), IL-1, plasminogen activator, and IL-6. Perricone et al. found that women with RPL have significantly lower levels of GM-CSF [25].

4.5 Other Alloimmune Factors

A rare immunologically mediated cause of RPL is alloimmunization to blood group antigen P [26]. Cytotoxic IgM or IgG3 antibody directed against the P and PK antigens has been associated with miscarriage in more than 50% of affected pregnancies, as well as fetal growth restriction in ongoing pregnancies. It was proposed that early plasmapheresis could be therapeutic.

4.6 Autoantibodies

The presence of autoantibodies, such as anticardiolipin antibodies, antinuclear antibodies (ANA), and anti-double-strand DNA antibodies, have often been reported in women with pregnancy loss even without overt autoimmune disease though these antibodies are also found in women with normal pregnancies [27].

There has been reported increase of the HLA-DQA1*0501 allele (now classified as 05:05) in women with recurrent pregnancy losses who are antiphospholipid (aPL) positive. Fetuses compatible with their mothers for this allele are autoimmune unacceptable to the mother, trigger development of aPL when the pregnancy fails, and are most prone to miscarriage in subsequent pregnancies. However, the few other authors could not confirm these findings [28].

4.7 Current Cellular Immunology Tests for RPL

Because of the critical role of NK in trophoblast damage, the diagnostic approach to alloimmune abortions is almost limited to the study of these cells. Their numbers and function are reflected in blood during pregnancy. These NK cells can be accurately measured in the blood and most accurately by cytotoxicity assays from NK cells that are present in women with RPL.

Several tests are available for prepregnancy diagnosis (prognosis) of RPL especially for NK cells like molecular assay of HLA-C group of receptors for NK cell regulation (KIR-HLA-C combinations). The detection of NK cell disturbances (increase of CD3−CD16+CD56+ cells) in the peripheral blood of unexplained RPL women is often used as a marker of the underlying alloimmune mechanism for miscarriage. Furthermore, monitoring of NK cells is used for the estimation of the effect of immunotherapy.

Another significant test in the peripheral blood cells of pregnant women is measurement of TNF-alpha (TNF-a) and other "TH1" cytokines by CD4+ T cells. When cells capable of producing TNF-a are activated and then quantitated by flow cytometry, the values are statistically significant in predicting RPL [29].

Evaluation of Th1/Th2 cytokine balance for detection of predominance of Th1 response can also be helpful. A significantly higher Th1/Th2 ratios of IFN-g/IL-4, TNF-a/IL-4, and TNF-a/IL-10 in CD4-TH1 cells are observed in women with RPL than in controls. The increased Th1 cytokine expression in these activated cells has been studied as the underlying immune etiology for reproductive failures, but regardless of the relationship to the pathophysiology of the disease, the levels can surely be used to diagnose and suggest possible treatment for these patients.

Many other tests, though having a doubtful diagnostic value, have also been described like partner's HLA typing for the detection of increased HLA sharing between them, detection of lymphocytotoxic antibodies against paternal cells (anti-paternal antibodies-APCA), and mixed lymphocyte cultures for the detection of blocking antibodies.

As the maternal age increases and the number of miscarriages also increases, so more testing may be indicated. Test groups 1, 2, and 3 could be utilized as suggested along with indicated age and number of abortions [30].

4.8 Immunotherapies

Both immune-stimulating and immunosuppressive therapies have been proposed for recurrent pregnancy loss depending on whether the maternal immune system is believed to be either hypo- or hyperresponsive to paternal-fetal antigens.

Immunization of potential mothers with paternal or third-party leukocytes to improve reproductive success was, in the past, a popular method of putatively improving live birth rates. The leukocyte immunization was thought to introduce a needed measure of immune recognition and stimulation. Few meta-analyses reported that therapies like white cell immunization does not improve the livebirth rate among those with unexplained recurrent miscarriage [31].

Treatment with intravenous immunoglobulin (IVIG) has also been proposed for unexplained pregnancy loss. In one study, IVIG significantly downregulated Th17 cells and upregulated CD4(+) Foxp3(+) T cells. In addition, Th17/CD4(+) Foxp3(+) T-cell ratio decreased in pregnancy. They concluded that intravenous immunoglobulin G treatment modulated imbalance of Th17 and Foxp3(+) Treg cells in pregnant RPL women with cellular immune abnormality [32]. However, meta-analysis of several trials concluded that there is insufficient evidence to recommend IVIG in routine practice for primary recurrent pregnancy loss; thus, this treatment is not recommended [33].

Other therapeutic possibilities available for recurrent pregnancy loss include anticoagulants (low-molecular-weight heparin, *aspirin*), hormones (progesterone), and immunomodulators (granulocyte-macrophage colony-stimulating factor [GM-CSF], human growth hormone [hCG], macrophage-colony stimulating factor [M-CSF]) [34].

A recent pilot randomized control trial (RCT)86 assessed the possibility of "screening and treating" women with recurrent miscarriage by demonstrating a high uterine NK density (>5%) 5–9 days after the LH surge and randomizing the treatment with prednisolone or placebo [35]. In relation of immunotherapy, pertaining to NK cells is currently confined to research because existing immunologic tests are either controversial or fail to provide substantive clinical decision making distinctions.

Systematic reviews have consistently found no beneficial effect of immunotherapy for treatment of RPL [36]. Immune therapy of RPL should be considered experimental and used only in the setting of a clinical trial regulated by an Institutional Review Board.

In the current scenario, there is no "immunotherapy" known to be beneficial in promoting improved pregnancy outcome, and appropriate use of such therapy remains unclear.

Key Points

- Increased decidual NK cell activity or numbers have been correlated with pregnancy losses.
- Increased Th17 cells and Th17 cytokines (e.g., IL-17 and IL-23) have been shown in unexplained RPL patients, while there is a decrease in CD4+CD25+ regulatory T (Treg) cells.
- Cytokine imbalance, i.e., increased production of Th1 cytokines leads to pregnancy loss.
- The allele sharing in HLA-B, HLA-DR, and HLA-DQ loci has been found with significantly higher frequency in RPL than control couples.
- The current immune tests available mainly focus on NK cell activity and measurement of TNF-alpha (TNF-a) and other "TH1" cytokines by CD4+ T cells mainly by using flow cytometry.
- There is insufficient evidence to recommend the routine use of immunotherapy in the form of IVIG, immune modulators, or NK cell therapy for treatment of RPL.

References

1. Robertson SA. Immune regulation of conception and embryo implantation-all about quality control? J Reprod Immunol. 2010;85:51.
2. Stoller M, Traupe T, Khattab AA, et al. Effects of coronary sinus occlusion on myocardial ischaemia in humans: role of coronary collateral function. Heart. 2013;99:548.
3. Mor G, Abrahams VM. The immunology of pregnancy. In: Creasy RK, Resnik R, Iams JD, et al., editors. Creasy and Resnik's maternal-fetal medicine: principles and practice. 7th ed. Philadelphia: Elsevier; 2014. p. 80.
4. Nagamatsu T, Schust DJ. The contribution of macrophages to normal and pathological pregnancies. Am J Reprod Immunol. 2010;63:460.
5. Zhang J, Chen Z, Smith GN, Croy BA. Natural killer cell-triggered vascular transformation: maternal care before birth? Cell Mol Immunol. 2011;8:1.
6. Lash GE, Robson SC, Bulmer JN. Review: functional role of uterine natural killer (uNK) cells in human early pregnancy decidua. Placenta. 2010;31(Suppl):S87.
7. Management of high-risk pregnancy. In: Queenan JT, Spong CY, Lockwood CJ, editors. Queenan's high-risk obstetrics. 6th ed. Malden: Blackwell Publishing; 2011.
8. Mjösberg J, Berg G, Jenmalm MC, Ernerudh J. FOXP3+ regulatory T cells and T helper 1, T helper 2, and T helper 17 cells in human early pregnancy decidua. Biol Reprod. 2010;82:698.

9. Rowe JH, Ertelt JM, Xin L, Way SS. Pregnancy imprints regulatory memory that sustains anergy to fetal antigen. Nature. 2012;490:102.
10. Kwiatek M, Gęca T, Krzyżanowski A, Malec A, Kwaśniewska A. Peripheral dendritic cells and CD4+CD25+Foxp3+ regulatory T cells in the first trimester of normal pregnancy and in women with recurrent miscarriage. PLoS One. 2015;10(5):e0124747.
11. Weaver CT, Harrington LE, Mangan PR, et al. Th17: an effector CD4 T cell lineage with regulatory T cell ties. Eur J Onstet Gynecol Reprod Biol. 2012;161:177–81.
12. Liu YS, Wu L, Tong XH, et al. Study on the relationship between Th17 cells and unexplained recurrent spontaneous abortion. Am J Reprod Immunol. 2011;65:503–11.
13. Saito S, Nakashima A, Shima T, Ito M. Th1/Th2/Th17 and regulatory T-cell paradigm in pregnancy. Am J Reprod Immunol. 2010;63:601.
14. Daher S, Mattar R, Gueuvoghlanian-Silva BY, et al. Genetic polymorphisms and recurrent spontaneous abortions: an overview of current knowledge. Am J Reprod Immunol. 2012;67:341–7.
15. Szekeres-Bartho J, Halasz M, Palkovics T. Progesterone in pregnancy; receptor-ligand interaction and signaling pathways. J Reprod Immunol. 2009;83:60.
16. Morales PJ, Pace JL, Platt JS, et al. Synthesis of beta(2)-microglobulin-free, disulphide-linked HLA-G5 homodimers in human placental villous cytotrophoblast cells. Immunology. 2007;122:179.
17. Varla-Leftherioti M. The significance of women's NK cell receptors' repertoire in the maintenance of pregnancy. Chem Immunol Allergy. 2005;89:84–95.
18. Menier C, Riteau B, Dausset J, et al. HLA-G truncated isoforms can substitute for HLA-G1 in fetal survival. Hum Immunol. 2000;61:1118–25.
19. Varla-Leftherioti M. Role of a KIR/HLA-C allorecognition system in pregnancy. J Reprod Immunol. 2004;62:19–27.
20. Meuleman T, Lashley LELO, Dekkers OM, van Lith JMM, Claas FHJ, Bloemenkamp KWH. HLA associations and HLA sharing in recurrent miscarriage: a systematic review and meta-analysis. Hum Immunol. 2015;76:362–73.
21. Holder BS, Tower CL, Forbes K, et al. Immune cell activation by trophoblast-derived microvesicles is mediated by syncytin 1. Immunology. 2012;136:184.
22. Lee KL, Na BJ, Kim JY, Hur SE, Lee M, Gilman-Sachs A, Kwak-Kim J. Determination of clinical cellular immune markers in women with recurrent pregnancy loss. Am J Reprod Immunol. 2013;70:398–411.
23. Lee SK, Kim JY, Hur SE, Kim CJ, Na BJ, Lee M, Gilman-Sachs A, Kwak-Kim J. An imbalance in interleukin-17-producing T and $Foxp3^+$ regulatory T cells in women with idiopathic recurrent pregnancy loss. Hum Reprod. 2011;26(11):2964–71.
24. Kwak-Kim JY, et al. Increased T helper 1 cytokine responses by circulating T cells are present in women with recurrent pregnancy losses and in infertile women with multiple implantation failures after IVF. Hum Reprod. 2003;18(4):767–73.
25. Perricone C, De Carolis C, Perricone R. Pregnancy and autoimmunity: a common problem. Best Pract Res Clin Rheumatol. 2012;26:47–60.
26. Hanafusa N, Noiri E, Yamashita T, et al. Successful treatment by double filtrate plasmapheresis in a pregnant woman with the rare P blood group and a history of multiple early miscarriages. Ther Apher Dial. 2006;10:498.
27. Christiansen OB. Reproductive immunology. Mol Immunol. 2013;55:8–15.
28. Varla-Leftherioti M, Keramitsopoulou T, Parapanissiou E, et al. HLA-DQA1*0505 sharing and killer immunoglobulin-like receptors in sub fertile couples: report from the 15th International Histocompatibility Workshop. Tissue Antigens. 2010;75:668–72.
29. Winger EE, Reed JL, Ashoush S, El-Toukhy T, Ahuja S, Taranissi M. Degree of TNF-a/IL-10 cytokine elevation correlates with IVF success rates in women undergoing treatment with Adalimumab (Humira) and IVIG. Am J Reprod Immunol. 2011;65:610–8.
30. Beaman KD, Ntrivalas E, Mallers TM, Jaiswal MK, Kwak-Kim J, Gilman-Sachs A. Immune etiology of recurrent pregnancy loss and its diagnosis. Am J Reprod Immunol. 2012;67:319–25. https://doi.org/10.1111/j.1600-0897.2012.01118.x.

31. Porter TF, LaCoursiere Y, Scott JR. Immunotherapy for recurrent miscarriage. Cochrane Database Syst Rev. 2006;(19):CD000112.
32. Kim DJ, Lee SK, Kim JY, Na BJ, Hur SE, Lee M, et al. Intravenous immunoglobulin G modulates peripheral blood Th17 and Foxp3(+) regulatory T cells in pregnant women with recurrent pregnancy loss. Am J Reprod Immunol. 2014;71(5):441–50.
33. Ata B, Tan SL, Shehata F, Holzer H, Buckett W. A systematic review of intravenous immunoglobulin for treatment of unexplained recurrent miscarriage. Fertil Steril. 2011;95:1080–5.
34. Matthiesen L, Kalkunte S, Sharma S. Multiple pregnancy failures: an immunological paradigm. Am J Reprod Immunol. 2012;67:334.
35. Tang AW, Alfirevic Z, Turner MA, et al. A feasibility trial of screening women with idiopathic recurrent miscarriage for high uterine natural killer cell density and randomizing to prednisolone or placebo when pregnant. Hum Reprod. 2013;28:1743–52.
36. Wong LF, Porter TF, Scott JR. Immunotherapy for recurrent miscarriage. Cochrane Database Syst Rev. 2014;(10):CD000112.

The Evolving Role of Genetics in Recurrent Pregnancy Loss

5

Bindiya Gupta and Pooja Singh

5.1 Introduction

Recurrent pregnancy loss (RPL) is defined as two or more consecutive clinical pregnancy loss before the pregnancy reaches 20 weeks of gestation [1]. The incidence of RPL is around 1–2% in couples who are desirous to conceive [2]. Various causes of RPL include advanced maternal age, uterine abnormalities, placental causes, incompetent cervix, parental chromosomal abnormalities, genetic abnormalities in the conceptus, immune disorders and/or endocrine imbalances. Recently, much attention is being paid to genetic causes involving changes in the parental or fetal chromosomes. Of recurrent miscarriages, 3–6% are due to chromosomal abnormalities of one of the two partners [3]. There is two to sevenfold increased risk of pregnancy loss in first-degree relatives of RPL couple as compared to the general population [4]. Among the genetic causes, the major factors are structural and numerical chromosomal abnormalities and allelic polymorphisms of some pro-thrombophilic genes [5].

5.2 Pathophysiology of Genetic Causes

It was Schmidt in 1962 who first identified a chromosomal abnormality, i.e., inherited translocation as a cause of recurrent pregnancy loss [6]. Of all the causes, chromosomal trisomies are the most common cause, while single most specific cause is monosomy X. The classification of various genetic causes of RPL and incidence is summarized in Table 5.1.

B. Gupta (✉) • P. Singh
Obstetrics and Gynecology, University College of Medical Sciences and GTB Hospital, Delhi, India
e-mail: dr_bindiya_gupta@yahoo.co.in; pooja.nrs@gmail.com

S. Mehta, B. Gupta (eds.), *Recurrent Pregnancy Loss*,
https://doi.org/10.1007/978-981-10-7338-0_5

Table 5.1 Classification of genetic causes of recurrent pregnancy loss

Genetic causes of RPL			
Chromosomal (accounts for 50% of first trimester loss)	Aneuploidy: of autosomes or sex chromosomes	Monosomy X (20%)	
		Trisomy (50%)	16 (31%)
			22 (11.4%)
			21 (10.5)
		Triploidy (15%)	
		Tetraploidy (5%)	
	Structural abnormality	Translocation (2–6%)	
		Inversion, ring chromosomes	
		Sex chromosome mosaicism	
Single-gene defect			
Multifactorial			

5.2.1 Aneuploidy

Meiotic nondisjunction in the germ cells of couples with normal parental karyotypes leads to numerical aneuploidy, and these are usually random nonrecurring events [7, 8]. Hence, prognosis for subsequent pregnancies in RPL couples is better after an aneuploid miscarriage than after an euploid miscarriage [9]. Studies have shown that fetal aneuploidies are present in up to 90% losses between 0 and 6 weeks of gestation, 50% between 8 and 11 weeks, and 30% from losses at 16–19 weeks of gestation [10]. After 20 weeks, only 6–12% are due to aneuploidies. Early pregnancy losses display unusual aneuploidies, while trisomies 21, 18, and 13 are more common in later losses [11]. Once a fetal heart rate is evident on ultrasound, the risk of aneuploidy is 5%.

Fifty percent of the cytogenetically abnormal abortus have been detected to have autosomal trisomies and out of them chromosomes 13, 16, and 21 have a possibility of viability. Trisomy 16, the most common autosomal trisomy in spontaneous abortion, is never seen in live-born babies. Trisomy-21 has 5% incidence in abortus but 1.15 per 1000 incidence in live borns. Trisomy-22 has also 5% incidence in abortus but no live births are possible. This implies 75% of trisomy conceptus are aborted spontaneously. Autosomal trisomies especially involving small chromosomes (8, 9, 10, 13, 14, 15, 18, 20, 21, and 22) are associated with advanced maternal age, whereas trisomy 16 is less closely correlated [12, 13]. The relationship of paternal age with aneuploidies is not well established.

5.2.2 Triploidy and Tetraploidy

Fertilization of a normal haploid ovum by dispermy leads to triploidy, while failure of an early cleavage division leads to tetraploid. Both these defects are not compatible with life. The primary pathogenic mechanism in 16% of abortion is triploidy [14]. Tetraploidy leads to around 8% of chromosomally abnormal abortions. Tetraploidy permits very little embryonic development, the majority of tetraploids being empty sacs or grossly abnormal embryos less than 5 mm long. Many specimens are incomplete, so only a limited examination is possible.

5.2.3 Chromosomal Structural Abnormality

Chromosomal structural abnormality is seen in 2–3% of cytogenetically abnormal conceptus, and the most common types are balanced and unbalanced translocations.

5.2.3.1 Translocations

It is defined as exchange of chromosomal material between two nonhomologous chromosomes. Translocation is present in 2.2% of couples after one miscarriage, 4.8% after two miscarriages, and 5.7% after three miscarriages [15]. In a recent study by Kocchar PK et al. in 788 pregnancies with RPL, chromosomal rearrangements were identified in 6.8% including 5.9% reciprocal translocations, 0.7% Robertsonian translocations, and 0.1% inversions. Out of subsequent 49 documented pregnancies in 2 years, 33% were miscarriages, of which 56.2% were euploid, 2% were trisomies, and 12.5% had an unbalanced translocation [16].

They are of two types: balanced and unbalanced. In **balanced translocation**, there is no gain or loss of any chromosomal material, and the chromosome aberrations cause no clinical symptoms in carriers but possibly induce the production of abnormal reproductive cells containing abnormal amounts of genetic material. In general population the frequency of carriers of balanced translocation is 0.2%, while in couples with recurrent miscarriage it is 2–5% [17]. In comparison to males, females are twice more common carriers of balanced translocation [18]. There is an increased incidence of spontaneous abortions, and 50% of fetuses may harbor an unbalanced chromosomal abnormality [19]. This risk is influenced by the size and the genetic content of the rearranged chromosomal segments.

In **unbalanced translocation**, the exchange of materials between the two chromosomes is not even; hence, a loss or gain of material occurs. **In reciprocal translocations**, there is an exchange of material between nonhomologous chromosomes. This may result in infertility due to production of unbalanced gametes and other mechanisms like translocation of X chromosome may lead to spermatogenic arrest [20]. They can also cause pregnancy loss because segregation during meiosis results in gametes with duplication or deficiency of chromosome segments [21]. This risk depends on the number of breakpoints during translocation.

When the translocation involves the short arm of the acrocentric chromosome (chromosome numbers 13, 14, 15, 21, and 22), they are termed as **Robertsonian translocation**. Robertsonian translocation results in trisomies and monosomies and hence contributes in pregnancy losses [22]. The incidence of Robertsonian translocations is 0.1% in the general population, 1.1% in patients with RPL [23]. Seventy-five percent of these translocations are seen in chromosomes 13 and 14 (der(13;14)(q10;q10)). Pregnancies from carriers of translocation can result in fetus with Patau syndrome (trisomy 13), but majority with der (13; 14) carriers result in early pregnancy loss [24]. Most of the unbalanced translocations result from abnormal segregation of Robertsonian translocations, while some arise de novo during gametogenesis. The incidence of Robertsonian translocation in newborn is 1 in 1000. The risk of miscarriage in Robertsonian translocation is low. There is a tenfold of excess of Robertsonian translocation in men with infertility. The risk of having abnormal baby (e.g., trisomy 21, trisomy 13) is more in female carriers (10–15%) in comparison to male carriers (5%).

Unbalanced paracentric inversions produce acentric or dicentric gametes that are not viable. However, unbalanced pericentric inversions can result in children with birth defects due to the presence of partial trisomy or partial monosomy. The overall risk for a carrier for pericentric inversion to have a child with an unbalanced chromosome rearrangement is estimated at 5–10% [25]. The risk is based on the size of the inverted region and becomes significant if it is more than 50%.

Other structural rearrangements include ring chromosomes, supernumerary marker chromosome, translocations, and complex rearrangements. These chromosomal abnormalities can be associated with congenital malformations and mental retardation, besides recurrent miscarriages. Other chromosome abnormalities include sex chromosome mosaicism.

Genetic counseling is needed for parents with structural chromosomal abnormality as the likelihood of a subsequent healthy live birth depends on the chromosomes involved and the type of rearrangement. Preimplantation genetic testing (PGT) and amniocentesis can be done to detect genetic abnormality in the offspring of a parent with structural genetic abnormality.

5.2.4 Single-Gene Defect

Single-gene defects may be responsible for multiple miscarriages, but will not be detected by a karyotype. They include musculoskeletal gene mutations including trinucleotide repeat disorders, genes involved in regulation of the immune system and implantation, thrombophilic gene mutations, and mutations in specific enzymes, including angiotensin-converting enzyme, ubiquitin-specific protease, and human alkaline phosphatase and sharing of HLA antigens, polymorphism in HLA G and HLA E antigen [26, 27].

The most common single-gene mutations seen in RPL with a relatively high prevalence include the genes associated with inherited thrombophilias, namely, factor V Leiden, prothrombin gene promoter mutations, activated protein C resistance, and mutations in methyl tetrahydrofolate reductase, plasminogen activator inhibitor, thrombomodulin, and annexin A5 genes [28]. Mutations in factor V Leiden is the most common genetic cause of thrombosis followed by Annexin V, both having a twofold higher prevalence in women with RPL compared with controls [29]. Screening for inherited thrombophilia in RPL can be done in patients who have a first-degree relative with a known or suspected thrombophilia or who report a personal history of venous thromboembolism [30].

In musculoskeletal defects, CTG repeats are excess in number in stillborn babies than live births. Polymorphisms in the HLA-G promoter region and presence of a null

Table 5.2 Single-gene defects, mode of inheritance, and presentations

Single-gene disorders associated with pregnancy loss		
Aicardi syndrome	X-linked dominant	Mental retardation, basal ganglia calcification, chronic cerebrospinal lymphocytosis
Chondrodysplasia punctata	X-linked dominant	Short limbs, punctuate calcification in epiphysis
Incontinentia pigmenti	X-linked dominant	Skin pigmentation, anodontia, nail dystrophy, retinal detachment
Orofacial digital syndrome	X-linked dominant	Oral frenula and cleft, hypoplasia of ala nasi, digital anomaly
Osteogenesis imperfecta	Autosomal recessive	Bowing or fracture of long bones, blue sclera, short stature
Rett syndrome	X-linked dominant	Autism, mental retardation, loss of purposeful hand movements, ataxia
Thalasemia major	X-linked dominant	Anemia, hepatosplenomegaly, thalassemic facies

allele for HLA-G isoform have been associated with recurrent miscarriage [31]. Polymorphisms in genes including p53, p72, leukemia-inhibiting factor (LIF), etc. may also lead to implantation failure. X-linked dominant disorders that are a major group of single-gene defects have been associated with pregnancy loss. In X-linked disorders, affected mother will pass the disease to 50% of their daughters and 50% to their sons. Affected father will pass the disease to 100% of their daughter and 0% to their son (i.e., there is no male to male transmission). The list of disorders is summarized in Table 5.2.

5.3 Diagnosis

For a complete evaluation of a couple with RPL, peripheral karyotyping of parents is recommended to detect any balanced and structural chromosomal abnormalities. However, there are certain controversies surrounding the need of a detailed genetic work-up of couple with RPL. Those in favor of genetic work-up say that it is beneficial for counseling of the couple regarding the recurrence risk as well as chances of having a fetus with unbalanced chromosomal rearrangements. On the other hand, the school of thought opposing the routine chromosomal analysis say that for a carrier couple the chances of having a successful pregnancy after two previous miscarriages are almost identical to that of a non-carrier couple with two previous miscarriages (83% and 84%, respectively). In this segment we will discuss the various methods of genetic analysis.

5.3.1 Karyotyping

Parental numeric and structural cytogenetic abnormalities can be detected by peripheral blood karyotyping, and this should be followed by genetic counseling [17]. Both the specific chromosome(s) affected and the types of rearrangement influence the probability of a future live birth. However, there is discrepancy in the detection and transmission of parental karyotypic abnormalities [9]. This disparity is due to the fact that majority of fetuses with karyotypic abnormalities do not survive pregnancy. Parents with balanced translocations are less likely to deliver a live-born affected child than would be predicted by transmission rates. Other samples for karyotyping include the specimens from prenatal testing such as chorionic villi and amniocytes. Standard G-banding karyotype is typically used to detect gross chromosome rearrangements which requires cells to be cultured to obtain a metaphase spread.

5.3.2 Cytogenetic Testing on Products of Conception

The product of conception is dried and rinsed of blood with physiological saline, before isolation of chorionic villi. If the fetal tissues are already well formed and visible, a fragment of the umbilical cord may be used for examination [32]. Miscarried material may also be analyzed in paraffin blocks. The main problem with analysis of product of conception is maternal contamination which often leads to false negative results. The various molecular and cytogenetic techniques available to analyze the material for the presence of genetic abnormalities are summarized in Table 5.3 [28, 33].

5.4 Management of Genetic Abnormalities

Once a genetic defect is identified, genetic counseling should be offered to the couple. The specifics of the result and its clinical risk must be explained, and the couple should be made aware of available strategies to minimize the risk of having an affected child, including preimplantation genetic screening and diagnosis. The various screening options in subsequent pregnancy include antenatal biochemical screen, ultrasound studies in first and second trimester for structural anomalies, noninvasive prenatal testing (NIPT) using cell-free fetal DNA in maternal circulation, and invasive procedures like chorionic villus sampling and amniocentesis.

5.4.1 Preimplantation Genetic Diagnosis and Screening (PGD/PGS)

Couples with recurrent pregnancy loss can also be given the option of in vitro fertilization (IVF) combined with PGD/PGS. Preimplantation genetic diagnosis (PGD) refers to testing for known heritable genetic abnormality present in one or both of the parents. Preimplantation genetic screening can be used in couples with idiopathic RPL for a global genetic assessment of the embryo [34]. Thus, healthy selected embryos are transferred in utero.

The use of PGD in RPL has been shown to be useful in translocation carriers or documented chromosomal inversion and has been shown to improve live-birth rates [28, 35, 36]. Fluorescence in situ hybridization (FISH) has traditionally been used

Table 5.3 Techniques for chromosomal analysis

Technique	Advantages	Limitations	Time taken for result
Conventional karyotype	Detects aneuploidy, polyploidies, marker chromosome, structural aberrations including inversion, deletion translocations	Requires culture, false negative because of culture contamination	2–3 weeks
FISH (probe is stained with fluorescent dye and then hybridized with prepared karyotype)	Diagnosis of aneuploidies, complex chromosomal structural aberrations, identification of marker chromosome, detects metaphase chromosomes, and interface nuclei	Specific changes can only be detected depending on probe used	14 days
Chromosomal microarray analysis (CMA)	Microdeletions and microduplications of chromosome segments – number abnormalities of chromosome (trisomy, monosomy) including Down syndrome – Unbalanced chromosomal rearrangements – Provides higher resolution		
Array comparative genomic hybridization (aCGH)	Changes in the number of chromosomes (aneuploidies, triploidies), unbalanced structural changes (such as duplications, deletions, and amplifications)	No detection of balanced translocations and inversions within the genome. For polyploidy flow cytometry has to be combined	Several days
MLPA	Chromosomal aneuploidies (deletions and duplications). Used mainly for identification of particular subtelomeric aberrations (i.e., aberrations within the chromosomal termini) as well as known microdeletion syndromes Simultaneous screening for multiple chromosome aberrations	Diagnostics of changes within the genetic material as defined in the intended use of the kit	2 days
QF-PCR	Aneuploidies within chromosomes 15, 16, 22 and 13, 18, 21, X, and Y Triploidies determination of the origin of the additional chromosome	Diagnostics of changes within the genetic material as defined in the intended use of the kit	1 day
BoBs	Common aneuploidies (13, 18, 21, X, Y). Deletions and duplications of particular regions	Diagnostics of changes within the genetic material as defined in the intended use of the kit	1 day

(continued)

Table 5.3 (continued)

Technique	Advantages	Limitations	Time taken for result
Next-generation sequencing (NGS)	GS facilitates sequencing of large genomic regions, high numbers of genes, or a high number of samples within a single test	Excessive information makes interpretation difficult to ascertain etiology	

to identify the presence of translocation imbalances, and recently microarrays have been used [37]. The G-banding technique which uses the metaphase chromosomes cannot be used for PGD as preimplantation embryo cells are caught in interphase and banding cannot be detected [20].

The role of PGS is more controversial. Fluorescent in situ hybridization (FISH) assays are used for PGS, which is limited by the number of probes that can be differentially labeled and discriminated at one time, thus analyzing only a subgroup of chromosomes; hence, false negative results are high. FISH evaluates between 5 and 14 chromosomes, while aneuploidy may occur in all 23 pairs [38, 39]. The most frequently used probes identify unbalanced translocations, trisomies, monosomies, and structural chromosome abnormalities, such as deletions [40]. Moreover, the day 3 embryo used for PGS has a high rate of mosaicism [41]. Studies have shown that the live-birth rates were similar among the PGS and control groups; however, pregnancy rates were significantly lower among patients undergoing genetic testing [42, 43].

As a result of these drawbacks, more laboratories are shifting to other techniques to analyze the whole chromosome and segmental defects which include single nucleotide polymorphism (SNP) microarray, array comparative genomic hybridization (CGH), etc. The resolution reported for CGH (10–20 Mb and 25–100 Mb), array CGH (2.5 and 2.8 Mb), and SNP microarrays (2.4 and 5 Mb) for these small segmental imbalances [44–46]. Currently more laboratories are shifting to next-generation sequencing (NGS) for whole chromosome aneuploidy screening in PGD, which includes a number of different modern sequencing technologies including Illumina (Solexa) sequencing, Roche 454 sequencing, Ion Torrent: Proton/PGM sequencing, and SOLiD sequencing. However the results are not yet clear compared to the array-based and FISH-based assays [20].

Alternatively, polar body biopsy of the oocyte, blastomere biopsy at the eight-cell stage of development (typically day 3 postfertilization), or trophectoderm biopsy of a blastocyst on day 5 or 6 postfertilization is being used for PGD or PGS [28]. Unlike others, polar body biopsy is useful to detect transmission of only maternal origin [47].

While counseling a patient for PGD/IVF, the clinician must keep in mind that the live-birth rates are not improved by PGD/IVF in a case of recurrent pregnancy loss, and the woman has to undergo further testing in pregnancy for confirmation. The practice committee recommendations of American Society of Assisted Reproductive

Medicine (ASRM) in 2008 stated that the routine implementation of PGS was ineffective in improving IVF pregnancy rates and in reducing miscarriage rates [48]. PGS was found to decrease take-home baby rates while subjecting patients and couples to invasive and costly therapy. The 2012 recommendations suggest supportive care and early pregnancy monitoring by ultrasound every 2 weeks in recurrent pregnancy loss [30].

Conclusions

Genetic abnormalities are among the leading etiologies for fetal loss. Karyotype of the couple and product of conception (POC) will help in counseling and prognostication of future pregnancies and increase chances of live birth using assisted reproduction. Recent advances in medical genetics and its application like use of array-based techniques and next-generation sequencing have significantly changed the approach toward evaluation of genetic causes of RPL. However, the cost-effectiveness and exact benefit of genetic evaluation is yet to be determined. The role of PGD/PGS still remains to be explored. Amidst the confusion and controversies, clinical genetics will become one of the disciplines physicians will be expected to use for the care of their patients. Moreover, it is very important that these interventions should be used by physicians in a responsible and ethical manner.

Key Points

- Aneuploidies especially trisomies are the most common cause of RPL, while monosomy X is the most specific cause.
- Chromosomal structural abnormality is seen in 2–3% of cytogenetically abnormal conceptus, and the most common types are balanced translocations.
- Karyotype of products of conception by cell culture or use of microarray technologies can be done. Microarray evaluations are capable of ruling out maternal cell contamination.
- The use of PGD in RPL has been shown to be useful in translocation carriers and documented chromosomal inversion.
- Routine implementation of PGS is ineffective in reducing miscarriage rates and antenatal screening, and early pregnancy monitoring by ultrasound every 2 weeks in recurrent pregnancy loss is recommended.

References

1. Practice Committee of American Society for Reproductive Medicine. Definitions of infertility and recurrent pregnancy loss: a committee opinion. Fertil Steril. 2013;99(1):63.
2. Ford HB, Schust DJ. Recurrent pregnancy loss: etiology, diagnosis, and therapy. Rev Obstet Gynecol. 2009;2(2):76–83.

3. Zastavna D, Sosnina K, Terpylyak O, Huleyuk N, Bezkorovayna H, Mikula M, Helner N. Cytogenetic and immunogenetic analysis of recurrent pregnancy loss in women. Tsitol Genet. 2014;48:44–50.
4. Christiansen OB. A fresh look at the causes and treatments of recurrent miscarriage, especially its immunological aspects. Hum Reprod Update. 1996;2(4):271–93.
5. Larsen EC, Christiansen OB, Kolte AM, Macklon N. New insights into mechanisms behind miscarriage. BMC Med. 2013;11:154.
6. Schmid W. A familial chromosome abnormality associated with repeated abortions. Cytogenetics. 1962;1:199–209.
7. Warren JE, Silver RM. Genetics of pregnancy loss. Clin Obstet Gynecol. 2008;51:84–95.
8. Suzumori N, Sugiura-Ogasawara M. Genetic factors as a cause of miscarriage. Curr Med Chem. 2010;17:3431–7.
9. Carp H, Guetta E, Dorf H, Soriano D, Barkai G, Schiff E. Embryonic karyotype in recurrent miscarriage with parental karyotypic aberrations. Fertil Steril. 2006;85:446–50.
10. Geraedts JPM. Chromosomal anomalies and recurrent miscarriage. Infertil Reprod Med Clin North Am. 1996;7:677–88.
11. Wapner RJ, Lewis D. Genetics and metabolic causes of stillbirth. Semin Perinatol. 2002;26:70–4.
12. Hassold TJ. A cytogenetic study of repeated spontaneous abortions. Am J Hum Genet. 1980;32:723–30.
13. Hassold T, Chiu D. Maternal age-specific rates of numerical chromosome abnormalities with special reference to trisomy. Hum Genet. 1985;70:11–7.
14. Zaragoza MV, Surti U, Redline RW, Millie E, Chakravarti A, Hassold TJ. Parental origin and phenotype of triploidy in spontaneous abortions: predominance of diandry and association with the partial hydatidiform mole. Am J Hum Genet. 2000;66(6):1807–20.
15. De Braekeleer M, Dao TN. Cytogenetic studies in couples experiencing repeated pregnancy losses. Hum Reprod. 1990;5:519–28.
16. Kochhar PK, Ghosh P. Reproductive outcome of couples with recurrent miscarriage and balanced chromosomal abnormalities. J Obstet Gynaecol Res. 2013;39(1):113–20.
17. Regan L, Backos M, Rai R. Green-top Guideline No 17. The investigation and treatment of couples with recurrent first-trimester and second-trimester miscarriage. London: Royal College of Obstetricians and Gynaecologists (RCOG); 2011.
18. Kavalier F. Investigation of recurrent miscarriages: a successful pregnancy is the most likely outcome. BMJ. 2005;331(7509):121–2.
19. Madan K, Nieuwint AW, van Bever Y. Recombination in balanced complex translocation of a mother leading to a balanced reciprocal translocation in the child. Review of 60 cases of balanced complex translocations. Hum Genet. 1997;99(6):806–15.
20. Morin SJ, Eccles J, Iturriaga A, Zimmerman RS. Translocations, inversions and other chromosome rearrangements. Fertil Steril. 2017;107(1):19–26.
21. Stephenson MD, Sierra S. Reproductive outcomes in recurrent pregnancy loss associated with a parental carrier of a structural chromosome rearrangement. Hum Reprod. 2006;21(4):1076–82.
22. Pourjafari B, Pour-Jafari H, Farimani M, Ghahramani S, Saleh EK. Genetic counseling in carriers of reciprocal translocations involving two autosomes. Indian J Hum Genet. 2012;18(2):250–3.
23. Fryns JP, van Buggenhout G. Structural chromosome rearrangements in couples with recurrent fetal wastage. Eur J Obstet Gynecol Reprod Biol. 1998;81:171–6.
24. Scriven PN, Flinter FA, Braude PR, Ogilvie CM. Robertsonian translocations—reproductive risks and indications for preimplantation genetic diagnosis. Hum Reprod. 2001;16:2267–73.
25. Martin RH, Chernos JE, Lowry RB, Pattinson HA, Barclay L, Ko E. Analysis of sperm chromosome complements from a man heterozygous for a pericentric inversion of chromosome 1. Hum Genet. 1994;93:135–8.
26. Vatin M, Bouvier S, Bellazi L, Montagutelli X, Laissue P, Ziyyat A, et al. Polymorphisms of human placental alkaline phosphatase are associated with in vitro fertilization success and recurrent pregnancy loss. Am J Pathol. 2014;184:362–8.

27. Wang Z, Wang P, Wang X, He X, Wang Z, Xu D, et al. Significant association between angiotensin-converting enzyme gene insertion/deletion polymorphism and risk of recurrent miscarriage: a systematic review and meta-analysis. Metabolism. 2013;62:1227–38.
28. Hyde KJ, Schust DJ. Genetic considerations in recurrent pregnancy loss. Cold Spring Harb Perspect Med. 2015;5(3):a023119.
29. Dizon-Townson D, Miller C, Sibai B, Spong CY, Thom E, Wendel G Jr, et al. The relationship of the factor V Leiden mutation and pregnancy outcomes for mother and fetus. Obstet Gynecol. 2005;106:517–24.
30. Practice Committee of the American Society for Reproductive Medicine. Evaluation and treatment of recurrent pregnancy loss: a committee opinion. Fertil Steril. 2012;98:1103–11.
31. Aldrich CL, Stephenson MD, Karrison T, Odem RR, Branch DW, Scott JR, et al. HLA-G genotypes and pregnancy outcome in couples with unexplained recurrent miscarriage. Mol Hum Reprod. 2001;7:1167–72.
32. Lathi RB, Milki AA. Tissue sampling technique affects accuracy of karyotype from missed abortions. J Assist Reprod Genet. 2002;19:536–8.
33. Kacprzak M, Chrzanowska M, Skoczylas B, Moczulska H, Borowiec M, Sieroszewski P. Genetic causes of recurrent miscarriages. Ginekol Pol. 2016;87(10):722–6.
34. Brezina PR, Kearns WG. The evolving role of genetics in reproductive medicine. Obstet Gynecol Clin North Am. 2014;41(1):41–55.
35. Brezina PR, Brezina DS, Kearns WG. Preimplantation genetic testing. BMJ. 2012;345:e5908.
36. Otani T, Roche M, Mizuike M, et al. Preimplantation genetic diagnosis significantly improves the pregnancy outcome of translocation carriers with a history of recurrent miscarriage and unsuccessful pregnancies. Reprod Biomed Online. 2006;13(6):869–74.
37. Du L, Brezina PR, Benner AT, et al. The rate of de novo and inherited aneuploidy as determined by 23-chromosome single nucleotide polymorphism microarray (SNP) in embryos generated from parents with known chromosomal translocations. Fertil Steril. 2011;96(3):S221.
38. Harper JC, Sengupta SB. Preimplantation genetic diagnosis: state of the art 2011. Hum Genet. 2012;131:175–86.
39. Brezina PR, Tobler K, Benner AT, et al. All 23 chromosomes have significant levels of aneuploidy in recurrent pregnancy loss couples. Fertil Steril. 2012;97(3):S7.
40. Fridstrom M, Ahrlund-Richter L, Iwarsson E, Malmgren H, Inzunza J, Rosenlund B, Sjoblom P, Nordenskjold M, Biennow E, Hovatta O. Clinical outcome of treatment cycles using preimplantation genetic diagnosis for structural chromosomal abnormalities. Prenat Diagn. 2001;21:781–7.
41. Munné S, Weier HU, Grifo J, et al. Chromosome mosaicism in human embryos. Biol Reprod. 1994;51:373–9.
42. Brigham SA, Conlon C, Farquharson RG. A longitudinal study of pregnancy outcome following idiopathic recurrent miscarriage. Hum Reprod. 1999;14:2868–71.
43. Platteau P, Staessen C, Michiels A, Van Steirteghem A, Liebaers I, Devroey P. Preimplantation genetic diagnosis for aneuploidy screening in patients with unexplained recurrent miscarriages. Fertil Steril. 2005;82:393–7.
44. Treff NR, Northrop LE, Kasabwala K, Su J, Levy B, Scott RT Jr. Single nucleotide polymorphism microarray-based concurrent screening of 24 chromosome aneuploidy and unbalanced translocations in preimplantation human embryos. Fertil Steril. 2010;95:1606–12.e1–2.
45. Fiorentino F, Spizzichino L, Bono S, Biricik A, Kokkali G, Rienzi L, et al. PGD for reciprocal and Robertsonian translocations using array comparative genomic hybridization. Hum Reprod. 2011;26:1925–35.
46. Johnson DS, Hill M, Abae M, Frederick J, Swanson M, Rabinowitz M. First clinical application of DNA microarrays for translocation and inversions. Fertil Steril. 2010;93:S13–4.
47. Montag M, van der Ven K, van der Ven H. Polar body biopsy. In: Harper JC, editor. Preimplantation genetic diagnosis. 2nd ed. Cambridge: Cambridge University Press; 2009. p. 166–74.
48. Practice Committee of the American Society for Reproductive Medicine. Preimplantation genetic testing: a Practice Committee opinion. Fertil Steril. 2008;90:S136–43.

Hormones in Recurrent Pregnancy Loss

6

Nutan Agarwal and Vidushi Kulshrestha

6.1 Introduction

Recurrent pregnancy loss (RPL) has traditionally been defined as three or more spontaneous and consecutive pregnancy losses, not including ectopic or molar pregnancy. The American Society for Reproductive Medicine (ASRM) has defined RPL as two or more failed clinical pregnancies [1]. Etiology of >two or three miscarriages is similar in contrast to sporadic miscarriages, and also the risk of another pregnancy loss after two miscarriages is only slightly lower than that of women with three or more spontaneous abortions [2]. Approximately 1–2% of women may suffer from RPL.

Successful growth and development of fetus depends on interplay of various hormones such as progesterone, estrogen, human chorionic gonadotrophin (HCG), prolactin, thyroid hormones, and androgens. Over- or underexpression of these hormones may result in failure of pregnancy. Endocrinal factors contribute to about 8–12% cases of RPL [3]. Therefore endocrinologic evaluation is a critical component of work-up of such women.

N. Agarwal (✉)
Professor, Fetal Medicine Division, Department of Obstetrics and Gynaecology,
All India Institute of Medical Sciences, New Delhi, India
e-mail: nutan_agarwal@yahoo.com

V. Kulshrestha
Assistant Professor, Department of Obstetrics and Gynaecology,
All India Institute of Medical Sciences,
New Delhi, India
e-mail: drvidushi.kul@gmail.com

S. Mehta, B. Gupta (eds.), *Recurrent Pregnancy Loss*,
https://doi.org/10.1007/978-981-10-7338-0_6

6.2 Hormones and RPL

6.2.1 Progesterone and RPL (Luteal Phase Defect or Deficiency or Insufficiency)

Adequate progesterone secretion by the corpus luteum is essential for maintenance of early pregnancy by preparing endometrium for implantation and promoting luteal phase support. Progesterone also modulates the immune response of the mother to prevent embryo rejection. It produces progesterone-induced blocking factor (PIBF) which inhibits NK cell activity. It also shifts the balance from unfavorable cytokines Th1 to favorable cytokines Th2. Progesterone enhances uterine quiescence and suppresses uterine contractions and cervical dilatation as well.

Removal of corpus luteum may result in failure of pregnancy. Inadequate or short duration of progesterone production leads to luteal phase defect (LPD). LPD has been associated with RPL, and the reported incidence of LPD in RPL varies between 12 and 28% [4], though lack of definite diagnostic criteria for LPD is a limitation. Identified causes of luteal phase defect include hyperprolactinemia, polycystic ovary syndrome, hypogonadotropic hypogonadism, poor ovarian reserve, stress, exercise, and extreme weight loss [5].

Gold standard for the diagnosis of LPD has been histopathological endometrial dating after timed biopsy which is not accurate due to intra- and interobserver variation in interpretation [6]. Luteal phase serum progesterone levels lower than 10 ng/mL suggests LPD. However, this also has flaws, as progesterone levels fluctuate due to pulsatile release of the luteinizing hormone (LH) and serum levels may not always correlate with the endometrial response to a given concentration. A criterion of luteal phase length less than 11 days can be useful for screening LPD [5]. Hence, there is lack of consensus for diagnosing LPD and routine endometrial biopsy for dating is not recommended [7].

6.2.2 Estrogen and RPL

Inadequate preovulatory estrogen stimulation may indicate poor oocyte quality and a poorly functioning corpus luteum [6].

6.2.3 Human Chorionic Gonadotrophin (HCG) and RPL

HCG is secreted by the trophoblastic cells. Besides maintaining corpus luteal function in early pregnancy, HCG also felicitates implantation and endometrial receptivity and prevents endometrial apoptosis [8, 9].

6.2.4 Prolactin and RPL

Hyperprolactinemia, though more commonly associated with anovulation and infertility due to impaired folliculogenesis and oocyte maturation, may lead to RPL by altering hypothalamic-pituitary-ovarian axis leading to short luteal phase [3]. Bromocriptine therapy is associated with a higher rate of successful pregnancy [10]. Often, hyperprolactinemia is secondary to medication use or primary hypothyroidism, and the underlying cause should be treated in such cases.

6.2.5 Thyroid Hormone and RPL

Untreated hypothyroidism, as defined by elevated thyroid-stimulating hormone (TSH) and decreased T4, may increase the risk of miscarriage and contribute to about 8% cases of RPL [11]. As TSH value increases, risk of pregnancy loss also increases [12]. Euthyroid patients with autoimmune thyroid disease, i.e., women with normal TSH and T4 levels with the presence of antithyroid antibodies (ATA), are also at higher risk for RPL [11]. In fact, ATA suggest more of an immune dysfunction due to abnormal T-cell function, rather than an endocrine disorder which may independently cause pregnancy loss [13].

Common causes of hypothyroidism in pregnancy include endemic iodine deficiency, chronic autoimmune thyroid diseases, postsurgery, post-radioiodine ablation, and secondary to pituitary diseases. Prevalence of autoimmune thyroid disorders in pregnancy is 5–20%, and reported prevalence of ATA in asymptomatic women is approximately 14% [13, 14]. Rate of RPL in women with TSH between 2.5 and 5 mIU/L in the presence of ATA is approximately 17% which is almost double with odds ratio of 2.5, compared to the ATA-negative women with RPL [15].

Autoimmune thyroid disease may diminish thyroid reserve so that excess demand of pregnancy is not met. Also, these women are older than healthy controls, and increased age is an independent risk factor for miscarriage. ATA are targeted against thyroperoxidase and thyroglobulin which are integral to T3 and T4 synthesis and, hence, may be associated with inappropriately low levels of thyroid hormones for the given gestational period, despite apparent biologic euthyroidism. Antibodies may also be marker for a generalized immune imbalance, which are independent risk factors for pregnancy loss [13].

Screening for patients with RPL may include TSH and thyroid peroxidase antibodies [16]. A randomized prospective study found higher pregnancy complications in women with TSH levels greater than 2.5 mIU/mL in the first trimester with and without the presence of thyroid antibodies, and correction of hypothyroidism before pregnancy restores pregnancy outcomes to the rate seen in euthyroid women [17, 18]. Some studies, however, contradict these findings.

Even though universal screening of healthy women for thyroid dysfunction before pregnancy is not recommended, RPL women may be screened with TSH and also tested for antibodies even if TSH is normal, as thyroid autoimmunity may be present for many years before hypothyroidism manifests [6, 16]. There are no clear recommendations in ATA-positive pregnancies with a normal TSH (TSH < 2.5 mIU/L), but common sense dictates that at the very least, close follow-up during pregnancy is warranted.

6.2.6 Hyperandrogenism, PCOS, and RPL

Women with polycystic ovarian syndrome (PCOS) have an increased risk of RPL although the exact prevalence is uncertain. Proposed mechanisms include elevated serum LH, hyperandrogenism, hyperinsulinemia, and also obesity seen in PCOS. Association between high LH and excess androgens with the risk of RPL remains unclear; as in studies, no difference was found in subsequent pregnancy outcome in RPL with high LH compared to normal LH and also suppressing LH levels had no benefit in outcome [19, 20]. Total testosterone in PCOS women who miscarried was also not different with those who had live birth in some studies, and in others, lower total testosterone and a lower free androgen index in non-RPL women had a successful pregnancy outcome after ovulation induction [19, 20]. A body mass index greater than 30 kg/m^2 increases the chance of miscarriage by 20% and more than triples the risk of RPL [21]. Insulin resistance in PCOS results in hyperinsulinemia which is a significant independent risk factor for miscarriage and is also the key link between PCOS/obesity and RPL. Increased insulin resistance is seen in approximately 27% women with unexplained RPL [22]. There is overlap of PCOS and type II diabetes, which is also an independent risk factor for pregnancy loss. Few authors have recommended estimation of insulin metabolism as part of the evaluation of RPL [22].

The link between obesity and hyperinsulinemia with miscarriage may involve plasminogen activator inhibitor-1, which inhibits plasmin formation during plasminogen activation, and may be an independent risk factor for pregnancy loss potentially through a thrombophilic effect [23].

6.2.7 Other Hormonal Conditions and RPL

6.2.7.1 Follicle-Stimulating Hormone (FSH)

Although increased FSH in early follicular phase is a marker of diminished ovarian reserve, but increased day 3 FSH level in women with RPL has been linked to worse prognosis [24]. Altered preovulatory estrogen stimulation reflecting poor oocyte quality has been implicated in poorly functioning corpus luteum, hence LPD. FSH testing may be advised in women older than 35 years with RPL [3].

6.2.7.2 Poorly Controlled Diabetes

It is associated with pregnancy loss whereas there is no increased risk of miscarriage in well-controlled diabetes. Early pregnancy loss correlates with elevated fasting glucose and glycosylated hemoglobin levels in the first trimester, and the increased risk is due to hyperglycemia, maternal vascular disease, associated congenital malformations, and possibly immunologic factors.

6.3 Role of Hormones in Treatment of RPL

Use of various hormones for treatment of RPL includes luteal phase supplementation with progestogen or human chorionic gonadotropin (hCG), correction of prolactin and thyroid levels, and control of diabetes.

6.3.1 Progestogen Therapy

There is no consensus, yet supplementing the luteal phase with exogenous progestogen has remained the most common therapy in abortions. Progesterone treatment does not decrease the risk of sporadic miscarriages. Even in RPL, scientific evidence is not very convincing regarding its therapeutic value, and many a times progesterone treatment is given as there is nothing else to offer to these women. Although conflicting data exist, a recent Cochrane review evaluating 15 trials, when did subgroup analysis of four studies with RPL, concluded that there was a benefit to the routine administration of progesterone in current pregnancy to all women with a history of RPL with 3 or more previous pregnancy losses [25].

Low serum progesterone levels have been linked to increased risk of first trimester abortion, and this risk increases as serum progesterone level decreases. At serum progesterone levels of >25 ng/mL, the abortion risk is 3% which is similar to the general risk in any pregnant woman. As the progesterone levels decline, risk of abortion increases: 7% for levels 20–25 ng/mL, 10% for 15–20 ng/mL, 30% for 10–15 ng/mL, steeply increasing to 80% for progesterone levels between 5 and 10 ng/mL, and 85% with <5 ng/mL [26]. Unfortunately progesterone levels are notoriously unreliable, and it is also not proved that exogenous progesterone may help in such cases.

This issue has been addressed in various Cochrane analyses. Initially in 2003, meta-analysis of four trials showed odds ratio (OR) of 0.3 in abortion rate following progesterone therapy [27]. Cochrane review 2013 Of 14 trials in 2158 cases showed no difference in abortion rate, but sub-analysis on basis of previous history of abortions, miscarriages in the index pregnancy reduced significantly with OR of 0.39 in women with ≥3 abortions [28]. An Indian study on 348 cases has shown reduction on abortion rate with dydrogesterone 20 mg daily with abortion rate of 6.9% vs. 16.8% in control group [8]. Recently the large multicentric trial with vaginal micronized progesterone in 836 women in first trimester did not find the benefit of therapy in RPL. Live birth rate after 24 weeks of gestation was 65.8% in progesterone group vs. 63.8% in placebo (RR 1.04) [29]. It is not known if treatment with intramuscular or oral micronized progesterone would improve the outcome. Study conducted by author on 90 cases showed the benefit of oral micronized progesterone in RPL, abortion rate being 3.3% in treatment group vs. 16.7% in non-treated group [30]. Also oral micronized progesterone led to increased rise of Th2 cytokines like IL6 ($p = 0.001$) and less rise of Th1 cytokines like TNF α ($p = 0.012$), indicating immunomodulating effect of progesterone [30]. However, outcomes with dydrogesterone are not modulated by Th1 and Th2 cytokine production [29].

6.3.1.1 Which Formulation and Which Route

Formulations, doses, timing, routes of administration, and duration of treatment remain contentious. There are numerous formulations given by various routes such as intramuscular 17-hydroxyprogesterone, oral dydrogesterone, and micronized progesterone that can be given as oral, intramuscular, and vaginal route. Oral progesterone is ineffective at increasing uterine progesterone levels. Intramuscular hydroxyprogesterone injections are very painful, its vehicle may induce labor, and few clinical trials have even shown increased risk of miscarriage [31]. Vaginal micronized progesterone was found effective in initial retrospective trials, but recent large trial has failed to show its efficacy in preventing abortion [29]. In Cochrane review 2011 on 421 cases of four trials, dydrogesterone was found better with reduction in abortion rate [32]. Indian study has also observed that oral dydrogesterone is effective in reducing abortion rate in RPL, 6.9% vs. 16.85 [29].

Efficacy of intramuscular and oral micronized progesterone is not known yet. Our pilot study on oral micronized progesterone has shown some promising effect; however, the study is not adequately powered [30]. More trials are needed for oral and injectable micronized progesterone.

6.3.1.2 When to Start and for How Long

Ideally progestogen supplementation should be started in the luteal phase, if LPD is suspected as a cause of RPL. Luteal initiation has added benefit because of immunomodulatory effect and improved endometrial gland development, which optimizes the local environment for early maintenance of pregnancy. Starting progesterone supplements after a positive pregnancy test may also provide adequate pregnancy support, whereby reducing costs, and the emotional toll of a delayed menses and negative pregnancy test.

Progesterone is started on the third day after LH surge and continued for 8–10 weeks [3]. In most studies, it is started after diagnosing pregnancy and has been given up to 16–24 weeks of gestation, with duration of treatment varying from 4 to 24 weeks. Treatment can be extended till 34 weeks in patients having history of preterm labor. In a study by the authors, oral micronized progesterone was started before 8 weeks of pregnancy and was given up to 16 weeks [30].

6.3.1.3 Fetal and Other Risks

There is a concern for pregnancy complications like intrahepatic cholestasis of pregnancy, but no increased maternal complications were found in trials. Virilization in fetus is also not reported in humans. Retrospective study on dydrogesterone showed some increased risk of cardiac defects, but it was not a well-designed study [32]. Larger trials with vaginal micronized progesterone found no increase in the risk of congenital malformations among offsprings [33]. We have large experience of treating these women with micronized progesterone and also their use is common in assisted reproduction, there is no report of increased risk of congenital malformations after therapy.

6.3.2 HCG Therapy

Systematic reviews suggest benefit from luteal phase HCG for recurrent loss [34]. Restoring a timely HCG signal during the window of implantation has been shown to improve corpus luteal rescue and improve the response of the corpus luteum in terms of progesterone output as well [35]. HCG treatment overcomes luteal phase inadequacy seen in gonadotrophin-stimulated cycles [36].

As with the progesterone support for RPL, treatment with HCG administered after the establishment of pregnancy may not have equal efficacy for the corpus luteum rescue compared to mid-luteal HCG administration, when receptivity of corpus luteum for HCG signal is at its peak [31]. Luteal HCG support increases ongoing pregnancy rate by approximately 2.5 times with number needed to treat being seven [9]. HCG improves outcomes in women with RPL by restoring synchrony and luteal support and preventing endometrial apoptosis [9].

6.3.3 Treatment of Hyperprolactinemia

Normalization of prolactin levels with a dopamine agonist improved subsequent pregnancy outcomes in patients with recurrent pregnancy loss, live-born rate being 85% in treated women compared to 52% in untreated group [10].

6.3.4 Treatment of Hypothyroidism

Thyroid hormone replacement therapy in pregnant women with hypothyroidism (TSH >2.5 mIU/L) and also in euthyroid pregnant women with antithyroid antibodies improves pregnancy outcome [37].

The Endocrine Society [16] and ASRM [1] recommend first trimester TSH less than 2.5 uIU/mL in patients with RPL. A starting dose of levothyroxine 50 mcg/day is recommended for TSH between 2.5 and 10 mIU/mL, and patients should be treated to become euthyroid (TSH between 1.0 and 2.5 uIU/mL for RPL) before attempting next pregnancy [1, 16]. Close monitoring in first trimester is important because of increasing thyroid demands often requiring increasing dose. There are no clear recommendations in antibody-positive pregnancies with a normal TSH <2.5 mIU/L, but close follow-up during pregnancy is warranted.

Endocrine Society practice guidelines for the "Management of Thyroid Dysfunction during Pregnancy and Postpartum" recommend screening of all at-risk women either before pregnancy or in early pregnancy when risk factors for thyroid dysfunction present, and test is repeated to confirm the assay result if prenatal

TSH level is >2.5 mIU/L [16]. TSH levels are monitored approximately every 4–6 weeks (minimum, once a trimester) with adjustments in doses for patients who are taking levothyroxine before conception. It also recommends to increase replacement by 30% to meet the demands of the fetus by taking two extra doses per week. Most women will return to their pre-pregnancy dose of thyroid replacement after delivery. As long as TSH levels are in the normal range, there is insufficient evidence to recommend screening for antithyroid antibodies.

6.3.5 Treatment of PCOS

Obesity or insulin resistance is associated with an increased risk of miscarriage; hence, such women should also be counseled regarding losing weight and diet modification which improves insulin sensitivity and appears to improve fertility and pregnancy outcome. The use of insulin-sensitizing agents such as metformin may reduce pregnancy loss in PCOS women with RPL when used before and throughout pregnancy [38]. Metformin has shown benefit in reducing the risk of miscarriage in women with a history of RPL and an abnormal glucose tolerance test result [39]. Metformin use during pregnancy does not appear to have any deleterious effects among exposed children during their first 18 months of life.

Key Points

- Endocrine disorders may contribute to RPL and this subset of causes of RPL are treatable.
- Progesterone is the most important hormone to maintain pregnancy and is indispensable for creating suitable environment for continuing pregnancy.
- Luteal phase defect is the most common endocrinologic cause of RPL. Other causes include hyperinsulinemia and hyperandrogenemia in PCOS, hyperprolactinemia, uncontrolled thyroid disease, uncontrolled diabetes, or diminished ovarian reserve.
- Evaluation of RPL should include TSH with antithyroid antibodies in selected cases, serum prolactin, glucose tolerance, and hemoglobin A1c and evaluation of ovarian reserve in women >35 years. Mid-luteal progesterone to diagnose luteal insufficiency is not recommended.
- Luteal phase supplementation with progestogen or HCG is beneficial. Progesterone additionally has an immunomodulatory effect which favors pregnancy.
- Management of insulin resistance in polycystic ovary syndrome with weight reduction or metformin reduces the risk of pregnancy loss.
- Safety of various progesterone formulations is established though evidence regarding efficacy is inconsistent. Their use is recommended in RPL but not in sporadic miscarriages.

References

1. The Practice Committee of the American Society for Reproductive Medicine. Evaluation and treatment of recurrent pregnancy loss: a committee opinion. Fertil Steril. 2012;98(5):1103–11.
2. Stirrat GM. Recurrent miscarriage. Lancet. 1990;336:673–5.
3. Brezina PA, Kutteh WH. Classic and cutting-edge strategies for the management of early pregnancy loss. Obstet Gynecol Clin North Am. 2014;41:1–18.
4. Li TC, Spuijbroek MD, Tuckerman E, et al. Endocrinological and endometrial factors in recurrent miscarriage. BJOG. 2000;107(12):1471–9.
5. Ke RW. Endocrine basis for recurrent pregnancy loss. Obstet Gynecol Clin North Am. 2014;41:103–12.
6. Smith ML, Schust DJ. Endocrinology and recurrent pregnancy loss. Semin Reprod Med. 2011;29:482–90.
7. Practice Committee of the American Society for Reproductive Medicine. The clinical relevance of luteal phase deficiency: a committee opinion. Fertil Steril. 2012;98:1112–7.
8. Licht P, Fluhr H, Neuwinger J, Wallwiener D, Wildt L. Is human chorionic gonadotropin directly involved in the regulation of human implantation? Mol Cell Endocrinol. 2007;269(1–2):85–92.
9. Lovely LP, Fazleabas AT, Fritz MA, McAdams DG, Lessey BA. Prevention of endometrial apoptosis: randomized prospective comparison of human chorionic gonadotropin versus progesterone treatment in the luteal phase. J Clin Endocrinol Metab. 2005;90(4):2351–6.
10. Hirahara F, Andoh N, Sawai K, et al. Hyperprolactinemic recurrent miscarriage and results of randomized bromocriptine treatment trials [comment]. Fertil Steril. 1998;70:246–52.
11. Stagnaro-Green A, Roman SH, Cobin RH, et al. Detection of at-risk pregnancy by means of highly sensitive assays for thyroid autoantibodies. J Am Med Assoc. 1990;19:1422–5.
12. Benhadi N, Wiersinga WM, Reitsma JB, et al. Higher maternal TSH levels in pregnancy are associated with increased risk for miscarriage, fetal or neonatal death. Eur J Endocrinol. 2009;160(6):985–91.
13. Glinoer D. Thyroidal and immune adaptation to pregnancy: focus on maternal hypo- and hyperthyroidism. In: Lazarus J, Pirags V, Butz S, editors. The thyroid and reproduction. New York: Thieme; 2009. p. 36–58.
14. Hollowell JG, Staehling NW, Flanders WD, et al. Serum TSH, T4, and thyroid antibodies in the United States population (1988 to 1994): national health and nutrition examination survey (NHANES III). J Clin Endocrinol Metab. 2002;87(2):489–99.
15. Chen L, Hu R. Thyroid autoimmunity and miscarriage: a meta-analysis. Clin Endocrinol. 2011;74:513–9.
16. De Groot L, Abalovich M, Alexander EK, et al. Management of thyroid dysfunction during pregnancy and postpartum: an Endocrine Society clinical practice guideline. J Clin Endocrinol Metab. 2012;97:2543–65.
17. Negro R, Schwartz A, Gismondi R, et al. Increased pregnancy loss rate in thyroid antibody negative women with TSH levels between 2.5 and 5.0 in the first trimester of pregnancy. J Clin Endocrinol Metab. 2010;95:E44–8.
18. Tan TO, Cheng YW, Caughey AB. Are women who are treated for hypothyroidism at risk of pregnancy complications? Am J Obstet Gynecol. 2006;194:e1–3.
19. Nardo LG, Rai R, Backos M, et al. High serum luteinizing hormone and testosterone concentrations do not predict pregnancy outcome in women with recurrent miscarriage. Fertil Steril. 2002;77:348–52.
20. Clifford K, Rai R, Watson H, et al. Does suppressing luteinising hormone secretion reduce the miscarriage rate? Results of a randomised controlled trial. BMJ. 1996;312:1508–11.
21. Lashen H, Fear K, Sturdee DW. Obesity is associated with increased risk of first trimester and recurrent miscarriage: matched case-control study. Humanit Rep. 2004;19(7):205–10.
22. Craig LB, Ke RW, Kutteh WH. Increased prevalence of insulin resistance in women with a history of recurrent pregnancy loss. Fertil Steril. 2002;78:487–90. Atiomo WU, Bates SA, Condon JE, et al. The plasminogen activator inhibitor system in women with polycystic ovary syndrome. Fertil Steril. 1998;69(2):236–41.

23. Sun L, Lv H, Wei W, et al. Angiotensin-converting enzyme D/I and plasminogen activator inhibitor-1 4G/5G gene polymorphisms are associated with increased risk of spontaneous abortions in polycystic ovarian syndrome. J Endocrinol Invest. 2010;33:77–82.
24. Hofmann GE, Khoury J, Thie J. Recurrent pregnancy loss and diminished ovarian reserve. Fertil Steril. 2000;74(6):1192–5.
25. Haas DM, Ramsey PS. Progestogen for preventing miscarriage. Cochrane Database Syst Rev. 2008;(2):CD003511.
26. Osmana M, Erdog I, Emina S, Karahan SC, et al. The diagnostic value of beta human chorionic gonadotropin, progesterone, CA-125 in prediction of abortion. J Obstet Gynaecol. 2010;30:288–93.
27. Oates-Whitehead RM, Haas DM, Carrier JA. Progestogen for preventing miscarriage. Cochrane Database Syst Rev. 2003;(4):CD003511.
28. Haas DM, Ramsey PS. Progestogen for preventing miscarriage. Cochrane Database Syst Rev. 2013;31(10):CD003511.
29. Kumar A, Begum N, Prasad S, Aggarwal S, Sharma S. Oral dydrogesterone treatment during early pregnancy to prevent recurrent pregnancy loss and its role in modulation of cytokine production: a double-blind, randomized, parallel, placebo-controlled trial. Fertil Steril. 2014;102(5):1357–63.
30. Agarwal N, Gupta S, Kumar R, Kriplani A, Bhatla N, Kulshrestha V. Cytokine levels and role of progesterone in recurrent pregnancy loss. Communicated.
31. Coomarasamy A, Williams H, Truchanowicz E, Seed PT, Small R, Quenby S, et al. A randomized trial of progesterone in women with recurrent miscarriages. N Engl J Med. 2015;373(22):2141–8.
32. Wahabi HA, Fayed AA, Esmaeil SA, Al Zeidan RA. Progestogen for treating threatened miscarriage. Cochrane Database Syst Rev. 2011;(12):CD005943.
33. Queisser-Luft A. Dydrogesterone use during pregnancy: overview of birth defects reported since 1977. Early Hum Dev. 2009;85(6):375–7.
34. Morley LC, Simpson N, Tang T. Human chorionic gonadotrophin (hCG) for preventing miscarriage. Cochrane Database Syst Rev. 2013;(1):CD008611.
35. Tay PY, Lenton EA. The optimum time for exogenous human chorionic gonadotropin to rescue the corpus luteum. J Assist Reprod Genet. 1999;16(9):495–9.
36. Peñarrubia J, Balasch J, Fábregues F, Creus M, Casamitjana R, Ballescá JL, et al. Human chorionic gonadotrophin luteal support overcomes luteal phase inadequacy after gonadotrophin-releasing hormone agonist-induced ovulation in gonadotrophin-stimulated cycles. Hum Reprod. 1998;13(12):3315–8.
37. Reid SM, Middleton P, Cossich MC, et al. Interventions for clinical and subclinical hypothyroidism pre-pregnancy and during pregnancy. Cochrane Database Syst Rev. 2013;(5):CD00752.
38. Sills ES, Perloe M, Palermo GD. Correction of hyperinsulinemia in oligoovulatory women with clomiphene-resistant polycystic ovary syndrome: a review of therapeutic rationale and reproductive outcomes. Eur J Obstet Gynecol Reprod Biol. 2000;91:135–41.
39. Zolghadri J, Tavana Z, Kazerooni T, et al. Relationship between abnormal glucose tolerance test and history of previous recurrent miscarriages, and beneficial effects of metformin in these patients: a prospective clinical study. Fertil Steril. 2008;90(3):727–30.

7 Anatomic Considerations in RPL

Anshuja Singla and Sonia Chawla

7.1 Introduction

Anatomic defects, both congenital and acquired of the uterus and the cervix, have been implicated in the etiology of recurrent pregnancy loss (RPL). These defects are listed in Table 7.1.

7.2 Congenital Uterine Anomalies

The exact contribution of congenital uterine anomalies to recurrent pregnancy loss (RPL) is not known. The reported prevalence in this population ranges between 1.8 and 37.6% [1]. This variability reflects the differences in the criteria and techniques used for diagnosis and the fact that available studies have included women with two, three, or more miscarriages in both the first and second trimester of pregnancy [2]. Generally, uterine malformations lead to second trimester abortions. Exact mechanism by which anatomic defects are thought to cause miscarriage is unclear, but it is attributed to decreasing effective intrauterine volume and abnormal and defective placentation.

Uterine defects causing RPL in decreasing order of frequency are septate (35%), bicornuate (25%), and arcuate uterus (20%) [3]. Other less common anomalies are didelphys and unicornuate uterus.

A. Singla (✉) • S. Chawla
Obstetrics and Gynecology, University College of Medical Sciences and GTB Hospital, Delhi, India
e-mail: dr.sonia0685@gmail.com; dranshuja@gmail.com

S. Mehta, B. Gupta (eds.), *Recurrent Pregnancy Loss*,
https://doi.org/10.1007/978-981-10-7338-0_7

Table 7.1 Anatomic defects associated with recurrent pregnancy loss

Congenital	Acquired
– Septate uterus – Bicornuate uterus – Arcuate uterus – Unicornuate uterus – Didelphys	– Leiomyoma – Intrauterine adhesions (Asherman's syndrome) – Cervical insufficiency

7.2.1 Septate Uterus

Septate uterus is by far the most common developmental anomaly (35%) [2] and is associated with poorest pregnancy outcomes [4]. It results from the failure of reabsorption of midline uterine septum between the two mullerian ducts. It could be complete if septum reaches up to internal os or partial if it falls short of internal os.

Poor reproductive outcomes are due to poor septal vascularization impairing placentation, increased amount of muscle tissue in the septum causing uncoordinated uterine contractions, and reduced effective length of uterine cavity.

Although septate uterus is not always associated with poor pregnancy outcomes, its detection in a patient of RPL warrants treatment [3, 5]. Treatment of choice is hysteroscopic septoplasty. It is a relatively safe and easy procedure and is associated with low morbidity. Significantly better reproductive outcomes have been reported with a reduction in RPL from 83 to 33% and an increase in live birth up to 67% [6]. Hysteroscopic septoplasty can be performed with laser, microscissors, or electrosurgical instruments. The septum is incised (rather than excision) just short of myometrium. The portion of the septum which is left retracts over itself. Procedure is considered complete when both the ostia are visualized simultaneously and hysteroscope can be moved freely between the two corneal recesses. Post-procedure, hormone therapy should be given for 2–4 months for endometrial regrowth [6].

7.2.2 Bicornuate Uterus

Bicornuate uterus is the second most common anomaly associated with RPL (25%). The etiology is incomplete fusion of mullerian ducts resulting in a deep fundal cleft and a common lower segment. It may be associated with a single cervix (Bicornuate unicollis) or two cervices (Bicornuate bicollis).

Surgery is generally not necessary until it is associated with RPL and no other etiologies are found. Strassman metroplasty is the procedure of choice for unification of two horns.

Data on reproductive outcomes after surgery with bicornuate uterus is limited. In one study of 22 patients with bicornuate uterus, 88% achieved live birth after Strassman metroplasty [7].

7.2.3 Arcuate Uterus

It is considered as a normal variant and is not associated with poor reproductive outcomes [8].

Other anomalies like uterus didelphys and unicornuate uterus though less common are associated with very poor pregnancy outcomes. Data on surgical treatment is very limited and cases have to be individualized.

7.3 Acquired Defects

7.3.1 Leiomyoma

Leiomyoma as a cause of RPL has always been debated. Several mechanisms have been proposed including:

- Mechanical compression of the fetus by the large fibroid.
- Large submucosal fibroid may cause distension of the uterine cavity.
- Increased contractility of the uterus.

Numerous studies have investigated the role of fibroid in causing pregnancy loss. Interestingly, majority of these studies have been conducted in patients undergoing in vitro fertilization (IVF) for infertility. Spontaneous miscarriage was higher in females having submucosal and intramural fibroids than with no fibroid [9]. No major difference was reported for pregnancy and delivery rate in women with subserosal fibroids [10, 11]. Thus, surgical removal of submucosal and intramural fibroids distorting cavity results in a better pregnancy outcome and live birth rate [11]. If a fibroid is subserosal or intramural and not distorting the uterine cavity, surgical treatment is not of much benefit, though the decision should be individualized for age, parity, site, size, number of fibroids, and other associated sign and symptoms.

7.3.2 Intrauterine Adhesions (Asherman's Syndrome)

Asherman syndrome usually causes infertility and menstrual problems but rarely can be associated with recurrent miscarriages. This is attributed to the decrease in functional intrauterine volume because of fibrotic bands. Common causes for intrauterine adhesions are vigorous postpartum curettage, endometrial tuberculosis, schistosomiasis, or other uterine surgery. It has been estimated that there is a 25% risk of developing Asherman's syndrome if dilatation and curettage is performed 1–4 weeks after delivery, 30.9% after missed abortion, and 6.4% after incomplete miscarriage [12–15].

March et al. [16] classified intrauterine adhesions as mild, moderate, and severe on hysteroscopy:

1. Mild: Less than three-fourth of the uterine cavity is involved. Adhesions are thin and flimsy. The fundus and the ostial areas are either minimally or not involved.
2. Moderate: One-fourth to three-fourths of the uterine cavity is involved. Adhesions are present but there is no agglutination of the walls. Fundus and ostial areas are only partially occluded.
3. Severe: More than three-fourths of the uterine cavity is involved. Thick bands and agglutination of the uterine walls are present. Ostial areas and the upper cavity are occluded.

Hysteroscopy is the mainstay in the diagnosis of intrauterine adhesions. Treatment includes hysteroscopic resection of the intrauterine adhesions and preventing regrowth of the fibrous tissue by supporting the endometrium with hormones.

7.3.3 Cervical Insufficiency

ACOG defines cervical incompetence as "inability of the uterine cervix to retain the pregnancy in second trimester in the absence of clinical contractions or labor or both." Cervical insufficiency affects 1% of pregnant females [17]. With cervical cerclage, improvement in pregnancy outcome has been reported. Studies have reported that improvement in pregnancy outcome occurred, with 68–78% of patients having term vaginal delivery after placement of cervical stitch [18, 19].

Causes of cervical insufficiency could be congenital or acquired (Table 7.2).

Diagnosis can be made either on the basis of history, examination findings, or investigations.

7.3.3.1 History-Based Diagnosis

- History of repeated second trimester losses associated with short painless labor and premature preterm rupture of membranes (PPROM)
- History of progressive early deliveries in subsequent pregnancies

Table 7.2 Causes of cervical insufficiency

Congenital causes	Acquired causes
(a) Connective tissue disorders (Marfan's syndrome, Ehlers-Danlos syndrome	(a) Forceful or repeated dilatation and curettage
(b) Uterine malformations like unicornuate, bicornuate, or didelphys uterus	(b) Cone biopsy
	(c) Unrepaired cervical tears
	(d) Instrumental delivery in a partially dilated cervix
	(e) Surgical procedure like Fothergill's operation, Duhrssen's incision

7.3.3.2 Examination

- Dilatation of the internal os with protruding membranes on per speculum examination
- Digital palpation—shortening of the length of the cervix
- Ultrasonographic assessment of the cervical length

7.3.3.3 Investigations

Inter-conceptional period:

- Passage of hegar dilator no.8 beyond the internal os without resistance and pain and absence of the snap upon withdrawal of the dilator
- Shirodkar's test—passage of uterine sound without resistance or pain

Various other tests using balloon of Foley's catheter have been postulated, but none of these can conclusively make or refute the diagnosis of incompetent cervix in nonpregnant state and should not be used [20].

During pregnancy:

Cervical length in general population is relatively stable after midtrimester. This fact may be helpful in serial evaluation of the cervical length for predicting preterm labor. Transvaginal sonography (TVS) is the most accurate method of measurement of cervical length, and transabdominal scan should not preferably be used for assessment of the cervix length [20]. Technique for USG measurement should be standardized so as to reduce the observational errors. Criteria proposed by Kagan are widely accepted and used [21].

Criteria for assessment of cervical length by TVS are:

- Patient's bladder must be empty.
- A longitudinal view of cervix should be obtained.
- The cervical canal and surrounding cervical mucosa should be identified.
- Pressure on the cervix should be minimal (as it elongates the cervical canal).
- Magnify the image, so that cervix should occupy 50–75% of the screen.
- The cervical length should be measured between the external and internal os.

With TVS, 25 mm length corresponds to tenth percentile and is suggested as the cut-off limit at 24-week period of gestation. Chances of preterm labor increase by sixfold if cervical length is <25 mm at 24 weeks [22, 23].

7.3.3.4 Management

As per RCOG guidelines, previous terminology of prophylactic, elective, or emergency cervical cerclage can be ambiguous [2]. Nomenclature based on indication is recommended and should be used.

- History-indicated cerclage
- Ultrasound-indicated cerclage
- Rescue cerclage

History-indicated cerclage: Women with three or more previous preterm births and/or second trimester losses are the candidates for cervical cerclage under this heading. It should not be routinely offered to women with two or fewer previous preterm births and/or second trimester losses.

Ultrasound-indicated cerclage: Women with history of one or more spontaneous midtrimester losses or preterm birth and who are undergoing ultrasound surveillance of cervical length should be offered cerclage, if cervix is 25 mm or less at or before 24 weeks of gestation. Cervical length screening is generally started at about 14 weeks in patients who are at high risk. There is no consensus on optimal timing or frequency of serial evaluation of cervical length. Repeat measurements should be at suitable intervals to minimize the observational errors with minimum interval being at least 1 week [20].

Timing of cerclage: Commonly performed around 12–14-week period of gestation for women with history-based diagnosis.

Procedure: Surgery of choice is cervical cerclage, which can be performed either by transvaginal route or by transabdominal route.

Prerequisites for surgery: Apart from routine antenatal investigations, first trimester ultrasound, screening to rule out congenital malformation, endocervical and high vaginal swab, and urine culture and sensitivity should be done.

7.3.3.5 Transvaginal Cerclage Operation

McDonald's Stitch

A purse-string suture using Mersilk or nylon is applied as high as possible at the cervicovaginal junction, below bladder. Four to five bites are taken and the knot is tied posteriorly. Stitch is removed after 37 completed weeks or when the patient goes into labor.

Shirodkar Stitch

In this procedure, the suture is placed at the level of internal os after retraction of the bladder. In the original technique, fascia lata was used for the stitch.

Steps of Shirodkar procedure:

- Transverse incision of about 2–3 cm is made on anterior vaginal wall at the cervicovaginal junction.
- Bladder is pushed up, well above the internal os.
- The cervix is pulled upward and an incision of about 2 cm is made on posterior vaginal wall at or above the internal os.
- A 5 mm Mersilene tape on a curved atraumatic needle is passed posteroanteriorly through the paracervical tissue and brought out through the anterior incision and then again anteroposteriorly so that knot ends up posteriorly avoiding the bladder.
- After the knot is tied, the band and the knot are anchored with the help of permanent stitch such as Mersilk or Prolene.

- Anterior and posterior incisions are closed with chromic catgut or any other absorbable suture.

Advantage

- It is high up, close to internal os, and most part of the suture is buried.

Disadvantages

- More chances of bleeding
- Difficult removal

7.3.3.6 Abdominal Cerclage

Indications

- Previous failed vaginal cerclage
- Extremely scarred or lacerated cervix due to previous surgeries like extensive cone biopsy or amputation
- Absent or hypoplastic cervix with history suggestive of cervical insufficiency

Procedure

- Abdomen is opened via transverse or vertical incision.
- Bladder flap is incised transversely till the level of internal cervical os.
- Mersilene tape is passed through the avascular space between the ascending and descending branches of uterine arteries.
- Tape is anchored to the uterine surface with the help of permanent sutures.
- Care should be taken not to twist the tape.

7.3.3.7 Laparoscopic Approach

Procedure is similar to transabdominal cerclage except that the procedure is done laparoscopically.

It has the added benefit of reduced blood loss, less postoperative pain, less adhesions, decreased hospital stay, and early recovery. The disadvantages of the procedure are high chances of ureteric injury and subsequent delivery is by cesarean section only.

7.3.3.8 Complications of Cerclage Operation

1. Infection
2. Hemorrhage
3. Preterm premature rupture of membranes
4. Cervical stenosis
5. Cervical dystocia and uterine rupture may also occur if there is delay in removal of stitch

7.4 Evidence-Based Management of Anatomic Abnormality in RPL

7.4.1 ASRM Committee Opinion

Congenital uterine abnormalities are generally associated with second trimester pregnancy losses and other pregnancy-related complications like preterm labor, malpresentation, and high chances of cesarean section. Role of uterine abnormalities in first trimester recurrent pregnancy loss is controversial, but assessment of uterine cavity is recommended.

The management of RPL patients with intrauterine synechiae and fibroid and polyp is debatable, and surgical correction of significant uterine defects should be considered.

7.4.2 RCOG Guidelines

The women with recurrent first trimester loss and one or more second trimester loss should be investigated by pelvic ultrasound for any possible uterine abnormality and if any abnormality is suspected, further investigations like hysteroscopy, laparoscopy, or 3D ultrasound should be done for confirmation. However, there is no conclusive evidence for supporting the benefits of surgical correction of the uterine abnormalities in improving pregnancy outcome.

Cervical cerclage is associated with potential risk of surgery and stimulation of uterine contractions. Therefore it should be considered in carefully selected cases.

Key Points

- Congenital uterine abnormalities are usually associated with second trimester pregnancy losses.
- In cases of recurrent second trimester losses assessment of uterine cavity should be done.
- Cerclage should be applied in carefully selected cases i.e. when indicated by history, ultrasound and emergent cases.

References

1. Practice Committee of the American Society for Reproductive Medicine. Evaluation and treatment of recurrent pregnancy loss: a committee opinion. Fertil Steril. 2012;98(5):1103–11.
2. Royal College of Obstetricians and Gynecologists. The investigation and treatment of couples with recurrent first-trimester and second-trimester miscarriage. Green-top Guideline No. 17; April 2011.
3. Grimbizis GF, Camus M, Tarlatzis BC, Bontis JN, Devroey P. Clinical implications of uterine malformations and hysteroscopic treatment results. Hum Reprod Update. 2001;7(2):161–74.

4. Homer HA, Li TC, Cooke ID. The septate uterus: a review of management and reproductive outcome. Fertil Steril. 2000;73(1):1–14.
5. Ghi T, De Musso F, Maroni E, Youssef A, Savelli L, Farina A, Casadio P, Filicori M, Pilu G, Rizzo N. The pregnancy outcome in women with incidental diagnosis of septate uterus at first trimester scan. Hum Reprod. 2012;27(9):2671–5.
6. Selvaraj P, Selvaraj K. Reproductive outcome of septate uterus following hysteroscopic septum resection. J Hum Reprod Sci. 2010;3(3):143–5.
7. Lolis DE, Paschopoulos M, Makrydimas G, Zikopoulos K, Sotiriadis A, Paraskevaidis E. Reproductive outcome after strassman metroplasty in women with a bicornuate uterus. J Reprod Med. 2005;50(5):297–301.
8. Raga F, Bauset C, Remohi J, Bonilla-Musoles F, Simón C, Pellicer A. Reproductive impact of congenital Müllerian anomalies. Hum Reprod. 1997;12(10):2277–81.
9. Pritts EA, Parker WH, Olive DL. Fibroids and infertility: an updated systematic review of the evidence. Fertil Steril. 2009;91(4):1215–23.
10. Klatsky PC, Tran ND, Caughey AB, Fujimoto VY. Fibroids and reproductive outcomes: a systematic literature review from conception to delivery. Am J Obstet Gynecol. 2008;198(4):357–66.
11. Casini ML, Rossi F, Agostini R, Unfer V. Effects of the position of fibroids on fertility. Gynecol Endocrinol. 2006;22(2):106–9.
12. Ahmadi F, Siahbazi S, Akhbari F, Eslami B, Vosough A. Hysterosalpingography finding in intra uterine adhesion (Asherman's syndrome): a pictorial essay. Int J Fertil Steril. 2013;7(3):155–60.
13. Salma U, Xu D, Sheikh MSA. Diagnosis and treatment of intrauterine adhesions. Bangladesh J Med Sci. 2011;2:72–82.
14. Adoni A, Palti Z, Milwidsky A, Dolberg M. The incidence of intrauterine adhesions following spontaneous abortion. Int J Fertil. 1982;27(2):117–8.
15. International Asherman's Association. http://www.ashermans.org/home/. Accessed on 28th June 2016.
16. March CM, Israel R, March AD. Hysteroscopic management of intrauterine adhesions. Am J Obstet Gynecol. 1978;130(6):653–7.
17. Callen PW. Ultrasonography in Obstetrics and Gynecology, 4th ed. Philadelpghia: Saunders Elsevier, 2000. p. 577–96.
18. Ikimalo JI, Izuchukwu KE, Inimgba N. Pregnancy outcome after cerclage for cervical incompetence at the University of Port Harcourt Teaching Hospital, Port Harcourt. Afr J Reprod Health. 2012;16(3):180–4.
19. Harger JH. Comparison of success and morbidity in cervical cerclage procedures. Obstet Gynecol. 1980;56(5):543–8.
20. Brown R, Gagnon R, Delisle MF, SOGC Maternal Fetal Medicine Committee. Cervical insufficiency and cervical cerclage. SOGC clinical practice guideline no. 301, December 2013. J Obstet Gynaecol Can. 2013;35:1115–27.
21. Kagan KO, Sonek J. How to measure cervical length? Ultrasound Obstet Gynecol. 2015;45(3):358–62.
22. Iams JD, Goldenberg RL, Meis PJ, Mercer BM, Moawad A, Das A, et al. The length of the cervix and the risk of spontaneous premature delivery. National Institute of Child Health and Human Development Maternal Fetal Medicine Unit Network. N Engl J Med. 1996;334(9):567–72.
23. Lee HJ, Park TC, Norwitz ER. Management of pregnancies with cervical shortening: a very short cervix is a very big problem. Rev Obstet Gynecol. 2009;2(2):107–15.

Antiphospholipid Antibody Syndrome

8

K. Aparna Sharma and Kavita Khoiwal

Antiphospholipid antibody syndrome (APS) is an acquired autoimmune disorder characterized by the presence of antiphospholipid antibodies (aPLs) with vascular thrombosis and/or recurrent pregnancy loss (RPL) or placental insufficiency. Antiphospholipid antibodies are autoantibodies that react with epitopes on proteins that are complexed with negatively charged phospholipids.

The incidence of APS in patients with RPL is 15% [1]. The prevalence of aPLs is less than 2% in low-risk obstetric women [2]. The chances of successful pregnancy outcome in women with aPLs are extremely poor, and without treatment, the live birth rate may be as low as 10% [3].

8.1 Classification of APS

APS can be classified as primary and secondary. It is referred as secondary APS when it is associated with the following underlying diseases (Table 8.1).

8.2 Pathophysiology of APS

Adverse pregnancy outcome such as pregnancy loss and restriction of fetal growth may be due to abnormal placentation, thrombosis of vessels in the placental bed, and local inflammatory destruction.

K.A. Sharma (✉)
Department of OBG, All India Institute of Medical Sciences, New Delhi, India
e-mail: kaparnasharma@gmail.com

K. Khoiwal
All India Institute of Medical Sciences, New Delhi, India
e-mail: kavita.kh27@gmail.com

S. Mehta, B. Gupta (eds.), *Recurrent Pregnancy Loss*,
https://doi.org/10.1007/978-981-10-7338-0_8

Table 8.1 Conditions associated with secondary APS

(a)	Autoimmune disease	(b)	Malignancies
	Systemic lupus erythematosus (SLE)		Carcinoma of ovary and cervix
	Rheumatoid arthritis		Leukemia
	Sjogren syndrome		Lymphoma
	Systemic sclerosis		
	Diabetes mellitus		
	Crohn disease		
	Autoimmune thyroid disease		
(c)	Infectious diseases	(d)	Drug-induced conditions
	Syphilis		Oral contraceptives
	Human immunodeficiency virus infection		

8.2.1 Abnormal Placentation

The most frequent histopathological finding in APS associated early pregnancy loss is defective decidual endovascular trophoblast invasion [4]. aPLs can inhibit trophoblast invasion directly or through an abnormal expression of integrins and cadherins and impair trophoblastic cellular differentiation, maturation, and induction of syncytiotrophoblast apoptosis [5].

8.2.2 Thrombosis

Thrombosis of vessels of placental bed could be the major causative factor for pregnancy loss and intrauterine growth restriction (IUGR). Thrombosis of vessels leads to placental infarction, placental insufficiency, and fetal hypoxia. Several studies supported this hypothesis by the finding of thrombosis and infarction in the placentas of women with APS who had first and second trimester abortions [6]. Figure 8.1 depicts pathogenesis of thrombosis in antiphospholipid antibody syndrome.

8.2.3 Complement Activation

During normal pregnancy, the maternal immune system is modified to prevent immune rejection of the fetoplacental unit. The interaction of aPLs to trophoblast cell membranes facilitates complement activation, specifically C3a and C5a [7]. Complement activation causes inflammatory tissue injury via tumor necrosis factor (TNF) and tissue factor (TF), eventually lead to thrombosis and pregnancy loss. Stone S revealed that placental tissue in pregnant women with primary APS show a clustering of inflammatory cells and macrophages around blood vessels on histopathology [8].

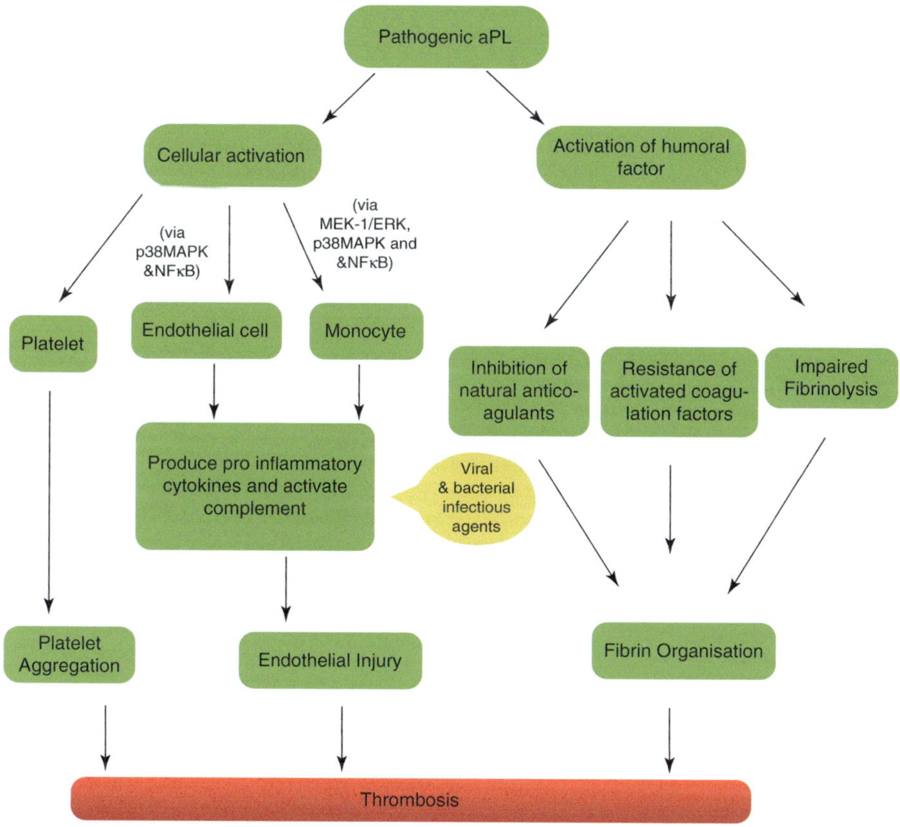

Fig. 8.1 Pathogenesis of thrombosis in antiphospholipid antibody syndrome. Abbreviations: *p38MAPK* p38 mitogen-activated protein kinase, *NFκB* nuclear factor κB

8.3 Diagnostic Criteria for APS

The diagnosis of APS should be considered if at **least one of the clinical criteria** and **one of the laboratory** criteria are met (as shown in Table 8.2).

8.3.1 Clinical Criteria

8.3.1.1 Vascular Thrombosis

Thrombosis is the most common and serious complications associated with APS. Venous thrombosis is more common than arterial thrombosis. The most common presentation of venous thrombosis in APS is lower limb deep vein thrombosis (DVT) and/or pulmonary embolism (PE). But any part of the venous system can be involved, including superficial, portal, renal, mesenteric, and intracranial veins, and

Table 8.2 Diagnostic criteria for APS

Clinical criteria	
1. Vascular thrombosis	Venous/arterial/microvascular
2. Pregnancy-associated morbidity	(a) Three or more unexplained consecutive spontaneous abortions before 10 weeks of gestation, provided there is no maternal anatomical or hormonal abnormalities or paternal and maternal chromosomal causes (b) One or more unexplained deaths of a morphologically normal fetuses beyond 10 weeks of gestation, diagnosed by ultrasound or direct examination of the fetus (c) One or more premature births of a morphologically normal neonate before 34 weeks of gestation caused by eclampsia, severe preeclampsia, or recognized features of placental insufficiency
Laboratory criteria	1. Lupus anticoagulant (LAC) present in plasma on two or more occasions at least 12 weeks apart [9] 2. Anticardiolipin (aCL) antibody of IgG or IgM isotype in serum or plasma present in medium or high titer (>40GPL units or MPL units or > the 99th percentile) on two or more occasions at least 12 weeks apart [9] 3. Anti-b2 glycoprotein-I antibody of IgG and/or IgM isotype in serum or plasma (in titer >the 99th percentile) present on two or more occasions at least 12 weeks apart [9]

Abbreviations: GPL units, IgG antiphospholipid units; MPL units, IgM antiphospholipid units. *IgG* immunoglobulin G, *IgM* immunoglobulin M

occlusions in unusual locations should prompt clinicians to consider the diagnosis of APS. Khamashta MA et al. found a thrombosis recurrence rate of 25% per year in untreated patients with APS and also showed that recurrence can be minimized with anticoagulation [10]. The risk of thrombosis is significantly increased by 5–12% during pregnancy or in the postpartum period in patients with APS [11]. de Groot et al. demonstrated that the strongest risk factors for DVT in a general population are the combination of LAC, anti-b2GP-I, and antiprothrombin antibodies [12].

The most frequent site of arterial thrombosis in APS is middle cerebral artery resulting in transient cerebral ischemia or stroke [13]. Myocardial infarction is less common, although subclinical myocardial ischemia may be under recognized [14]. It can occur in atypical sites, such as the retinal, subclavian, digital, or brachial arteries. Antiphospholipid antibodies are present in 4–6% of patients with stroke who are younger than 50 years [15]. Individuals with unexplained arterial thrombosis, stroke, amaurosis fugax, or transient ischemic attacks should undergo testing for aPLs. Other medical conditions associated with aPLs include autoimmune thrombocytopenia, autoimmune hemolytic anemia, livedo reticularis, cutaneous ulcers, chorea gravidarum, multi-infarct dementia, and transverse myelitis.

In general, among aPLs, the specificity for thrombosis is higher for LAC than aCL or anti-b2GP-I and greater for higher than lower titer aCL [16].

Despite these clear associations between aPLs and thrombosis, APS makes only a minor contribution to the overall burden of disease from venous thromboembolism and stroke.

Microvascular thrombosis in APS is least common but may manifest as the potentially lethal "catastrophic antiphospholipid syndrome" (CAPS) which constitutes progressive thrombosis and multi-organ failure [17].

8.3.1.2 Antiphospholipid Antibodies (aPLs) and Pregnancy Morbidity

The women with circulating aPLs are at increased risk of recurrent and late pregnancy loss [18]. In the meta-analysis by Opatrny et al. [19], LAC has a stronger association with pregnancy loss than the other antiphospholipid antibodies, and both IgG and IgM aCL were associated with recurrent fetal loss, while the importance of anti-b2GP-I and pregnancy loss is uncertain. There is an association between preeclampsia, placental abruption and IUGR, and the presence of aPLs, but this association is less strong than with recurrent pregnancy loss [20].

Recurrent Pregnancy Loss

According to American Society of Reproductive Medicine, RPL is defined as two or more failed clinical pregnancies as documented by ultrasonography or histopathologic documentation of products of conception and recommended a thorough evaluation of RPL after two or more clinical losses [21]. The risk of abortion in subsequent pregnancies is 30% after 2 losses and 45% after 3 losses in patients without a history of live birth. Antiphospholipid antibodies are found in approximately 7–25% of early RPL. Although all three of the laboratory criteria for diagnosis of APS (LAC, aCL, and Anti-b2GP-I) [22] have been linked with RPL, LAC is the most specific, found in 1–5% of patients [23].

Fetal Loss

Late fetal loss (after 10 weeks of pregnancy) associated with aPL antibodies is one of the diagnostic criteria for APS. In a study by Ruffatti A et al. among patients with APS and without hereditary thrombophilia, test positive for all three including LAC, aCL, and Anti-b2GP-I had a risk of late fetal loss of 52.6% compared with a loss rate of 2.2% when only two tests were positive [24].

Severe Preeclampsia Before 34 Weeks

Severe preeclampsia is another clinical criterion of the APS. A recent review of APS and preeclampsia in 2011 reported a rate of 20% of patients with severe preeclampsia before 34 weeks having at least one aPL test positive compared with 6% in late-onset (after 34 weeks' gestation) preeclampsia [25].

Severe Placental Insufficiency

Severe placental insufficiency usually manifests as IUGR and placental abruption at or before 34 weeks' gestation. IUGR complicates 15–30% of pregnancies in women with APS [26]. Because IUGR is most commonly seen in the presence of preeclampsia, actual causality is difficult to establish. Although there are no prospective trials studying the association between abruption and APS, Alfirevic and colleagues [27] noted an association between abruption and aCL IgG antibodies in a systematic review.

8.3.2 Laboratory Criteria

The most widely accepted tests are lupus anticoagulant (LAC), anticardiolipin antibody (aCL), and anti-b2 glycoprotein I (anti-b2GP-I).

LAC is more specific but less sensitive than the aCL and anti-b2GP-I [28]. Some patients with APS have all the three antibodies. Because transient positive test results may occur, the diagnosis of APS requires two positive aPL test results at least 12 weeks apart.

8.3.2.1 Lupus Anticoagulant

Irrespective the name, LAC is associated with thrombosis not with anticoagulation. Two test systems of different principles should be used to improve specificity. Patient is considered to have LAC if one or both tests are positive. The presence of LAC is assessed indirectly, and a series of tests are needed for the laboratory diagnosis. The initial laboratory screening test for LAC is performed using a combination of sensitive clotting assays, such as activated partial thromboplastin time and dilute Russell's viper venom time. Lupus anticoagulants paradoxically block phospholipid-dependent clotting assays by interfering with the assembly of the prothrombin complex. Because prolonged clotting times in these assays can result from factors other than lupus anticoagulant, such as improperly processed specimens, anticoagulant medications, clotting factor deficiencies, and factor-specific inhibitors, plasma suspected of containing lupus anticoagulant based on a prolonged clotting time is subjected to additional testing. If the prolonged clotting time is caused by a factor deficiency, the addition of normal plasma (containing the missing factor) results in a normal clotting time on repeat testing. In contrast, if an inhibitor such as lupus anticoagulant is present, the clotting time remains prolonged despite the addition of normal plasma. A second confirmatory test, which involves the addition or removal of phospholipid from the assay, has been recommended. For example, preincubation of plasma with phospholipid binds and removes lupus anticoagulant from the sample being tested and normalizes clotting time. Regardless of the assays used, lupus anticoagulant cannot be quantified and is reported only as present or absent.

8.3.2.2 Anticardiolipin Antibodies

Anticardiolipin antibodies are most commonly detected using enzyme-linked immunosorbent assays. It is recommended that immunoglobulin G (IgG) and immunoglobulin M (IgM) isotypes are to be measured. The clinical relevance of immunoglobulin A aCL antibodies remains uncertain. Standard, reference reagents for aCL antibodies are available, and results are typically reported in international standard units, designated "GPL" for IgG phospholipid and "MPL" for IgM phospholipid. Current consensus guidelines suggest that a positive aCL result is greater than 40 GPL or 40 MPL (i.e., greater than the 99th percentile) [22].

8.3.2.3 Anti-β2-Glycoprotein-I Antibodies

As with aCL antibodies, anti-β2GP-I antibodies are most commonly detected using enzyme-linked immunosorbent assays. Both IgG and IgM anti-β2-glycoprotein-I isotypes should be measured. Anti-β2-GP-I antibodies are reported most commonly in international standard units known as "SGU" or "SMU" for IgG and IgM, respectively. Current consensus guidelines suggest that a positive result is greater than the 99th percentile [22].

Practice points for laboratory testing [29]:

- In patients with thrombosis, measuring IgM antibodies does not add useful information.
- In patients with pregnancy morbidity, the role of IgM antibodies is unclear.
- Testing for IgA antibodies is not recommended.

Testing for aPLs should be performed in women with a prior unexplained arterial or venous thromboembolism, or a new arterial or venous thromboembolism during pregnancy, or a history of venous thromboembolism who have not been tested previously. Obstetric indications for aPLs testing include a history of one fetal loss more than 10 weeks, three or more recurrent embryonic or fetal losses less than 10 weeks, preterm severe preeclampsia, and early-onset placental insufficiency.

8.4 Management of APS

The main objective of treatment is to improve maternal and fetal-neonatal outcome. Women with APS are prone to develop thrombosis and hence require anticoagulation during pregnancy. Adverse pregnancy outcomes like abortion, preeclampsia, and intrauterine deaths can occur secondary to the underlying pathology. The treatment protocol should take into account the individual clinical scenarios as shown in Fig. 8.2.

Several treatments have been proposed till date, including a single low-dose aspirin per day, aspirin and low-dose or high-dose prednisone, aspirin and unfractionated heparin (UFH), aspirin and low molecular weight heparin (LMWH), and intravenous immunoglobulin (IVIg).

8.4.1 Drugs in Management of APS

The combination of UFH with low-dose aspirin provides the highest success rate [30].

Aspirin (75–150 mg) improves the pregnancy outcome by selective inhibition of thromboxane A2 production, thereby restoring the balance with prostaglandin. It should be started preconceptionally.

Fig. 8.2 Therapeutic protocols in various clinical scenarios in women with APS

APS with prior thrombosis
Non Pregnant
- Warfarin
- Switch to the rapeutic LMWH in pregnancy

APS with Pregnancy Morbidity
- Low Dose Aspirin preconception
- prophylactic LMWH at confirmation of pregnancy(UPT)

APLA without thrombosis or pregnancy Morbidity
- Low Dose Aspirin

Dose of UFH is 5000 U (7500 U if patient weigh >80 kg) subcutaneously twice a day from the day pregnancy test is positive. It is important to obtain a baseline platelet count and partial thromboplastin time. Heparin does not cross the placenta; there is no potential to cause fetal hemorrhage or teratogenicity. Heparin is associated with maternal complications such as bleeding, hypersensitivity reactions, heparin-induced thrombocytopenia, osteopenia, and vertebral fractures on long-term use. So, these patients should be advised calcium 600 mg orally twice a day along with vitamin D 400 IU twice daily to optimize absorption of calcium and to reduce the risk of osteopenia. The incidence of heparin-induced thrombocytopenia is less than 1%. The heparin dosage should be adjusted or an alternative therapy to be given if platelet counts decreased dramatically during pregnancy. Patients should be clearly instructed about the proper administration of subcutaneous heparin to minimize complications.

LMWH is an effective alternative to UFH [31]. It is as safe as UFH and has potential advantages over UFH during pregnancy. It can be administered once daily, less intensive monitoring required, and is associated with a lower risk of heparin-induced thrombocytopenia and osteoporosis [32].

LMWH is emerging as the treatment of choice for RPL associated with APS. The usual prophylactic dose is 40 mg subcutaneously once a day.

The mechanism of action of heparin to prevent pregnancy complications in obstetric APS is by inhibiting the binding of aPL to trophoblastic cell membranes, modulating trophoblast apoptosis, promoting trophoblast cell invasiveness, and reducing complement activation with the ensuing inflammatory response at the decidual-placental interface [33]. These mechanisms are independent of heparin's known anticoagulant property.

Neither corticosteroids nor IVIg therapy improve the live birth rate of women with recurrent miscarriage associated with APS compared with other treatment modalities. Their use may lead to significant maternal and fetal morbidity [34].

8.4.2 Antepartum Surveillance

All women with APS should undergo routine antepartum testing, based on their previous obstetric history. It is usual to perform serial ultrasounds weekly until the patients have progressed beyond the point of their prior early pregnancy losses. Antepartum assessment including daily fetal kick counts, twice weekly nonstress test, and weekly biophysical profile is to be done after period of viability. Serial USG for fetal growth monitoring is also recommended. Platelet count should be checked every week for 2 weeks initially, 1 week following any adjustment in dose, and each trimester throughout pregnancy to evaluate for heparin-induced thrombocytopenia.

8.4.3 Peripartum Management

Aspirin should be discontinued 4 weeks before the expected date of delivery, around 36 weeks. Heparin should be continued until the patient goes into spontaneous labor or until the night before any scheduled induction or operative delivery. Heparin therapy must be stopped temporarily during the immediate peripartum period to minimize the risk of hemorrhage and to allow for the option of regional anesthesia.

The American Society of Regional Anesthesia [35] states that subcutaneous UFH prophylaxis is not a contraindication to neuraxial regional anesthesia. But in case of LMWH, it can be considered safe at least 12 h after the last prophylactic dose and 24 h after the last therapeutic dose. If the patient is fully anticoagulated and delivery is emergent, 1% protamine sulfate can be administered intravenously over 10 min (2.5 mg protamine per 1000 U heparin, maximum 50 mg protamine).

8.4.4 Postpartum Management

Women who had a vaginal delivery should ambulate as soon as possible. Women who had a cesarean delivery should continue to use pneumatic compression stockings until they are fully ambulating. Low-dose aspirin and heparin should be restarted and to be continued for 4–6 weeks postpartum [9]. In general, this recommendation includes women with and without a prior history of thrombosis. Supplemental calcium should be continued as long as the patient is on heparin. There is no contraindication for breast-feeding.

Patients should not use estrogen-containing birth control pills for contraception. Figure 8.3 summarizes the obstetric management in women APS.

8.5 Long-Term Implications of APS

Once the diagnosis is made with appropriate clinical and laboratory criteria, this should be considered to be a diagnosis that they carry for life even if the test results returned to normal in later life. Long-term risks for women with APS include

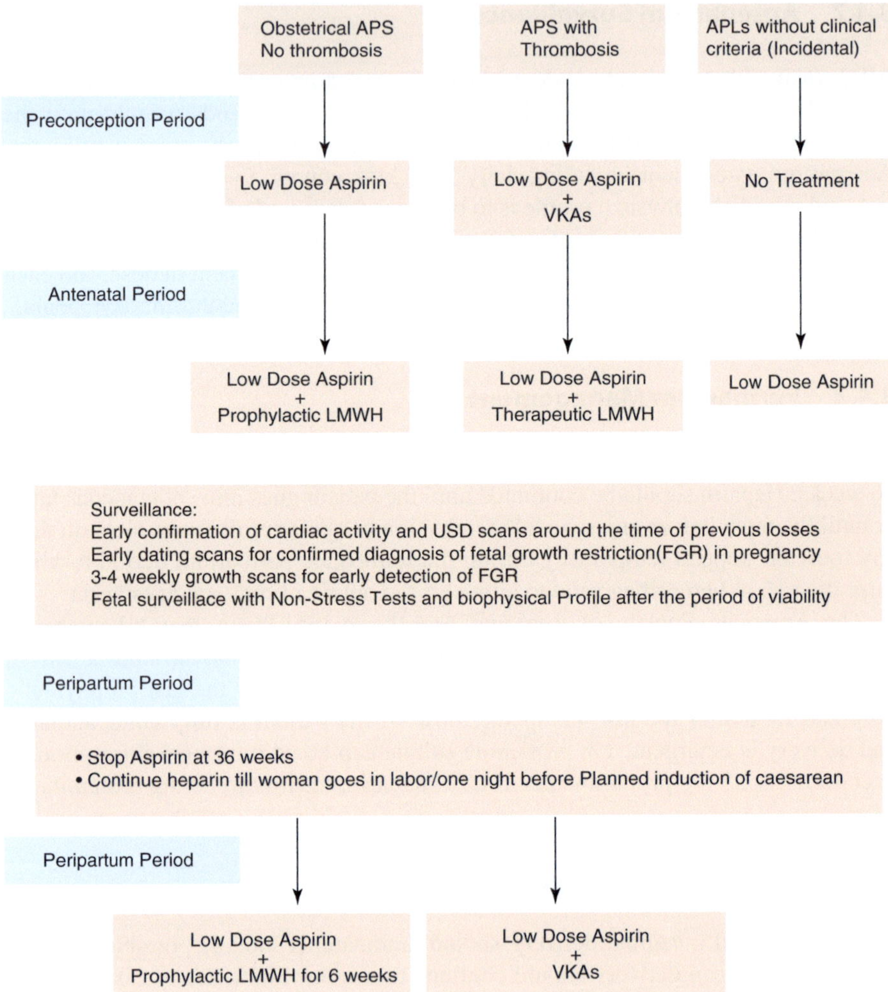

Fig. 8.3 Obstetrical APS: management flow chart (VKA, vitamin K antagonist)

thrombosis and stroke. In studies of women with APS with or without prior thrombosis, almost 50% developed thrombosis during 3–10 years of follow-up and 10% developed systemic lupus erythematosus [13]. Therefore, for long-term management postpartum, patients with APS should be referred to a physician with expertise in treatment of the syndrome, such as an internist, hematologist, or rheumatologist. Pregnancy and the use of estrogen-containing oral contraceptives appear to increase the risk of thrombosis in women with APS. So, women with APS should not use estrogen-containing oral contraceptive pills but should use progestin-only pills, barrier methods, or intrauterine devices [36]. They should similarly not use tobacco products and should maintain a normal weight. Any correctable risk factors for future thrombosis, such as increased cholesterol, should also be corrected. These women should use lifelong aspirin 81 mg per day unless it is contraindicated for other reasons [37]. In general, these individuals should live a healthy lifestyle.

Key Points

- Women with RPL before 10 weeks of gestation or one fetal loss >10 weeks of gestation should be screened for aPLs.
- Testing for aPLs should be performed in women with a prior unexplained venous thromboembolism, a new venous thromboembolism during pregnancy, or in those with a history of venous thromboembolism but not tested previously.
- For women with APS with pregnancy morbidity, antenatal administration of heparin combined with low-dose aspirin is recommended throughout pregnancy and 6 weeks postpartum.
- Incidental finding of aPLs (without any clinical criterion) can be considered for low-dose aspirin in pregnancy.
- For long-term management, postpartum patients with APS should be referred to a physician with expertise in treatment of the syndrome, such as an internist, hematologist, or rheumatologist.
- Women with APS should not use estrogen-containing contraceptives.

References

1. Rai RS, Regan L, Clifford K, Pickering W, Dave M, Mackie I, et al. Antiphospholipid antibodies and beta-2-glycoprotein-I in 500 women with recurrent miscarriage: results of a comprehensive screening approach. Hum Reprod. 1995;10:2001–5.
2. Pattison NS, Chamley LW, McKay EJ, Liggins GC, Butler WS. Antiphospholipid antibodies in pregnancy: prevalence and clinical association. Br J Obstet Gynaecol. 1993;100:909–13.
3. Rai RS, Clifford K, Cohen H, Regan L. High prospective fetal loss rate in untreated pregnancies of women with recurrent miscarriage and antiphospholipid antibodies. Hum Reprod. 1995;10:3301–4.
4. Ornoy A, Yacobi S, Matalon ST, et al. The effects of antiphospholipid antibodies obtained from women with SLE/APS and associated pregnancy loss on rat embryos and placental explants in culture. Lupus. 2003;2:573–8.
5. Di Simone N, Castellani R, Calandro D, et al. Antiphospholipid antibodies regulate the expression of trophoblast cell adhesion molecules. Fertil Steril. 2002;77:805–11.
6. Hanly JG, Gladman DD, Rose TH, et al. Lupus pregnancy. A prospective study of placental changes. Arthritis Rheum. 1988;31:358–66.
7. Salmon JE, Girardi G. The role of complement in the antiphospholipid syndrome. Curr Dir Autoimmun. 2004;7:133–48.
8. Stone S, Pijnenborg R, Vercruysse L, et al. The placental bed in pregnancies complicated by primary antiphospholipid syndrome. Placenta. 2006;27:457–67.
9. Branch DW, Holmgren C, Goldberg JD. Antiphospholipid syndrome. American College of Obstetricians and Gynecologists Practice Bulletin Number 132. Obstet Gynecol. 2012;120:1514–21.

10. Khamashta MA, Cuadrado MJ, Mujic F, Taub NA, Hunt BJ, Hughes GR. The management of thrombosis in the antiphospholipid-antibody syndrome. N Engl J Med. 1995;332:993–7.
11. Lima F, Khamashta MA, Buchanan NM, Kerslake S, Hunt BJ, Hughes GR. A study of sixty pregnancies in patients with the antiphospholipid syndrome. Clin Exp Rheumatol. 1996;14:131–6.
12. de Groot PG, Lutters B, Derksen RH, Lisman T, Meijers JC, Rosendaal FR. Lupus anticoagulants and the risk of a first episode of deep venous thrombosis. J Thromb Haemost. 2005;3:1993–7.
13. Silver RM, Draper ML, Scott JR, Lyon JL, Reading J, Branch DW. Clinical consequences of antiphospholipid antibodies: an historic cohort study. Obstet Gynecol. 1994;83:372–7.
14. Sacre K, Brihaye B, Hyafil F, Serfaty JM, Escoubet B, Zennaro MC, et al. Asymptomatic myocardial ischemic disease in antiphospholipid syndrome: a controlled cardiac magnetic resonance imaging study. Arthritis Rheum. 2010;62:2093–100.
15. Ferro D, Quintarelli C, Rasura M, Antonini G, Violi F. Lupus anticoagulant and the fibrinolytic system in young patients with stroke. Stroke. 1993;24:368–70.
16. Pengo V, Ruffatti A, Legnani C, Gresele P, Barcellona D, Erba N, et al. Clinical course of high-risk patients diagnosed with antiphospholipid syndrome. J Thromb Haemost. 2010;8:237–42.
17. Asherson RA, Cervera R, Piette JC, Font J, Lie JT, Burcoglu A, et al. Catastrophic antiphospholipid syndrome. Clinical and laboratory features of 50 patients. Medicine. 1998;77:195–207.
18. Robertson B, Greaves M. Antiphospholipid syndrome: an evolving story. Blood Rev. 2006;20:201–12.
19. Opatrny L, David M, Kahn SR, Shrier I, Rey E. Association between antiphospholipid antibodies and recurrent fetal loss in women without autoimmune disease: a metaanalysis. J Rheumatol. 2006;33:2214–21.
20. Robertson L, Wu O, Langhorne P, Twaddle S, Clark P, Lowe GD, Walker ID, Greaves M, Brenkel I, Regan L, Greer IA. Thrombophilia in pregnancy: a systematic review. Br J Haematol. 2006;132:171–96.
21. The Practice Committee of the American Society for Reproductive Medicine. Evaluation and treatment of recurrent pregnancy loss. Fertil Steril. 2012;98:1103–11.
22. Miyakis S, Lockshin MD, Atsumi T, Branch DW, Brey RL, Cervera R, et al. International consensus statement on an update of the classification criteria for definite antiphospholipid syndrome (APS). J Thromb Haemost. 2006;4:295–306.
23. Allison J, Schust D. Recurrent first trimester pregnancy loss: revised definitions and novel causes. Curr Opin Endocrinol Diabetes Obes. 2009;16:446–50.
24. Ruffatti A, Tonello M, Cavazzana A, et al. Laboratory classification categories and pregnancy outcome in patients with primary antiphospholipid syndrome prescribed antithrombotic therapy. Thromb Res. 2009;123:482–7.
25. Heilmann L, Schorsch M, Hahn T, et al. Antiphospholipid syndrome and preeclampsia. Semin Thromb Hemost. 2011;37:141–5.
26. Caruso A, De Carolis S, Ferrazzani S, Valesini G, Caforio L, Mancuso S. Pregnancy outcome in relation to uterine artery flow velocity waveforms and clinical characteristics in women with antiphospholipid syndrome. Obstet Gynecol. 1993;82:970–7.
27. Alfirevic Z, Roberts D, Martlew V. How strong is the association between maternal thrombophilia and adverse pregnancy outcome? A systematic review. Eur J Obstet Gynecol Reprod Biol. 2002;101:6–14.
28. Galli M, Luciani D, Bertolini G, Barbui T. Lupus anticoagulants are stronger risk factors for thrombosis than anticardiolipin antibodies in the antiphospholipid syndrome: a systematic review of the literature. Blood. 2003;101:1827–32.
29. David K, Ian M, Gary WM, Ian AG, Michael G. Guidelines on the investigation and management of antiphospholipid syndrome. Br J Haematol. 2012;157:47–58.
30. Ziakas PD, Pavlou M, Voulgarelis M. Heparin treatment in antiphospholipid syndrome with recurrent pregnancy loss: a systematic review and meta-analysis. Obstet Gynecol. 2010;115:1256–62.

31. Stephenson MD, Ballem PJ, Tsang P, et al. Treatment of antiphospholipid antibody syndrome (APS) in pregnancy: a randomized pilot trial comparing low molecular weight heparin to unfractionated heparin. J Obstet Gynaecol. 2004;26:729–34.
32. Greer IA, Nelson-Piercy C. Low-molecular-weight heparins for thromboprophylaxis and treatment of venous thromboembolism in pregnancy: a systematic review of safety and efficacy. Blood. 2005;106:401–7.
33. Franklin RD, Kutteh WH. Effects of unfractionated and low molecular weight heparin on antiphospholipid antibody binding in vitro. Obstet Gynccol. 2003;101:4555–62.
34. Empson M, Lassere MB, Craig J, Scott J. Prevention of recurrent miscarriage for women with antiphospholipid antibody or lupus anticoagulant. Cochrane Database Syst Rev. 2005;(2):CD002859.
35. Horlocker TT, Wedel DJ, Benzon H, et al. Regional anesthesia in the anticoagulated patient: defining the risks (the second ASRA Consensus Conference on Neuraxial Anesthesia and Anticoagulation). Reg Anesth Pain Med. 2003;28:172–97.
36. Erkan D, Patel S, Nuzzo M, Gerosa M, Meroni PL, Tincani A, et al. Management of the controversial aspects of the antiphospholipid syndrome pregnancies: a guide for clinicians and researchers. Rheumatology. 2008;47(3):iii23–7.
37. Erkan D, Merrill JT, Yazici Y, et al. High thrombosis rate after fetal loss in antiphospholipid syndrome: effective prophylaxis with aspirin. Arthritis Rheum. 2001;44:1466–7.

Recurrent Pregnancy Loss and Inherited Thrombophilia

9

Sumeet Singla and Sandhya Jain

RPL affects 1% of couples; various causes include anatomical defects of the female reproductive tract, chromosomal aberrations in the foetus, endocrine factors, infections and immunological factors and thrombophilias [1]. RPL can traumatise the affected couple, both emotionally and financially. Advancing maternal age and fecundity puts stress on mother and obstetrician alike for successful pregnancy outcomes. If the definition of RPL is broadened to include two or more spontaneous miscarriages, 5% of the couples will be affected [2, 3]. Hence, efforts to find and remedy the underlying cause(s) should be pursued in every case of RPL.

Pregnancy is a state of hypercoagulability, which is further increased in various thrombophilias. This abnormal, enhanced thrombotic tendency leads to adverse pregnancy outcomes such as miscarriage, abruption, intrauterine growth restriction (IUGR), and pre-eclampsia. The purported mechanisms include thrombosis of the decidual vessels, impaired trophoblast invasion and formation of placental microthrombi.

Among the prothrombotic states, antiphospholipid syndrome (APS) is an established (and treatable) cause of RPL. However, for reasons to be discussed, the same cannot be said for inherited thrombophilia (IT). Although treatment with aspirin and heparin for management of APS is well documented, its role in IT is not clearly established.

For the purpose of this chapter, the discussion shall be limited to examining the available evidence about the role of IT, and benefit of anticoagulation, for women

S. Singla (✉)
Department of Medicine, Maulana Azad Medical College and Associated Lok Nayak Hospital, New Delhi, India
e-mail: sumeetsingla555@gmail.com

S. Jain
Department of Obstetrics and Gynecology, University College of Medical Sciences and Associated Guru Teg Bahadur Hospital, New Delhi, India
e-mail: drsandy2015@gmail.com

S. Mehta, B. Gupta (eds.), *Recurrent Pregnancy Loss*,
https://doi.org/10.1007/978-981-10-7338-0_9

with RPL. Further, the role of IT and its management *vis-a-vis* venous thromboembolism (VTE) in pregnancy shall not be discussed as there are succinct evidence-based guidelines for the same, and women who require it, would already be on thromboprophylaxis for VTE during pregnancy.

9.1 What Is Inherited Thrombophilia?

A genetically determined tendency towards thrombosis is defined as thrombophilia. The various IT are shown in Table 9.1. All the thrombophilic states alter the delicate balance of prothrombotic and antithrombotic factors in the blood, towards excessive and abnormal clotting. However, it is very important to remember that clotting in prothrombotic states does not happen without a precipitating cause, pregnancy being the usual immediate cause in nearly all cases. All the IT are also well-known

Table 9.1 Inherited thrombophilias

Defect	Association with RPL	Testing method	Comments
Factor V Leiden mutation	++[a]	APCR assay, followed by PCR-based DNA analysis	Reported as heterozygotes or homozygotes for the mutation, PCR testing can be done while on anticoagulation (not for APCR assay)
Prothrombin gene 20210A mutation	++[a]	PCR-based DNA analysis	Reported as heterozygotes or homozygotes for the mutation, PCR testing can be done while on anticoagulation
Antithrombin III deficiency	+/−	ELISA	Cannot be tested while on anticoagulation and during acute thrombosis
Protein C deficiency	+	ELISA-based functional assay	Cannot be tested while on anticoagulation and during acute thrombosis
Protein S deficiency	++[b]	ELISA-based functional assay	Testing during pregnancy not reliable. Use pregnancy specific cut-offs or retest 3 months after delivery Cannot be tested while on anticoagulation and during acute thrombosis
MTHFR polymorphism	+/−	PCR-based DNA analysis	PCR testing can be done while on anticoagulation
Plasminogen activator inhibitor - 1 (PAI-1) mutation	++[b]	PCR-based DNA analysis	PCR testing can be done while on anticoagulation

MTHFR methylenetetrahydrofolate reductase, *PCR* polymerase chain reaction, *ELISA* enzyme-linked immunosorbent assay, *APCR* activated protein C resistance

[a]This association is weaker in Indian studies

[b]This association is stronger in Indian studies

predisposing factors for venous thrombosis including pulmonary thromboembolism.

9.2 Pathophysiology of RPL in Inherited Thrombophilia

It is hypothesised that a hypercoagulant state causes micro-thrombosis in the placental vascular bed leading to placental infarction, thus compromising the feto-maternal circulatory system, with eventual pregnancy loss. During the pre-embryonic stage, IT could disrupt the formation of early vascular communication channels, the trophoblast spaces, between the trophoblast and maternal endometrium. This will lead to defective and failed implantation. During the embryonic and foetal periods, disruption of maternal blood flow due to utero-placental vessel thrombosis can lead to miscarriage.

The protein C deactivates factors Va and VIIIa, with protein S as cofactor. Protein C also enhances trophoblast viability and growth and plays a role in trophoblast apoptosis [4]. Hence, a deficiency of protein C or protein S results in procoagulant activity in utero-placental circulation. Many women with RPL have a prothrombotic state due to chronic endothelial cell stimulation and associated activation of the coagulation system. This is evidenced by the high circulating levels of thrombin-antithrombin complexes in the blood of women with RPL as compared to controls [5]. Women with RPL were found to have excess production of thromboxane and deficiency of prostacyclin during weeks 4 to 11 of pregnancy [6]. The shift in the thromboxane/prostacyclin ratio in favour of the prothrombotic agent thromboxane may lead to vasospasm and platelet aggregation in the trophoblast, causing the development of microthrombi and placental necrosis.

Finally, many women with RPL are at higher risk of IUGR, pre-eclampsia and foetal death, which suggests that these entities share a common origin, viz. placental ischaemia due to microthrombus formation [5].

9.3 What Is the Evidence Linking Inherited Thrombophilia and RPL?

The prevalence of IT can be seen in up to 15% of general population, but its aetiological role in RPL is not yet clearly proven. The evidence for IT being the underlying cause of RPL shall be examined on three basic tenets, namely: (a) whether there is increased prevalence of IT in women experiencing RPL, (b) whether there is higher incidence of RPL among women with IT and (c) whether there is benefit of using thromboprophylaxis to prevent RPL among women with IT.

9.4 Evidence from Studies Among Women with IT and RPL

The retrospective European Prospective Cohort on Thrombophilia (EPCOT) study showed that overall risk of pregnancy loss was increased with an odds ratio (OR) of 1:35 in thrombophilia [7]. The risk was highest with late foetal loss and in women with combined defects. In the TREATS (Thrombosis: Risk and Economic Assessment of Thrombophilia Screening) study, the authors examined the association between thrombophilia and early and late pregnancy loss [8]. In early losses, significant associations were observed with homozygous and heterozygous factor V (FV) Leiden mutation, prothrombin gene mutation heterozygosity, acquired activated protein C resistance and hyperhomocysteinemia. There was an increased risk of late pregnancy loss, in FV Leiden mutation heterozygotes, prothrombin G mutation heterozygotes and protein S deficiency. Due to heterogeneous data, the authors suggested a modest association.

In a recent meta-analysis, FV Leiden mutation was associated with early and late RPL and late nonrecurrent foetal loss; prothrombin G mutation was associated with early RPL and late nonrecurrent loss; protein S deficiency was associated with late nonrecurrent foetal loss; protein C deficiency and antithrombin III deficiency were not significantly associated with any type of pregnancy loss [9].

Among all inherited thrombophilias, FV Leiden mutation is most common among women with RPL, ranging from 3 to 42%. Thrombophilia is more common in women with three or more losses and late pregnancy loss [10, 11]. Combined defects are more common, 21% compared to 5.5% in controls [12]. Prothrombin mutation carriers are more common in RPL as compared to controls, while prevalence of MTHFR mutation is similar between the groups [13–17]. Various studies have studied the association between IT like FV Leiden mutation, MTHFR and RPL, but the causative association is not well established [18–22].

Hyperhomocysteinemia is a documented risk factor, and the pooled OR for elevated homocysteine was 2.7 (1.5–5.2), for afterload homocysteine 4.2 (2.0–8.8) and for MTHFR 1.4 (1.0–2.0) [23].

Evidence of association between RPL and prothrombin mutation is conflicting [24–27]. Deficiency of antithrombin, protein S and protein C and dysfibrinogenemia can also lead to miscarriage in 20–30% cases [28–30].

9.5 Thrombophilia and Late Foetal Loss

Positive tests for IT are seen in 21% of patients with second-trimester loss compared to 3.9% of controls, with an odds ratio of 5.5 with stillbirth. Recognised IT factors in stillbirth are protein S deficiency and FV Leiden mutation. Homozygous genotype of C677T mutation in the MTHFR gene was strongly associated with late foetal loss.

The prevalence of thrombophilias in women with late trimester losses (>20 weeks) ranges from 20 to 50% [31–33]. The relative risk is increased to 3.2–3.3 in carriers of the FV and prothrombin mutation.

To summarise, whereas meta-analyses and retrospective studies have revealed an association between IT and RPL, prospective cohort studies have not found such an association. Most of the literature is based on observational or case-control studies. Also, the results vary between the studies. This reflects the fact that most studies have included small numbers of women, were prone to selection bias and had varying definitions of early and late foetal losses. Ethnic variability and the ensuing differences in prevalence of IT (especially FV Leiden and Prothrombin G mutation) have also been a major confounding factor while interpreting the results of these studies. Further confounding factors include lack of standardisation of the thrombophilia testing, inclusion of undiagnosed APS and lack of population specific cut-offs for diagnosing thrombophilias.

9.6 Evidence for Thromboprophylaxis

Often, the final validation of the role of any therapy in a disease is the ability to consistently demonstrate a positive (or negative) outcome in high-quality prospective, randomised controlled trials. A similar reasoning can be applied to evaluate the role of thromboprophylaxis to prevent RPL in women with IT. Based on the most obvious pathogenetic mechanism, i.e. utero-placental thrombosis, and the success in women with RPL due to antiphospholipid syndrome, thromboprophylaxis has been evaluated in women with IT and RPL. However, use of anticoagulation in thrombophilia to improve pregnancy outcomes is controversial.

There is paucity of good quality evidence to ascertain the role of anticoagulation in women with thrombophilia to improve pregnancy outcome in RPL. Majority of these studies are underpowered, not placebo controlled or randomised, and have methodological flaws and biases, and the applicability of the results is not universally accepted.

A retrospective study with an inherited thrombophilia (FV Leiden or prothrombin G mutations or AT, PC or PS deficiency) found a live birth rate of 100% in the group that received unfractionated heparin (UFH) (5000 units twice daily) compared to 59% in the placebo group. However, the true benefit of UFH was uncertain as only five women had history of RPL and 35% had obstetric complications in both arms [34]. Similarly, another non-randomised trial showed superior efficacy of low molecular weight heparin (LMWH) with a live birth rate of 70% versus 44% in controls [35]. Another study showed a threefold higher live birth rate with enoxaparin, but it had several methodological flaws as it included only women who had a single prior loss (not RPL, as per definition) and there was no placebo group [36].

A multicentre study (LIVE-ENOX) compared pregnancy outcomes following low-dose LMWH (40 mg enoxaparin) and high dose (80 mg enoxaparin) with multiple thrombophilic defects and showed a live birth rate of 84% and 78%, respectively [37]. However, the study was not randomised and did not have placebo or low dose aspirin (LDA) group. In another non-randomised study, pregnant women with high risk for venous thromboembolism (with either AT, PC or PS deficiency) use of UFH, LMWH or vitamin K antagonists had a superior live birth rate of 98% vs. 42% [38]. However, majority of the women recruited for this study were not having RPL (only 5% had prior pregnancy losses). This study was not designed to assess usefulness of anticoagulation in improving outcomes of pregnancy in women with RPL, but was a cohort study, among women at high risk for venous thromboembolism, based on family history of VTE.

In a study by Deligiannidis et al., all of the subjects had RPL and IT. The women in the study group received a combination of LMWH and LDA, while the control group received no treatment [39]. There was a significantly lower miscarriage rate among the women who received LMWH plus LDA when compared with those who received no treatment. However, the study was not randomised.

There are few well-conducted placebo-controlled trials to that have studied the role of anticoagulation in RPL in women with thrombophilia. Live birth rates were similar between 67% and 70% in the placebo, aspirin alone, and aspirin with LMWH arms in the ALIFE (Anticoagulant for Living Foetus) study, while in the SPIN (Scottish Pregnancy Intervention) study, the rates were also similar around 78% [40, 41]. The Thrombophilia in Pregnancy Prophylaxis Study (TIPPS) was a randomised, multicentre trial in 292 women with known thrombophilias, exploring the effect of prophylactic dose dalteparin compared with no dalteparin on live births, and it did not show a benefit in the subgroups with either early or late RPL [42]. All the three major trials concluded that LMWH should not be used indiscriminately.

In Visser et al.'s prospective Low Molecular Weight Heparin and/or Aspirin in Prevention of Habitual Abortion (HABENOX) study, a randomised, double-blind, multicentre study, 207 women with RPL were recruited [43]. All women were randomised to receive either LMWH (40 mg of enoxaparin) plus a placebo, LMWH (40 mg of enoxaparin) plus 100 mg of aspirin or 100 mg of aspirin alone. The live birth rate was 71% in women who received LMWH plus a placebo, 65% for those who received LMWH plus LDA and 61.5% in those who received LDA alone, the difference being not statistically significant.

The heparin and aspirin (HepASA) trial studied 88 pregnant women with RPL who were either antiphospholipid positive or who had IT or antinuclear antibodies [44]. Women were randomised into two groups, with group one receiving LMWH plus LDA while group two received LDA alone. The live birth rate was 77.8% in group 1 and 79.1% in group 2. It was concluded that LMWH plus LDA showed no benefit over LDA alone in women with RPL.

In an industry-funded study (from the makers of dalteparin, Pfizer Pharma) among 449 women with unexplained RPL, there were no differences in the live birth rates between the women who received dalteparin 5000 IU (86%) and those who did not receive it (86.7%) [45]. However, the study was not blinded and did not use placebo. But, it was interesting because it is rare to see a negative result from an industry-funded study.

In conclusion, all the high-quality studies point towards the futility of using anticoagulation to prevent RPL in women with thrombophilia. However, the off-label use of heparin has been advocated by expert opinion, consensus panels and the small, lower-quality non-randomised studies suggesting benefit. It must be realised that heparin is not a benign intervention; it can be complicated by heparin-induced thrombocytopenia and precludes use of epidural analgesia, increased bleeding, allergic reactions, hepatotoxicity and risk of induction of labour. Also, the woman may have to take up to 400 subcutaneous heparin injections per term pregnancy, which is a daunting and costly task. The bottom line is that we need further research to explore whether anticoagulation can improve live birth rates in women with IT. However, until this research is completed, heparin should not be offered to women with (except APS) or without thrombophilias outside of clinical trials, based on the weak association highlighted above and the lack of good-quality evidence to support benefit.

9.7 Epidemiology of Inherited Thrombophilia and RPL: Indian Studies

Most of the Indian data is acquired from prevalence studies, i.e. by studying prevalence of various IT in women experiencing RPL. In a study by Vora et al., 381 women with more than 1 unexplained pregnancy loss were studied for the presence of thrombophilias. 37.5% of the women had at least one IT marker, and 10.8% had two or more IT markers. 3.4% of the patients were positive for FV Leiden mutation, 5.5% were found to have Protein C deficiency, 15.2% were deficient for protein S and 2.1% were deficient for antithrombin III. Prothrombin G mutation was not found in this group of women. The risk of pregnancy loss was the greatest with protein S deficiency (OR = 17.8) followed by protein C deficiency (OR = 5.8) [46]. In another study by Jayasree and Joydeb, 53 women with RPL were studied and compared with 47 women with no pregnancy complications. Thrombophilic defect was present in 64% of the women in study group. The most common IT was protein S deficiency at 51%, followed by elevated factor VIII levels in 26.4% and protein C deficiency in 15% women. Combined defects were seen in 28.3% women [47]. In a study by Jyotsna P et al., 30 pregnant women with two or more RPL were studied for the presence of IT markers. It was found that 33.3% of the women had low protein C levels and 23.3% of the women had low protein S levels. Four patients showed combined IT defects [48]. In a study by Patil et al., 587 women with two or more RPL were recruited and tested for the presence of IT markers. They found that 41.5% of the patients were positive for at least one IT marker. The prevalence of IT markers was as follows: PAI-1 mutation, 23%; protein S deficiency, 16%; protein C deficiency, 6%; antithrombin III deficiency, 2.6%; and FV Leiden mutation, 3.5% [49]. Patil et al., in another study, concluded that the presence of a chronic continued endothelial damage and activation is shown by elevated endothelial, tissue factor and phosphatidylserine-expressing microparticles. This may get exaggerated at the time of pregnancy leading to utero-placental thrombosis and pregnancy loss [50].

From these studies, it can be surmised that (a) IT are common in Indian women with RPL; (b) protein S deficiency, PAI-1 mutation and protein C deficiency are the commonest IT markers detected; (c) FV Leiden and prothrombin G mutation are rarely found; and (d) none of these were prospective cohort studies which looked at the outcomes of pregnancies among women with known IT.

9.8 What Do the Guidelines Say?

A summary of the recommendations from various international expert groups pertaining to thrombophilia testing and thromboprophylaxis for pregnant women with RPL is tabulated in Tables 9.2 and 9.3.

Table 9.2 Summary of recommendations from different expert groups for testing of inherited thrombophilias in women with recurrent pregnancy loss[a]

Society	Guideline	Recommendations	Grade	LOE
RCOG	Greentop Guideline no. 17; 2011 [51]	• Women with second-trimester miscarriage should be screened for inherited thrombophilias including factor V Leiden, factor II (prothrombin) gene mutation and protein S	Grade D	2++
ASRM	Evaluation and treatment of recurrent pregnancy loss: a committee opinion; 2012 [52]	• Routine testing of women with RPL for inherited thrombophilias is not currently recommended • Screening for inherited thrombophilias (specifically, factor V Leiden and the prothrombin gene mutations, protein C, protein S and antithrombin deficiencies) may be clinically justified when a patient has a personal history of venous thromboembolism in the setting of a non-recurrent risk factor (such as surgery) or a first-degree relative with a known or suspected high-risk thrombophilia • Although an association between hereditary thrombophilias and foetal loss has been suggested, prospective cohort studies have failed to confirm this	–	–
ACOG	Clinical management guidelines for Obstetrician–Gynecologists; 2013 [53]	• Testing for inherited thrombophilias in women who have experienced recurrent foetal loss or placental abruption is not recommended because it is unclear if anticoagulation therapy reduces recurrence • Because of the lack of association between either heterozygosity or homozygosity for the MTHFR C677T polymorphism and any negative pregnancy outcomes, including any increased risk for venous thromboembolism, screening with either MTHFR mutation analyses or fasting homocysteine levels is not recommended	Grade B Grade B	–
ESHRE	Evidence-based guidelines for the investigation and medical treatment of recurrent miscarriage; 2006 [54]	• Most women with recurrent pregnancy loss probably have several risk factors for miscarriage • Thrombophilia screening of couples for recurrent miscarriage to be done in the context of a clinical trial only	–	–

Table 9.2 (continued)

Society	Guideline	Recommendations	Grade	LOE
BSH-BCSH	Clinical guidelines for testing for heritable thrombophilias; 2010 [55]	• Testing asymptomatic women before assisted conception and those with ovarian hyperstimulation syndrome is not indicated	–	1B
ACCP	Venous thromboembolism, thrombophilia, Antithrombotic therapy, and pregnancy; 2008 [56]	• Most studies included in systematic reviews and meta-analysis are case control in design and, therefore, may overestimate the magnitude of association • Late unexplained foetal loss has also been associated with maternal thrombophilia, although results of case control studies have again been inconsistent with some reporting an association and others identifying no association with thrombophilia • Given the uncertainty associated with the magnitude of risk, the uncertainty associated with any benefits of prophylaxis in women with heritable thrombophilia and the uncertainty about the effect on anxiety and well-being in women screened vs. not screened, whether screening for congenital thrombophilias is in the best interests of women with pregnancy complications remains uncertain	–	–
CNGOF	Pregnancy loss: French clinical practice guidelines; 2016 [57]	• Neither a thrombophilia work-up nor a genetic polymorphism study (Grade C) is recommended in cases of unexplained recurrent pregnancy loss • Testing for hereditary thrombophilia (mutations of factor V or factor II, deficiency of protein S) is not recommended for women with a history of early miscarriage	Grade C Grade B	4 4

RCOG Royal College of Obstetricians and Gynaecologists, *ASRM* American Society of Reproductive Medicine, *ACOG* American College of Obstetricians and Gynaecologists, *ESHRE* European Society of Human Reproduction and Embryology, *BSH-BCSH* British Society of Haematology—British Committee for Standards in Haematology, *ACCP* American College of Chest Physicians, *CNGOF* Collège National des Gynècologues Obstètriciens Français (French College of Gynaecologists and Obstetricians)

[a]Wherever, in the table, blanks have been left, it signifies that the guideline did not specify the grade of recommendation or level of evidence for the recommendation

Table 9.3 Summary of recommendations from different expert groups for prophylaxis of inherited thrombophilias in women with recurrent pregnancy loss[a]

Society	Guideline	Recommendations	Grade	LOE
RCOG	Greentop Guideline no. 17; 2011	• There is insufficient evidence to evaluate the effect of heparin in pregnancy to prevent a miscarriage in women with recurrent first-trimester miscarriage associated with inherited thrombophilia • Heparin therapy during pregnancy may improve the live birth rate of women with second-trimester miscarriage associated with inherited thrombophilias • Women with unexplained recurrent miscarriage have an excellent prognosis for future pregnancy outcome without pharmacological intervention if offered supportive care alone in the setting of a dedicated early pregnancy assessment unit	Grade C Grade A Grade B	3 1+ 2+
ASRM	Evaluation and treatment of recurrent pregnancy loss: a committee opinion; 2012	• No specific recommendation	–	–
ACOG	Clinical management guidelines for Obstetrician–Gynecologists; 2015 [58]	• The use of aspirin, heparin or both has not been shown to reduce the risk of early pregnancy loss in women with thrombophilias except in those with antiphospholipid syndrome	Level A	–
ESHRE	Evidence-based guidelines for the investigation and medical treatment of recurrent miscarriage; 2006	• Tender loving care and health advice are the only interventions that do not require more RCTs • Aspirin and/or LMW heparins require more RCTs for women with recurrent miscarriage	–	–
BSH-BCSH	Clinical guidelines for testing for heritable thrombophilias; 2010	• Antithrombotic therapy should not be given to pregnant women with a history of pregnancy complications based on testing for heritable thrombophilia, pending results of prospective trials of anticoagulant use in women with recurrent pregnancy loss	–	–

Table 9.3 (continued)

Society	Guideline	Recommendations	Grade	LOE
ACCP	Venous thromboembolism, thrombophilia, antithrombotic therapy and pregnancy; 2008	• The data surrounding the use of antithrombotic therapy in women with hereditable thrombophilia and pregnancy loss is less convincing and consists predominantly of small uncontrolled trials or observational studies • Evidence that LMWH may improve the pregnancy outcome in women with heritable thrombophilia and recurrent pregnancy loss or loss after 10 weeks has important methodological limitations and firm recommendations cannot be made regarding the use of antithrombotic therapy in this patient population	–	–
CNGOF	Pregnancy loss: French clinical practice guidelines; 2016	• It is recommended that the following treatments should not be used to prevent recurrence of unexplained recurrent pregnancy loss: aspirin, low molecular weight heparin (LMWH) • A combination of aspirin and LMWH is only recommended for women with both late miscarriage and antiphospholipid syndrome • This combination is not recommended to prevent recurrence in women with both recurrent pregnancy loss and genetic thrombophilia without thromboembolic events	Grade B Grade A Grade B	–

RCOG Royal College of Obstetricians and Gynaecologists, *ASRM* American Society of Reproductive Medicine, *ACOG* American College of Obstetricians and Gynaecologists, *ESHRE* European Society of Human Reproduction and Embryology, *BSH-BCSH* British Society of Haematology—British Committee for Standards in Haematology, *ACCP* American College of Chest Physicians, *CNGOF* Collège National des Gynècologues Obstètriciens Français (French College of Gynaecologists and Obstetricians)

[a]Wherever, in the table, blanks have been left, it signifies that the guideline did not specify the grade of recommendation or level of evidence for the recommendation

9.9 The Way Forward

In the end, the questions facing most obstetricians would be (1) whether to test women with RPL for IT or not and (2) whether to initiate a woman with RPL on thromboprophylaxis, more so if the results of IT testing are negative?

There are no straightforward answers at the moment, but the way forward can be as follows:

- Both doctors and patients should be counselled that with supportive care alone, the overall chance of a successful pregnancy can be as high as 70–75% following RPL [59]. Patients should be made aware that IT are just that, a genetic tendency to thrombosis; that additional factors are also involved, namely, family history, acquired thrombophilias and newer hitherto unrecognised factors; and that empirical prophylaxis with heparin/LMWH is not without risks and costs and may not always lead to successful pregnancy outcome.
- Women with combination of two or more thrombophilia factors (acquired or inherited), those with history of previous unprovoked VTE and those with family history of VTE in a first-degree relative may be offered thrombophilia testing and, then, depending upon the results of testing, prophylactic anticoagulation, however, with caveat as in point 1 above.
- Testing/treatment of women without any risk factors, as in point 2 above, should be employed only as part of investigational protocols for studies.
- Large, randomised, multicentric, multi-ethnic, prospective cohort studies to accurately assess causality between RPL and IT are urgently required.
- Diagnostic criteria and laboratory protocols for thrombophilia must be standardised.
- Cytogenetic analysis of the abortus is essential and must be incorporated in future studies evaluating causes of RPL, to exclude genetic anomalies as causes of RPL.
- There should be a paradigm shift in emphasis from the monofactorial concept of prothrombotic tendency towards a multifactorial risk assessment of women based on individual genetic, phenotypic and other factors—perhaps a risk score, akin to that for VTE risk, is warranted. Future studies must assess prothrombotic risk, both genetic and phenotypic. Assess newer risk factors like global coagulability among women with RPL using newer methods like thromboelastography and calibrated automated thrombography.
- Inherited thrombophilia must be looked at as just one factor in the complex cascade which leads to pregnancy loss in a woman. Other factors must be working in tandem with the genetic risk to produce the adverse pregnancy outcome. These factors could be stress, diet, hormones, inflammation, chemicals or autoimmunity. Future studies must address these questions.

Key Points

- Women with recurrent miscarriage should be not be routinely screened for inherited thrombophilias including factor V Leiden, factor II (prothrombin) gene mutation and protein S unless it is a clinical trial, h/o thromboembolism, high risk for thrombosis.
- Routine treatment with aspirin and/ or heparin is not recommended of been shown to reduce the risk of early pregnancy loss in women with thrombophilias except in those with antiphospholipid syndrome.
- More RCT are needed to evaluate the role of inherited thrombophilia in RPL.

References

1. Younis JS, Ohel G, Brenner B, Ben-Ami M. Familial thrombophilia—the scientific rationale for thromboprophylaxis in recurrent pregnancy loss? Hum Reprod. 1997;12(7):1389–90.
2. Stirrat GM. Recurrent miscarriage. Lancet. 1990;336(8716):673–5.
3. Rai R, Clifford K, Regan L. The modern preventative treatment of recurrent miscarriage. Br J Obstet Gynaecol. 1996;103(2):106–10.
4. Isermann B, Sood R, Pawlinski R, Zogg M, Kalloway S, Degen JL, et al. The thrombomodulin-protein C system is essential for the maintenance of pregnancy. Nat Med. 2003;9(3):331–7.
5. Regan L, Rai R. Thrombophilia and pregnancy loss. J Reprod Immunol. 2002;55(1–2):163–80.
6. Tulppala M, Viinikka L, Ylikorkala O. Thromboxane dominance and prostacyclin deficiency in habitual abortion. Lancet. 1991;337(8746):879–81.
7. Preston FE, Rosendaal FR, Walker ID, Briët E, Berntorp E, Conard J, et al. Increased fetal loss in women with heritable thrombophilia. Lancet. 1996;348(9032):913–6.
8. Robertson L, Wu O, Langhorne P, Twaddle S, Clark P, Lowe GD, et al. Thrombophilia in pregnancy: a systematic review. Br J Haematol. 2006;132(2):171–96.
9. Rey E, Khan SR, David M, Shrier I. Thrombophilic disorders and fetal loss: a meta-analysis. Lancet. 2003;361:901–8.
10. Brenner B, Sarig G, Weiner Z, Younis J, Blumenfeld Z, Lanir N. Thrombophilic polymorphisms are common in women with fetal loss without apparent cause. Thromb Haemost. 1999;82(1):6–9.
11. Ridker PM, Miletich JP, Buring JE, Ariyo AA, Price DT, Manson JE, Hill JA, Factor V. Leiden mutation as a risk factor for recurrent pregnancy loss. Ann Intern Med. 1998;128(12 Pt 1):1000–3.
12. Sarig G, Younis JS, Hoffman R, Lanir N, Blumenfeld Z, Brenner B. Thrombophilia is common in women with idiopathic pregnancy loss and is associated with late pregnancy wastage. Fertil Steril. 2002;77(2):342–7.
13. Finan RR, Tamim H, Ameen G, Sharida HE, Rashid M, Almawi WY. Prevalence of factor V G1691A (factor V-Leiden) and prothrombin G20210A gene mutations in a recurrent miscarriage population. Am J Hematol. 2002;71(4):300–5.
14. Foka ZJ, Lambropoulos AF, Saravelos H, Karas GB, Karavida A, Agorastos T, et al. Factor V Leiden and prothrombin G20210A mutations, but not methylenetetrahydrofolate reductase C677T, are associated with recurrent miscarriages. Hum Reprod. 2000;15(2):458–62.

15. Reznikoff-Etiévan MF, Cayol V, Carbonne B, Robert A, Coulet F, Milliez J. Factor V Leiden and G20210A prothrombin mutations are risk factors for very early recurrent miscarriage. BJOG. 2001;108(12):1251–4.
16. Alonso A, Soto I, Urgellés MF, Corte JR, Rodríguez MJ, Pinto CR. Acquired and inherited thrombophilia in women with unexplained fetal losses. Am J Obstet Gynecol. 2002;187(5):1337–42.
17. Grandone E, Margaglione M, Colaizzo D, d'Addedda M, Cappucci G, Vecchione G, et al. Factor V Leiden is associated with repeated and recurrent unexplained fetal losses. Thromb Haemost. 1997;77(5):822–4.
18. Kutteh WH, Park VM, Deitcher SR. Hypercoagulable state mutation analysis in white patients with early first-trimester recurrent pregnancy loss. Fertil Steril. 1999;71(6):1048–53.
19. Dizon-Townson DS, Kinney S, Branch DW, Ward K. The factor V Leiden mutation is not a common cause of recurrent miscarriage. J Reprod Immunol. 1997;34(3):217–23.
20. Deitcher SR, Park VM, Kuttert WH. Methylene tetrahydrofolate reductase C677T mutation analysis in Caucasian women with early first trimester recurrent pregnancy loss. Blood. 1998;92:117b.
21. Komberg A, Razid A, Rahimini-Lavene N. Hypercoagulability and recurrent abortion. Blood. 1998;92:121b.
22. Nelen WL, Blom HJ, Thomas CM, Steegers EA, Boers GH, Eskes TK. Methylenetetrahydrofolate reductase polymorphism affects the change in homocysteine and folate concentrations resulting from low dose folic acid supplementation in women with unexplained recurrent miscarriages. J Nutr. 1998;128(8):1336–41.
23. Nelen WL, Blom HJ, Steegers EA, den Heijer M, Eskes TK. Hyperhomocysteinemia and recurrent early pregnancy loss: a meta-analysis. Fertil Steril. 2000;74(6):1196–9.
24. Souza SS, Ferriani RA, Pontes AG, Zago MA, Franco RF. Factor V Leiden and factor II G20210A mutations in patients with recurrent abortion. Hum Reprod. 1999;14(10):2448–50.
25. Pickering W, Marriott K, Regan L. G20210A prothrombin gene mutation: prevalence in a recurrent miscarriage population. Clin Appl Thromb Hemost. 2001;7(1):25–8.
26. Deitcher SR, Park VM, Kuttert WH. Prothrombin 20210GA mutation analysis in Caucasian women with early first trimester recurrent pregnancy loss. Blood. 1998;92:118b.
27. Pihusch R, Buchholz T, Lohse P, Rübsamen H, Rogenhofer N, Hasbargen U, Hiller E, Thaler CJ. Thrombophilic gene mutations and recurrent spontaneous abortion: prothrombin mutation increases the risk in the first trimester. Am J Reprod Immunol. 2001;46(2):124–31.
28. Sanson BJ, Friederich PW, Simioni P, Zanardi S, Hilsman MV, Girolami A, ten Cate JW, Prins MH. The risk of abortion and stillbirth in antithrombin-, protein C-, and protein S-deficient women. Thromb Haemost. 1996;75(3):387–8.
29. Brenner B. Inherited thrombophilia and fetal loss. Curr Opin Hematol. 2000;7(5):290–5.
30. Gris JC, Quéré I, Monpeyroux F, Mercier E, Ripart-Neveu S, Tailland ML, et al. Case-control study of the frequency of thrombophilic disorders in couples with late foetal loss and no thrombotic antecedent—the Nîmes Obstetricians and Haematologists Study5 (NOHA5). Thromb Haemost. 1999;81(6):891–9.
31. Kupferminc MJ, Eldor A, Steinman N, Many A, Bar-Am A, Jaffa A, et al. Increased frequency of genetic thrombophilia in women with complications of pregnancy. N Engl J Med. 1999;340(1):9–13.
32. Martinelli I, Taioli E, Cetin I, Marinoni A, Gerosa S, Villa MV, et al. Mutations in coagulation factors in women with unexplained late fetal loss. N Engl J Med. 2000;343(14):1015–8.
33. Many A, Elad R, Yaron Y, Eldor A, Lessing JB, Kupferminc MJ. Third-trimester unexplained intrauterine fetal death is associated with inherited thrombophilia. Obstet Gynecol. 2002;99(5 Pt 1):684–7.
34. Ogueh O, Chen MF, Spurll G, Benjamin A. Outcome of pregnancy in women with hereditary thrombophilia. Int J Gynaecol Obstet. 2001;74(3):247–53.
35. Carp H, Dolitzky M, Inbal A. Thromboprophylaxis improves the live birth rate in women with consecutive recurrent miscarriages and hereditary thrombophilia. J Thromb Haemost. 2003;1(3):433–8.

36. Gris JC, Mercier E, Quéré I, Lavigne-Lissalde G, Cochery-Nouvellon E, Hoffet M, et al. Low-molecular-weight heparin versus low-dose aspirin in women with one fetal loss and a constitutional thrombophilic disorder. Blood. 2004;103(10):3695–9.
37. Brenner B, Hoffman R, Carp H, Dulitsky M, Younis J, LIVE-ENOX Investigators. Efficacy and safety of two doses of enoxaparin in women with thrombophilia and recurrent pregnancy loss: the LIVE-ENOX study. J Thromb Haemost. 2005;3(2):227–9.
38. Folkeringa N, Brouwer JL, Korteweg FJ, Veeger NJ, Erwich JJ, Holm JP, et al. Reduction of high fetal loss rate by anticoagulant treatment during pregnancy in antithrombin, protein C or protein S deficient women. Br J Haematol. 2007;136(4):656–61.
39. Deligiannidis A, Parapanissiou E, Mavridis P, Tabakoudis G, Mavroudi A, Papastavrou T, et al. Thrombophilia and antithrombotic therapy in women with recurrent spontaneous abortions. J Reprod Med. 2007;52(6):499–502.
40. Kaandorp SP, Goddijn M, van der Post JA, Hutten BA, Verhoeve HR, Hamulyák K, et al. Aspirin plus heparin or aspirin alone in women with recurrent miscarriage. N Engl J Med. 2010;362(17):1586–96.
41. Clark P, Walker ID, Langhorne P, Crichton L, Thomson A, Greaves M, et al. SPIN (Scottish Pregnancy Intervention) study: a multicenter, randomized controlled trial of low-molecular-weight heparin and low-dose aspirin in women with recurrent miscarriage. Blood. 2010;115(21):4162–7.
42. Rodger MA, Hague WM, Kingdom J, Kahn SR, Karovitch A, Sermer M, et al. Antepartum dalteparin versus no antepartum dalteparin for the prevention of pregnancy complications in pregnant women with thrombophilia (TIPPS): a multinational open-label randomised trial. Lancet. 2014;384(9955):1673–83.
43. Visser J, Ulander VM, Helmerhorst FM, Lampinen K, Morin-Papunen L, Bloemenkamp KW, et al. Thromboprophylaxis for recurrent miscarriage in women with or without thrombophilia. HABENOX: a randomised multicentre trial. Thromb Haemost. 2011;105(2):295–301.
44. Laskin CA, Spitzer KA, Clark CA, Crowther MR, Ginsberg JS, Hawker GA, et al. Low molecular weight heparin and aspirin for recurrent pregnancy loss: results from the randomized, controlled HepASA Trial. J Rheumatol. 2009;36(2):279–87.
45. Schleussner E, Kamin G, Seliger G, Rogenhofer N, Ebner S, Toth B, et al. Low-molecular-weight heparin for women with unexplained recurrent pregnancy loss: a multicenter trial with a minimization randomization scheme. Ann Intern Med. 2015;162(9):601–9.
46. Vora S, Shetty S, Salvi V, Satoskar P, Ghosh K. Thrombophilia and unexplained pregnancy loss in Indian patients. Natl Med J India. 2008;21(3):116–9.
47. Jayasree H, Joydeb R. Study of thrombophilia in recurrent pregnancy loss. J Obstet Gynaecol India. 2012;62:536–40.
48. Jyotsna PL, Sharma S, Trivedi SS. Coagulation inhibitors and activated protein C resistance in recurrent pregnancy losses in Indian women. Indian J Pathol Microbiol. 2011;54(4):752–5.
49. Patil R, Ghosh K, Vora S, Shetty S. Inherited and acquired thrombophilia in Indian women experiencing unexplained recurrent pregnancy loss. Blood Cells Mol Dis. 2015;55(3):200–5.
50. Patil R, Ghosh K, Satoskar P, Shetty S. Elevated procoagulant endothelial and tissue factor expressing micro-particles in women with recurrent pregnancy loss. PLoS One. 2013;8(11):e81407.
51. Royal College of Obstetrician and Gynaecologists. The investigation and treatment of couples with recurrent first trimester and second trimester miscarriage. Greentop Guideline No. 17. London: RCOG; 2011.
52. Practice Committee of the American Society for Reproductive Medicine. Evaluation and treatment of recurrent pregnancy loss: a committee opinion. Fertil Steril. 2012;98(5):1103–11.
53. ACOG Practice Bulletin No. 138: Inherited thrombophilias in pregnancy. American College of Obstetricians and Gynecologists Women's Health Care Physicians. Obstet Gynecol. 2013;122(3):706–17.
54. Jauniaux E, Farquharson RG, Christiansen OB, Exalto N. Evidence-based guidelines for the investigation and medical treatment of recurrent miscarriage. Hum Reprod. 2006;21(9):2216–22.

55. Baglin T, Gray E, Greaves M, Hunt BJ, Keeling D, Machin S, et al. Clinical guidelines for testing for heritable thrombophilia. Br J Haematol. 2010;149(2):209–20.
56. Bates SM, Greer IA, Pabinger I, Sofaer S, Hirsh J, American College of Chest Physicians. Venous thromboembolism, thrombophilia, antithrombotic therapy, and pregnancy: American College of Chest Physicians Evidence-Based Clinical Practice Guidelines (8th Edition). Chest. 2008;133(6 Suppl):844S–86S.
57. Beucher G, Lavoue V, Carcopino X, Lemery D. Pregnancy loss: French clinical practice guidelines. Eur J Obstet Gynecol Reprod Biol. 2016;201:18–26.
58. Early pregnancy loss. Practice Bulletin No. 150. American College of Obstetricians and Gynecologists. Obstet Gynecol. 2015;125:1258–67.
59. Brigham SA, Conion C, Farquharson RG. A longitudinal study of pregnancy outcome following idiopathic recurrent miscarriage. Hum Reprod. 1999;14:2868–71.

Microbiology of Recurrent Pregnancy Loss

10

Nilanchali Singh and Komal Rastogi

10.1 Introduction

Clinically recognized pregnancy loss occurs in 15–20% of pregnancies [1]. Infections are considered to cause recurrent pregnancy loss in 4% of cases [2]. Recurrent pregnancy loss is defined as the occurrence of two or more clinical pregnancy losses before 20 weeks from last menstrual period.

Ureaplasma urealyticum, *Mycoplasma hominis*, *Listeria monocytogenes*, chlamydia, *Toxoplasma gondii*, cytomegalovirus, rubella and herpes virus have been frequently identified in serum and cervical and vaginal cultures of women with sporadic miscarriages. All microorganisms can cause acute infection and occasional abortion, but only those causing chronic maternal disease are responsible for recurrent abortions. The role of infections in recurrent pregnancy loss is not clear due to lack of prospective studies. In this chapter we will discuss the infectious causes of recurrent pregnancy loss, their pathogenesis, diagnosis and therapeutic management.

10.2 Organisms Associated with Recurrent Pregnancy Loss

The organisms responsible for recurrent pregnancy loss are bacterial, viral and parasitic as enumerated in Table 10.1.

N. Singh (✉) • K. Rastogi
Obstetrics and Gynecology, Maulana Azad Medical College and Lok Nayak Hospital, Delhi, India
e-mail: nilanchalisingh@gmail.com

S. Mehta, B. Gupta (eds.), *Recurrent Pregnancy Loss*,
https://doi.org/10.1007/978-981-10-7338-0_10

Table 10.1 Pathogens in recurrent abortions

Bacteria	Viruses	Parasites	Spirochetes
Bacterial vaginosis	Cytomegalovirus	*Toxoplasma gondii*	*Treponema pallidum*
Listeria monocytogenes	Herpes simplex	*Plasmodium falciparum*	
Ureaplasma urealyticum	Rubella		
Mycoplasma hominis	Human immunodeficiency virus		
Chlamydia trachomatis			

10.3 Pathogenesis

Pathogens lead to the recruitment of macrophages and T cells into the endometrium and secrete excessive amount of Th1 cytokines, which are detrimental to implantation and maintenance of successful pregnancy [3]. IL-1, IL-6 and TNF-alpha attract neutrophils to the site of infection along with chemokine IL-8 [4]. Production of toxins and cytokines induces uterine contractions and damage to feto-placental unit. This mechanism is common to all pathogens. Bacteria in addition to this produce proteins with an amino terminal N-formylated methionine, which activates complement fragments and receptors for chemokines [5].

Viral infections like CMV downregulate cytotrophoblast molecules (integrins and MMP-9) which are responsible for placental invasion of uterine tissue and foetal development [6]. Interaction between CMV and decidual NK cells may cause NK cell activation and miscarriage [7]. The various mechanisms are summarized in Fig. 10.1.

10.4 Bacterial Infections

10.4.1 Bacterial Vaginosis

Bacterial vaginosis is characterized by an overgrowth of predominantly anaerobic bacteria along with a reduction or absence of lactobacilli within the vagina [8]. Bacterial vaginosis may be asymptomatic or may result in a vaginal discharge, which is grey in colour and has a 'fishy' odour. The diagnosis is made on the presence of 'clue cells' on microscopic examination of vaginal swab sample. According to various studies, bacterial vaginosis has been predominantly associated with late miscarriages [9, 10]. However, according to a study by Donders et al. [11], an increased risk of miscarriage during early pregnancy was found amongst women with bacterial vaginosis. *Gardnerella vaginalis*, *Ureaplasma urealyticum* or

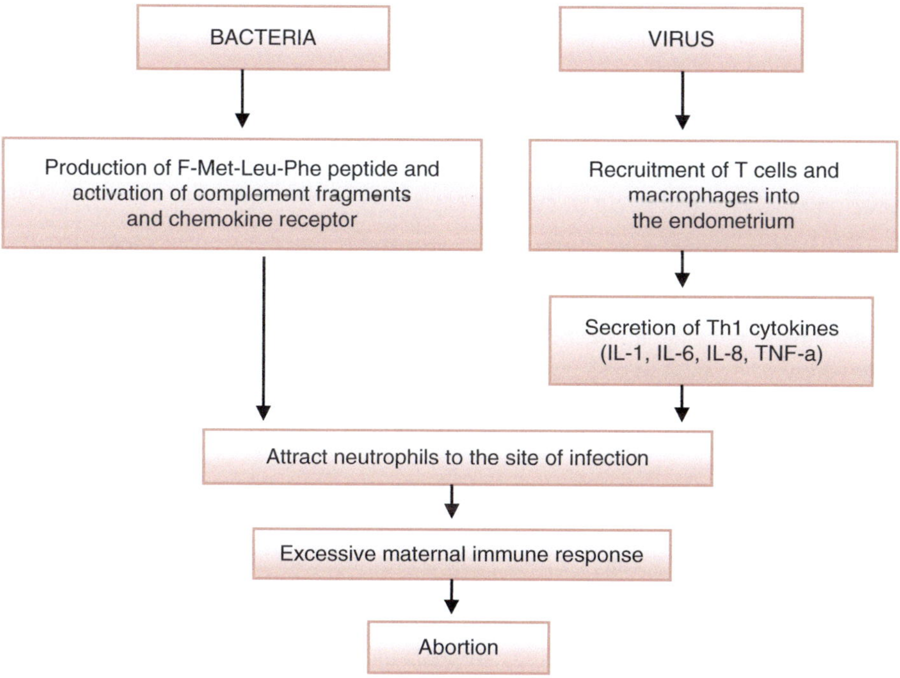

Fig. 10.1 Mechanism for induction of abortion by microorganisms

Mycoplasma hominis were cultured at first visit from 48% of women with early pregnancy loss as compared to 8.2% of control females ($p < 0.0001$).

However, the management is still uncertain. According to a meta-analysis by Guise et al. [12], there is no benefit of routine bacterial vaginosis screening, but there may be a benefit of treatment for bacterial vaginosis for preventing preterm deliveries <37 weeks. A recent Cochrane review including 7847 women in 21 trials also found decreased risk of late miscarriage when antibiotic treatment was administered [13]. CDC recommends either metronidazole 250 mg oral TDS for 7 days or clindamycin 300 mg BD for 7 days [14].

10.4.2 *Mycoplasma hominis* and *Ureaplasma urealyticum*

The genital mycoplasmas, *M. hominis* and *U. urealyticum*, have been associated with increased risk of recurrent pregnancy loss, preterm labour and preterm premature rupture of membranes. According to a study, endometrial colonization by these organisms was more frequent in patients with recurrent pregnancy loss (27.6%) as compared to controls (9.7%) ($p < 0.05$) [15]. Antibiotic treatment for women colonized with mycoplasmas has been seen to prevent recurrent spontaneous miscarriages.

10.4.3 *Chlamydia trachomatis*

Chlamydia is an obligate intracellular bacteria and is the most common sexually transmitted bacterial disease worldwide. Chlamydia infection is mostly asymptomatic but may result in acute urethral syndrome, cervicitis and pelvic inflammatory disease. Diagnosis is made on PCR on vaginal swab samples, and treatment includes administration of antibiotics such as tetracycline and azithromycin. Various studies have reported an association between *Chlamydia trachomatis* and recurrent pregnancy loss [16, 17]. Persisting chlamydial infection may lead to pregnancy loss by stimulating either foetal inflammatory response or evoking maternal immunogenic reaction to chlamydial heat-shock protein 60 antigen [18, 19]. According to a recent study, chlamydia was more often detected by PCR in patients with previous abortion (11.8%) as compared to controls ($p = 0.029$) [20], hence confirming its role in recurrent spontaneous miscarriages.

10.4.4 *Listeria monocytogenes*

Listeria monocytogenes enters through gastrointestinal tract leading to bacteremia and transplacental spread to the foetus. Ascending infection through introduction of *Listeria* into the vagina and cervix also may occur. *Listeria* may interfere with immune tolerance to foetus in pregnancy resulting in pregnancy loss. *Listeria* causes intrauterine infection in third trimester and leads to preterm labour, neonatal infection or stillbirth.

Romana et al. proposed that latent listeriosis may cause recurrent pregnancy loss [21]. Another Iranian study demonstrated high seroprevalence of *Listeria monocytogenes* in patients with previous spontaneous abortion as compared to controls [22]. However, Manganiello and Yearke [23] in their study on patients with two or more foetal losses demonstrated that *Listeria monocytogenes* contributes to foetal loss but not on recurrent basis as none of the patients with recurrent pregnancy loss were found to harbour *Listeria* in their genital tract and concluded that routine culturing for *Listeria monocytogenes* and therapy in patients with recurrent pregnancy loss is not needed.

10.4.5 Other Bacterial Infections

Acute brucellosis caused by *Brucella melitensis* has been considered as a cause of recurrent miscarriages in humans. It is transmitted via consumption of unpasteurized dairy products. However, acute brucellosis rarely causes miscarriage as human placenta does not contain erythritol, which is a substrate for brucella adhesion and spread to foetus [24]. Another organism *Borrelia duttonii* causing relapsing fever is also believed to be a common cause of abortion in sub-Saharan Africa. *Klebsiella pneumoniae* has also been reported as a cause of abortions due to seminal contamination by the organism. Syphilis caused by *Treponema pallidum* has also been implicated as a cause of recurrent spontaneous abortions. It is transmitted sexually or by coming in contact with blood of an infected person. Diagnosis is made using PCR. A study conducted in South Africa demonstrated a reduction in perinatal death and a reduced risk of pregnancy loss by treatment with benzathine penicillin

[25]. Another study conducted in China by Hong et al. reported a decrease in miscarriages after a screening programme to prevent mother to child transmission of syphilis. *Campylobacter jejuni* may also be considered as a differential diagnosis of recurrent miscarriages especially in women with diarrheal disease.

10.5 Viral Infections

10.5.1 Cytomegalovirus

Cytomegalovirus (CMV) is a member of *Herpesviridae* family. Infection with CMV is very common with seropositivity rates ranging from 40% in developed countries to 100% in developing countries. Symptomatic disease occurs mostly in immunocompromized hosts or when immunocompetent host is critically ill. Congenital CMV may occur due to primary infection during pregnancy or due to reactivation of previously acquired CMV. During pregnancy CMV reaches placenta from cervix or by viremia causing tissue damage, vascular insufficiency and foetal infection. Abortion can occur as a result of placental detachment and foetal death.

According to a study, CMV antigen pp65 was detected in decidua of 35% of patients with spontaneous abortions [26]. Another study demonstrated a higher percentage of vaginal CMV DNA detection in women with miscarriages as compared to controls [7]. Radcliffe et al. [27] proposed that patients with unexplained recurrent abortions have an immune difficulty in responding to CMV and such patients should be considered for immunotherapy.

10.5.2 Herpes Simplex Virus

HSV causes subclinical intrauterine endometrial infection leading to transplacental embryo infection and spontaneous abortion. Kapranos reported on the role of HSV in early pregnancy loss and its detection by nested PCR, which allowed appropriate antiviral therapy and successful future pregnancy [28].

Other herpes viruses, Epstein–Barr virus, varicella-zoster virus and human herpesvirus-6 have been associated with occasional abortions.

10.5.3 Other Viral Infections

Parvovirus B19 has also been implicated as a cause of foetal loss. The virus infects the erythroid precursors inhibiting erythropoiesis and causes non-immune hydrops. An Egyptian study demonstrated a significantly higher rate of B19 IgM in women with recurrent miscarriages as compared to controls and proposed it as a cause of recurrent spontaneous abortions [29]. Another virus, the adeno-associated parvovirus (AAV) belonging to *Parvoviridae* family, has also been reported to be associated with recurrent miscarriages. HIV though not associated with recurrent abortions may act as a predisposing factor for development of chronic infections leading to adverse pregnancy outcomes.

Table 10.2 Treatment options for infections associated with recurrent miscarriage

Bacterial	Bacterial vaginosis	Metronidazole Clindamycin
	Mycoplasma Ureaplasma Chlamydia	Tetracycline Azithromycin
	Listeria	Ampicillin + Gentamycin
	Brucella	Doxycycline + Gentamycin
Virological	Herpes simplex virus	Valganciclovir
	Cytomegalovirus	Acyclovir
	Parvovirus B-19	Intravenous Immunoglobulin

10.6 Protozoan Infections

Toxoplasma gondii can cause pregnancy loss during primary infection, but recurrent infection is highly unlikely in subsequent pregnancies except in immunocompromized host, where it may result in abortion, prematurity, growth restriction or stillbirth. *Plasmodium falciparum* infection causes stillbirth or miscarriage by proliferating in intervillous space of the placenta. Screening for malaria in women with recurrent abortions should be considered in endemic areas and in symptomatic patients.

10.7 Treatment for Patients with Recurrent Miscarriages

Although routine screening of infections is not recommended in women with RPL, therapeutic options can be considered in case the infection is persistent as summarized in Table 10.2.

10.8 Recommendations for Screening and Treatment of Infections in RPL

According to the American Society of Reproductive Medicine, due to lack of convincing data and prospective studies linking infectious agents and recurrent miscarriages, testing for these infectious agents and routine antibiotic treatment is not recommended. RCOG also does not recommend TORCH screening in patients with recurrent pregnancy loss.

Conclusion

In all patients with recurrent spontaneous abortions, personal risk of infections should be assessed by history, physical and laboratory examination, and chronic infections should be excluded. Immunological investigations including immunoglobulin levels, T and B lymphocyte levels, and NK cytotoxic activity may also be carried out as risk of developing placental and foetal infection depends upon immune reactivity of pregnant women. Specific antibiotic or antiviral therapy should be used for eradication of persistent bacterial and viral infections.

Key Points

- Infections (bacterial, viral, protozoal) are associated only with sporadic miscarriages and are rarely associated with recurrent pregnancy loss.
- Mechanism of abortion includes complement activation and production of inflammatory cytokines.
- Routine testing for infectious agents and routine antibiotic treatment is not recommended in recurrent pregnancy loss.

References

1. Kutteh WH. Recurrent pregnancy loss: an update. Curr Opin Obstet Gynecol. 1999;56:247–53.
2. Summers PR. Microbiology relevant to recurrent miscarriage. Clin Obstet Gynecol. 1994;37:722–9.
3. Bricker L, Farquharson RG. Types of pregnancy loss in recurrent miscarriage: implications for research and clinical practice. Hum Reprod. 2002;17:1345–50.
4. Wegmann TG, Lin H, Guilbert L, Mosmann TR. Bidirectional cytokine interactions in the maternal fetal relationship: is successful pregnancy a TH2 phenomenon? Immunol Today. 1993;14:353–6.
5. Sugiura-Ogasawara M, Nozawa K, Nakanishi T, Hattori Y, Ozaki Y. Complement as a predictor of further miscarriage in couples with recurrent miscarriages. Hum Reprod. 2006;21:2711–4.
6. Yamamoto-Tabata T, McDonagh S, Chang H-T, Fisher S, Pereira L. Human cytomegalovirus interleukin-10 downregulates matrix metalloproteinase activity and impairs endothelial cell migration and placental cytotrophoblast invasiveness in vitro. J Virol. 2004;78:2831–40.
7. Tanaka K, Yamada H, Minami M, Kataoka S, Numazaki K, Minakami H, Tsutsumi H. Screening for vaginal shedding of cytomegalovirus in healthy pregnant women using real-time PCR: correlation of CMV in the vagina and adverse outcome of pregnancy. J Med Virol. 2006;78:757–9.
8. Viniker DA. Hypothesis on the role of sub-clinical bacteria of the endometrium (bacteria endometrialis) in gynaecological and obstetric enigmas. Hum Reprod Update. 1999;5:373–85.
9. Ralph SG, Rutherford AJ, Wilson JD. Influence of bacterial vaginosis on conception and miscarriage in the first trimester: cohort study. BMJ. 1999;319:220–3.
10. Oakeshott P, Hay P, Hay S, Steinke F, Rink E, Keny S. Association between bacterial vaginosis or chlamydial infection and miscarriage before 16 weeks gestation: prospective community based cohort study. BMJ. 2002;325:1334–8.
11. Donders GG, Van Bulck B, Caudron J, Londers L, Vereecken A, Spitz B. Relationship of bacterial vaginosis and mycoplasma to the risk of spontaneous abortion. Am J Obstet Gynecol. 2000;183:431–7.
12. Guise JM, Mahon SM, Aickin M, Helfand M, Peipert JF, Westhoff C. Screening for bacterial vaginosis in pregnancy. Am J Prev Med. 2001;20(Suppl 3):62–72.
13. Brocklehurst P, Gordon A, Heatley E, Milan S. Antibiotics for treating bacterial vaginosis in pregnancy. Cochrane Database Syst Rev. 2013;(1):CD000262. doi: 10.1002/14651858.CD000262.pub4.
14. Centres for Disease Control and Prevention. Sexually transmitted diseases treatment guidelines 2002. MMWR Morb Mortal Wkly Rep. 2002;51:1–80.
15. Narssens A, Foulon W, Cammu H, Goossens A, Lauwers S. Epidemiology and pathogenesis of ureaplasma urealyticum in spontaneous abortion and early preterm labour. Acta Obstet Gynecol Scand. 1987;66:513–6.
16. McGregor JA, French CNN. Chlamydia trachomatis infection during pregnancy. Am J Obstet Gynecol. 1991;164:1782–4.
17. Centres for Disease Control and Prevention. Sexually transmitted disease surveillance 2007, Chlamydia Prevalence Monitoring Project Annual Report, Atlanta; 2007.

18. Stirrat GM. Recurrent pregnancy loss. II. Clinical associations, causes, and management. Lancet. 1990;336:728–33.
19. Witkin S. Immune pathogenesis of asymptomatic Chlamydia trachomatis in the female genital tract. Infect Dis Obstet Gyneol. 1995;3:169–74.
20. Wilkowska-Trojniel M, Zdrodowska-Stefanow B, Ostaszewska-Puchalaska I, Redzko S, Przepiesc J, Zdrodowski M. The influence of Chlamydia trachomatis infection on spontaneous abortions. Adv Med Sci. 2009;54:86–90.
21. Romana C, Salleras L, Sage M. Latent listeriosis may cause habitual abortion, intrauterine deaths, fetal malformations. When diagnosed and treated adequately normal children will be born. Acta Microbiol Hung. 1989;36:171–2.
22. Jamshidi M, Jahromi AS, Davoodian P, Amirian M, Zangeneh M, Jadcareh F. Seropositivity for listeria monocytogenes in women with spontaneous abortion: a case control study in Iran. Taiwan J Obstet Gynecol. 2009;48:46–8.
23. Manganiello PD, Yearke RR. A 10-year prospective study of women with a history of recurrent fetal losses fails to identify Listeria monocytogenes in female genital tract. Fertil Steril. 1991;56:781–2.
24. Kochar DK, Gupta A, Gupta BK, Kalla A, Nayak KC. Hospital based case series of 175 cases serologically confirmed brucellosis. J Assoc Physicians India. 2007;55:271–5.
25. Myer L, Abdool Karim SS, Lombard C, Wilkinson D. Treatment of maternal syphilis in rural South Africa: effect of multiple doses of benzathine penicillin on pregnancy loss. Trop Med Int Health. 2004;9:1216–21.
26. Van Lijnschoten G, Stals F, Evers JCH, Bruggeman CA, Havenith MH, Geraedts JPM. The presence of cytomegalovirus antigens in karyotyped abortions. Am J Reprod Immunol. 1994;32:211–20.
27. Radcliffe JJ, Hart CA, Francis WJ, Johnson PM. Immunity to cytomegalovirus in women with unexplained recurrent spontaneous abortion. Am J Reprod Immunol Microbiol. 1986;12:103–5.
28. Kapranos NC, Kotronias DC. Detection of herpes simplex virus in first trimester pregnancy loss using molecular techniques. In Vivo. 2009;23:839–42.
29. el-Sayed Zaki M, Goda H. Relevance of parvovirus B19, herpes simplex virus 2, and cytomegalovirus virologic markers in maternal serum for diagnosis of unexplained recurrent abortions. Arch Pathol Lab Med. 2007;131:956–60.

Male Factor in Recurrent Pregnancy Loss 11

Ritu Khatuja and Latika Chawla

11.1 Introduction

Miscarriage is defined as spontaneous pregnancy loss before the fetus reaches the period of viability. Recurrent miscarriage was traditionally defined as the loss of three or more consecutive pregnancies [1]. But the latest guideline by the American Society for Reproductive Medicine (ARSM) considers at least two consecutive embryo miscarriages within the first or early second trimester as RPL [2]. Around 1% of the couples trying to conceive may suffer from RPL [1]. Most research available till date has been focused on the female partner in an attempt to search for causes of RPL. Immunologic factors (20–50%), endocrine factors (17–20%), anatomic factors (12–16%), genetic factors (3.5–5%), infectious causes (0.5–5%), and other factors like altered uterine receptivity and environmental toxins have been implicated as the various causes. But even after thorough investigation, the factor may remain unknown in almost one third of the couples [3, 4]. Not much however is known so far about the contribution of the male partner in the occurrence of RPL in spite of that it is responsible for half of the embryo. It may be speculated that various factors in the male partner could be responsible for pregnancy losses where no cause is found in the female partner.

R. Khatuja (✉)
Department of Obstetrics and Gynecology,
Dr. BSA Medical College and Hospital, Delhi, India
e-mail: drritu.kj@gmail.com

L. Chawla
Department of Obstetrics and Gynecology, All India Institute of Medical Sciences,
Rishikesh, Uttrakhand, India

S. Mehta, B. Gupta (eds.), *Recurrent Pregnancy Loss*,
https://doi.org/10.1007/978-981-10-7338-0_11

11.2 Male Factor and RPL

As already stated, male factor has been relatively poorly evaluated with respect to RPL. The hypothesized causes so far include:

- Semen factor: Abnormal sperm morphology and abnormal sperm function tests
- Genetic Factors: Cytogenetic abnormalities (Sperm chromosomal abnormalities & Gene mutations) and sperm DNA damage
- Others: Seminal oxidative stress, advanced parental age, environmental factors, antiphospholipid antibodies, domestic violence, and mannan-binding protein

11.3 Semen Factors

The first step in the evaluation of a male, be it infertility or recurrent pregnancy loss, entails semen analysis. Conventional semen analysis involves analysis of the total sperm concentration, number, motility, morphology, and vitality along with the volume, pH, and leucocyte count. The evidence of association of conventional semen analysis with RPL is still debatable [5], but studies [6, 7] show poorer sperm number, motility, and morphology in the male partners of couple with RPL.

Sperm Morphology: A morphologically abnormal sperm will result in an abnormal nonviable embryo despite successful fertilization of a healthy oocyte. Such embryos have difficulty in implantation and nidation, finally resulting in pregnancy losses. In IVF-ET there is increased risk of RPL due to abnormal sperm morphology [5].

Sperm Function tests: Sometime in spite of normal sperm morphology, there may be alteration in membrane constitution, loss of chromatin condensation or abnormal acrosomal reaction may occur due to minor cytogenic defect. So it is important to carry out sperm function tests along with semen analysis in cases of RPL [8, 9].

11.4 Genetic Factors

The genetic factors implicated in the male partners may be subcategorized as below:

11.4.1 Sperm Chromosome

1. Structural abnormality
2. Numerical abnormality

11.4.2 Gene Mutations

1. HLA-G polymorphisms
2. Thrombophilia mutations
3. Micro-deletions of the Y chromosome

11.4.3 Sperm DNA Damage

Sperm chromosome: The sperm contributes to half of the genomic material of the embryo and thus plays an important role in placental and embryonic development [10]. So any abnormality in structural arrangement of the sperm genome or numerical change in sperm chromosome may lead to genetically defective embryo, difficult implantation, and placentation thus leading to a miscarriage.

Sperm chromosomal abnormality can be of the following types:

Structural: This involves a normal number (23 pairs or 46 chromosomes) of sperm chromosomes but with an abnormal arrangement of the chromosomes. A study [11] observed that the rate of chromosomal structural rearrangements in couples with a history of RPL was 4.7%. A chromosomal translocation is an abnormality caused by rearrangement of parts between nonhomologous chromosomes. It may be balanced (even simple exchange of material with no loss or gain of genetic information) or unbalanced (where exchange of chromosome material is unequal resulting in extra or missing genes). Translocation can be reciprocal (balanced or unbalanced) and nonreciprocal (balanced or unbalanced). A reciprocal translocation involves the exchange of material between nonhomogenous chromosomes, whereas in nonreciprocal translocation there is transfer of genes from one chromosome to another nonhomogenous chromosome. In this situation all the genetic material is present but at abnormal places. So they may produce the gamete with normal, balanced, or unbalanced translocation depending on the breakpoints and on the chromosomes involved.

Unbalanced chromosome results in embryos that will not result in progress of pregnancy and will finally abort. The individual having balanced translocation may not have clinical or physical findings. They are diagnosed only after karyotype. Robertsonian translocations are caused by breaks at or near the centromeres of two acrocentric chromosomes. This is found in the general population with an incidence of 0.1%. The prevalence of it is as high as 8% in couples with RPL [12]. Pericentric inversion (crossing over during meiotic division that may result in deletion or duplication of a chromosome segment) has also been found to be associated with RPL [13].

Many studies in the past have suggested that in couples with RPL, role of chromosomal abnormalities in women is more significant than male carriers [14, 15]. However, another study suggests that higher miscarriage rates are associated with the male as the carrier of the abnormal karyotype [16].

Numerical abnormality: Chromosomal abnormalities with an abnormal number of chromosomes typically results in a miscarriage. Men with an extra chromosome generally have significant abnormalities that are clinically detectable by history and physical examination. The more common of these disorders include Down's syndrome (trisomy 21; incidence 1 in 600) and Klinefelter's syndrome (47, XXY; incidence 1 in 2000). Men with these syndromes are thought to have significantly reduced fertility or sterility and high miscarriage rates. With improvement in techniques in form of FISH (fluorescent in situ hybridization), TUNEL assay, and FCCE (flow cytometric chromatin evaluation), we can study karyotype of gametes and analyze germ line, i.e., individual sperm chromosome as well as the DNA basis of RPL. Also it is found that sperm aneuploidy is higher in cases of RPL [17].

Gene mutations: Gene mutations may occur in any gene. The mutations may be a single point mutation thereby resulting in an amino acid change, or they may be deletions, substitutions, or insertions. The common gene mutations associated with miscarriages are:

1. HLA-G polymorphisms: A study shows the relation between HLA-G (a nonclassical human leukocyte antigen expressed primarily in fetal tissues at the maternal–fetal interface) genotype polymorphisms and unexplained recurrent miscarriages [18]. HLA-G expression is thought to play an important role in establishing and maintaining the feto-placental unit in early pregnancy, possibly via natural killer cells. They found that HLA-G carriers are higher in couple with RPL. But it is still controversial and more studies are required in this field.
2. Thrombophilia mutations: The role of genetic thrombophilic mutations as potential causes for recurrent miscarriages has been studied in the past [19]. The miscarriage rate was higher when the male carried more than one thrombophilic mutation than when the female carried more than one thrombophilic mutation, but the numbers in this study are small.
3. Y chromosome micro-deletions: The association of Y chromosome micro-deletions and infertility has been well documented in literature, but the association with recurrent pregnancy loss is still controversial. Micro-deletions on the long arm of Y chromosome may occur on at least three regions known as the azoospermia factor (AZFa, AZFb, AZFc) [20]. These regions are imperative for normal spermatogenesis, and their deletion is associated with poor sperm quality and has negative impact on sperm function. Y chromosome micro-deletions are found in around 7% of men with oligozoospermia [20], and compared with the general population, a higher frequency of spontaneous abortions has been observed in couples with infertility. A recent study observed significantly higher number of Y chromosome micro-deletions in the male partner of couple with RPL as compared to fertile couple [21]. This was similar to what was observed in another study which demonstrated that the prevalence of the Y chromosome micro-deletions in the proximal AZFc region was higher in men of RPL couples as compared to fertile or infertile couples [22]. On contrary, it has also been reported that Y chromosome micro-deletions are not associated with RPL and therefore testing for the same in such couples may not be recommended [23].

Sperm DNA Damage: The concept of sperm DNA fragmentation, its association with male infertility, and prediction of success with ART procedures has been a matter of great interest over the last few decades. Since sperm DNA contributes to half of the genome of the embryo, therefore fertilization and early embryonic development can be considered to be dependent upon the integrity of sperm DNA. Defective sperm DNA could lead to defective genome of the embryo, and thus such a couple is more likely to have recurrent miscarriages. Association of sperm DNA fragmentation with RPL is a relatively newer concept. Sperm DNA damage can happen due to testicular and post testicular causes. Testicular causes include exposure to environmental toxins, radiation, and chemotherapy [24]. Post-testicular DNA fragmentation is induced mainly due to reactive oxygen species (ROS) during the transport of sperm through the seminiferous tubules and the epididymis [24].

11.5 Other Factors

Oxidative Stress: It is a state of homeostatic imbalance with cellular damage due to oxygen derivatives which overpower the bodies' antioxidant defense mechanisms. Reactive oxygen species (ROS) are highly reactive oxidizing moieties that belong to the class of free radicals. They are extremely unstable and can react with lipids, amino acids, carbohydrates, proteins, and DNA, thus causing damage. The human sperm is very rich in polyunsaturated fatty acids which make it susceptible to attack by ROS. It leads to altered sperm membrane permeability, affects sperm motility, leads to mid piece damage, and alters sperm capacitation and acrosome reaction. Besides this, ROS causes strand breaks, cross-linking in the DNA, and oxidation of the sperm DNA bases and –SH groups, all leading to Sperm DNA fragmentation and thus contributing to RPL.

Parental Age: As in female, age of the male partner also increases the chance for mutation or an aneuploidy in the developing embryo, and decrease in seminal parameters (particularly motility) results in a decrease in conception rate, an increase in miscarriage rate, and an increase in birth defects and fetal demise. It has also been suggested that men of more than 40 years of age have an increased frequency of chromosomal abnormality [25].

Environment and anatomical factors: External factors like ionization radiation, air pollution, chemotherapy, smoking, alcoholism, and occupational risk like exposure to heavy metals and polycyclic aromatic hydrocarbons can cause mutation and alteration in the genes. As spermatogenesis is a continuous process so it can be affected very much by these environmental factors [6]. Men with anatomical abnormalities such as cyst in the head of the epididymis, varicocele, and small right testis had a normal count with subnormal motility [26].

The role of antiphospholipid antibodies: A recent study also suggests the role of the presence of antiphospholipid antibodies in males and RPL [27].

Domestic violence: Alcohol and tobacco intake in the male partner may be associated with domestic violence, which in turn may lead to early pregnancy losses [28].

Mannan-binding protein (MBP): MBP still remains an enigmatic entity, and there is controversy regarding the reproducibility of its effect in different populations. It has been observed that a deficiency in this protein is associated with recurrent miscarriages [29]. This initial study suggested therefore that low MBP within the feto-placental unit increases the risk of fetal loss, possibly due to an infection-induced placental cytokine imbalance.

11.6 Diagnosis

Although there are no guidelines, investigating the male partner in couples with RPL involves conventional semen analysis, sperm function test, chromosomal and genetic evaluation, sperm DNA fragmentation analysis, and oxidative stress measurement.

1. Sperm morphology and function
   (a) Conventional semen analysis
   (b) Sperm function tests which include nuclear chromatin condensation test (NCDT), hypoosmotic swelling test (HOST), and acrosomal intactness (AIT)
2. Chromosomal and genetic evaluation
   (a) Karyotype
   (b) Preimplantation genetic diagnosis (PGD)
   (c) High magnification ICSI
3. Sperm DNA fragmentation analysis
   (a) Acridine orange test (AO)
   (b) Sperm chromatin structure assay (SCSA)
   (c) Comet assay/single gel electrophoresis (SGE)
   (d) Terminal deoxynucleotidyl transferase (TdT) dUTP end labeling (TUNEL)
   (e) Sperm chromatin dispersion (SCD) test

11.6.1 Sperm Morphology and Function

Semen analysis: The first step in assessment of the male is based upon conventional semen analysis which has been revised relatively recently [30]. This analysis is based on gross visual determination of sperm number, motility, vitality, and morphology as measured by light microscopy. Table 11.1 shows the reference values of semen analysis according to WHO 2010 laboratory manual.

Table 11.1 Semen analysis according to WHO 2010 laboratory manual

Semen parameter	Lower reference limit	5th centile, 95% Confidence Interval (CI)
Semen volume	1.5 mL	1.4–1.7
Total motility (progressive + Nonprogressive)	40%	38–42%
Progressive motility	32%	31–34%
Vitality	58%	55–63%
Total sperm concentration	15 million/mL	12–16 million/mL
Total sperm number	39 million/mL	33–46 million/mL
Normal morphology	4%	3.0–4.0%
Peroxidase positive cells	1 million/mL	No reference range

The role of conventional semen analysis and RPL is still controversial, but as this is an inexpensive and noninvasive method and provides a general view of sperm morphology as well, this should always be a part of the investigation panel.

Sperm function tests:

Qualitative tests like nuclear chromatin condensation test, hypoosmotic swelling test, and acrosomal intactness test are done to evaluate the functional capacity of the sperm.

(a) Nuclear chromatin condensation test (NCDT): This test is carried out to check the ability of nuclear material to decondense in spermatozoa. The more the condensation of nuclear chromatin is, the poorer is the sperm quality and the more chances of early pregnancy losses [31].
(b) Hypoosmotic swelling test (HOST): Integrity of plasma membrane is performed using this test. The semen is incubated with a hypoosmotic solution and then examined under microscope for coiled tail. Low HOS test score relates with RPL [8].
(c) Acrosomal intactness test (AIT): Quality of the enzyme in the acrosome was analyzed using this test. The principal of this test is that acrosome of sperm contains proteases which help in penetration of sperm into oocytes. Lower score of test is related with RPL [31].

11.6.2 Chromosomal and Genetic Evaluation

(a) Karyotype: The karyotype is an important investigation for the evaluation of RPL as it gives review of chromosomal abnormalities in sperm.
(b) High magnification ICSI: Newer techniques such as "high magnification ICSI" may help to overcome some paternal effects.

11.6.3 Sperm DNA Fragmentation Analysis

(a) Acridine orange (AO) test: Acridine orange is a nucleic acid-specific, fluorescent dye which interacts with DNA and RNA. On binding to double-stranded DNA, it has an emission maximum at 525 nm (green in color). When it binds to single-stranded DNA produced by single-stranded DNA breaks, the emission maximum shifts to 650 nm (red). The acridine orange tests utilize this metachromatic shift phenomenon for testing sperm DNA integrity. The number of cells with red fluorescence is a representative of the DNA-damaged sperm in the sample. The technique utilizes fluorescence microscope and is rapid, simple, and inexpensive.
(b) Sperm chromatin structure assay: It is a flow cytometric assay of the abnormal sperm chromatin which leads to physical induction of partial DNA denatur-

ation in situ. This test works upon the same principle as that of the acridine orange test but requires flow cytometry for the analysis of the fragmentation index. By this assay, we can analyze many thousand spermatozoa at a time. This test is currently considered to be the "gold standard" for assessing DNA fragmentation.

(c) Comet assay/single cell gel electrophoresis (SCGE): In this method, sample sperm suspension is mixed with low melting point agarose and spreads onto a microscope glass slide. Following lysis of cells with detergent at high salt concentration, sperm are subjected to electrophoresis. The movement of fragmented DNA from a damaged sperm chromatin becomes visible as a comet with tail. The staining intensity and length of the comet tail represents the amount of migrated DNA, indicating different degrees of DNA fragmentation. Intact sperm does not create comets because high-molecular-weight DNA does not mobilize well. The major drawback of this method is that it is very labor intensive, has observer subjectivity, and requires experience to evaluate the comets.

(d) TUNEL (terminal deoxynucleotidyl transferase (TdT) dUTP end labeling): This test provides a direct measure of the DNA breaks. The dUTP gets incorporated into the unequal DNA ends that represent the DNA breaks. The intensity of luminescence corresponds to the number of incorporated dUTP thus correlating with the number of nicks in the sperm DNA. The number of TUNEL-positive sperm divided by the total number of sperms in the sample is expressed as a percentage. The advantages of this technique are that it requires less than 200 sperms to measure the DNA damage as well as detects single- and double-stranded DNA end breaks simultaneously and this technique can use both bright-field and fluorescence microscopy; also flow cytometry can be used. But due to lack of thresholds and non-validated data, it is not used in routine tests.

(e) Sperm chromatin dispersion (SCD) assay: In this method, the intact sperm in an agarose matrix is treated with an acid solution to denature DNA that contains breaks, followed by treatment with lysis buffer to remove membranes and proteins. Removal of nuclear proteins results in nucleoids with a central core and a peripheral halo of dispersed DNA loops. This test is based on the quality of intact DNA without chromatin proteins to loop around the sperm nucleus carcass. When fluorescent staining is used, sperm nuclei with elevated DNA fragmentation produce very small or no halos of DNA dispersion, whereas those sperm with low levels of DNA fragmentation release their DNA loops forming large halos [32]. The halos may be visualized using bright-field microscopy after Diff-Quick staining or Wright's stain. This technique is a relatively simple procedure; however, there is a high interobserver variability in characterization of the halos, which is an important drawback. It has been seen that the SCD test is in good concordance with the gold standard procedure (SCSA).

11.7 Management

Management strategies for abnormalities in the male partner in RPL are limited, and no consensus has been achieved so far. Antioxidants can be presumed to be helpful in the couples with higher seminal antioxidant stress levels or with higher sperm DNA damage levels, but the evidence in this context is still limited. Donor semen insemination or donor semen ART cycles can be an option when the male partner has significant sperm chromosomal abnormalities. Couples with high sperm fragmentation may be benefited by ART-ICSI cycles. Preimplantation genetic diagnosis (PGD) can be useful in couples where either partner has chromosomal abnormalities. Using this method in an assisted reproduction cycle, the embryos can be evaluated for aneuploidy, and only the normal embryos are transferred in the uterine cavity.

Key Points

- Sperm contributes to half of the genetic material of the embryo. So evaluation of the male factor is important.
- The male factors contributing to RPL are broadly categorized into semen factor, chromosomal and genetic factor, and many other factors which contribute directly or indirectly in pregnancy losses.
- Semen factors include the sperm morphology and sperm function, although abnormal morphology and function lead to fertilization with normal ovum but can cause nonviable fetus and difficulty in implantation of embryo which may lead to RPL.
- Chromosomal defect in form of structural abnormality or numerical abnormality leads to genetically defective embryo, difficult implantation, and placentation leading to pregnancy losses.
- Genetic mutation like HLA-G polymorphism, thrombophilia mutations, or Y chromosome micro-deletion leads to change in amino acids which leads to change in basic structure of embryo and RPL.
- Sperm DNA fragmentation is one of the causes of defective genome of the embryo, and such couples are more likely to have recurrent miscarriage.
- Other male factors include oxidative stress, parental age, environment and anatomical factor, antiphospholipid antibodies, and domestic violence.
- There is a battery of investigations to find out the causative male factor, but none of these have been approved for RPL.
- Antioxidants, donor IUI, donor ART cycle, ART–ICSI cycles, and preimplantation genetic diagnosis may be used in suitable candidates.

References

1. Stirrat GM. Recurrent miscarriage. Lancet. 1990;336:673–5.
2. American Society for Reproductive Medicine (ASRM). Recurrent pregnancy loss: patient fact sheet. 2008. http://www.asrm.org/Guidelines/.
3. Alberman E. The epidemiology of repeated abortion. In: Beard RW, Sharp F, editors. Early pregnancy loss: mechanisms and treatment. New York: Springer; 1988. p. 9–17.
4. Stephenson MD. Frequency of factors associated with habitual abortion in 197 couples. Fertil Steril. 1966;66:24–9.
5. Hill JA, Abbott AF, Politch JA. Sperm morphology and recurrent abortion. Fertil Steril. 1994;61(4):776–8.
6. Wang R, Zhou H, Zhang Z, et al. The impact of semen quality, occupational exposure to environmental factors and lifestyle on recurrent pregnancy loss. J Assist Reprod Genet. 2013;30:1513–8.
7. Saxena P, Misro MM, Roy S, Chopra K, Sinha D, Nandan D, Trivedi S. Possible role of male factors in recurrent pregnancy loss. Indian J Physiol Pharmacol. 2008;52(3):274–82.
8. Buckett WM, Luckas MJ, Aird IA, et al. The hypo-osmotic swelling test in recurrent miscarriage. Fertil Steril. 1997;68:506–9.
9. Gopalkrishnan K, Padwal V, Meherji PK. Poor quality of sperm as it affects repeated early pregnancy loss. Arch Androl. 2000;45(1):111–7.
10. Vigodner M, Shrivastava V, Gutstein LE, Schneider J, Nieves E, Goldstein M, Feliciano M, Callaway M. Localization and identification of sumoylated proteins in human sperm: excessive sumoylation is a marker of defective spermatozoa. Hum Reprod. 2013;28(1):210–23.
11. De Braekeler M, Dao TN. Cytogenetic studies in couples experiencing repeated pregnancy losses. Hum Reprod. 1990;5:519–28.
12. Morel F, Roux C, Bresson JL. FISH analysis of chromosomal status of spermatozoa from three men with 45,XY,der(13;14)(9q10;q10) karyotype. Mol Hum Reprod. 2001;7:483–8.
13. Fauth C, Bartels I, Haaf T, Speicher MR. Additional dark G-band in the p-arm of chromosome 19 due to a paracentric inversion with a breakpoint in the pericentromeric heterochromatin. Am J Med Genet. 2001;103:160–2.
14. Kochhar PK, Ghosh P. Reproductive outcome of couples with recurrent miscarriage and balanced chromosomal abnormalities. J Obstet Gynaecol Res. 2013;39:113–20.
15. Gonçalves RO, Santos WV, Sarno M, Cerqueira BA, et al. Chromosomal abnormalities in couples with recurrent first trimester abortions. Rev Bras Ginecol Obstet. 2014;36:113–7.
16. Sugiura-Ogasawara M, Ozaki Y, Sato T, et al. Poor prognosis of recurrent aborters with either maternal or paternal reciprocal translocations. Fertil Steril. 2004;81:367–73.
17. Carrell DT, Wilcox AL, Lowy L, et al. Elevated sperm aneuploidy and apoptosis in patients with unexplained recurrent pregnancy loss. Obstet Gynecol. 2003;101:1229–35.
18. Aldrich CL, Stephenson MD, Karrison T, et al. HLA-G genotypes and pregnancy outcome in couples with unexplained recurrent miscarriage. Mol Hum Reprod. 2001;7:1167–72.
19. Jivraj S, Rai R, Underwood J, Regan L. Genetic thrombophilic mutations among couples with recurrent miscarriage. Hum Reprod. 2006;21:1161–5.
20. Ferlin A, Arredi B, Speltra E, Cazzadore C, Selice R, Garolla A, et al. Molecular and clinical characterization of Y chromosome microdeletions in infertile men: a 10-year experience in Italy. J Clin Endocrinol Metab. 2007;92:762–70.
21. Agarwal S, Agarwal A, Khanna A, Singh K. Microdeletion of Y chromosome as a cause of recurrent pregnancy loss. J Hum Reprod Sci. 2015;8(3):159–64.
22. Dewan S, Puscheck EE, Coulam CB, Wilcox AJ, Jeyendran RS. Y-chromosome microdeletions and recurrent pregnancy loss. Fertil Steril. 2006;85:441–5.
23. Ghorbian S, Saliminejad K, Sadeghi MR, Javadi G. The association between Y chromosome microdeletion and recurrent pregnancy loss. Iran Red Crescent Med J. 2012;14(6):358–62.
24. Sakkas D, Alvarez JG. Sperm DNA fragmentation: mechanisms of origin, impact on reproductive outcome, and analysis. Fertil Steril. 2010;93:1027–36.

25. Kleinhaus K, Perrin M, Friedlander Y, et al. Paternal age and spontaneous abortion. Obstet Gynecol. 2006;108:369–77.
26. Kavitha P, Malini SS. Positive association of sperm dysfunction in the pathogenesis of recurrent pregnancy loss. J Clin Diagn Res. 2014;8(11):OC07–10.
27. Panton JA, Kilpatrick DC. Anti-cardiolipin antibodies in sexual partners of recurrent aborters. Hum Reprod. 1997;12(3):464–7.
28. Hedin LW, Janson PO. Domestic violence during pregnancy: the prevalence of physical injuries, substance use, abortions and miscarriage. Acta Obstet Gynecol Scand. 2000;79:625–30.
29. Kilpatrick DC, Bevan BH, Liston WA. Association between mannan binding protein deficiency and recurrent miscarriage. Hum Reprod. 1995;10:2501–5.
30. WHO laboratory manual for the examination and processing of human semen. 5th ed. 2010.
31. Gopalkrishnan K, Padwal D, Balaiah V. Efficiency of routine semen analysis to predict functional and structural integrity of human spermatozoa. Indian J Exp Biol. 1995;33(9):652–4.
32. Fernández JL, Muriel L, Goyanes V, Segrelles E, Gosálvez J, MaríaEnciso M, LaFromboise M, Jonge CD. Simple determination of human sperm DNA fragmentation with an improved sperm chromatin dispersion test. Fertil Steril. 2005;84:833–42.

Unexplained Recurrent Miscarriage: A Dilemma

12

Shalini Rajaram, Vasudha Gupta, and Bindiya Gupta

12.1 Introduction

According to the American Society of Reproductive Medicine (ASRM), recurrent pregnancy loss is defined as two or more miscarriages [1], whereas according to the European Society for Human Reproduction and Embryology (ESHRE), three or more miscarriages are considered as recurrent pregnancy loss (RPL) [2]. According to ASRM, only those pregnancy losses should be included in the definition which is documented by ultrasonography or histopathological examination [1]. Biochemical pregnancies are very common in general population. It has been seen that 20% women in general population may experience three biochemical losses attributed to chance alone, most of which do not need any further investigation. Overall, RPL affects ~1% of the general population, range between 0.4 and 3% depending on the age group [3–5].

Recurrent early pregnancy loss suggests two or more miscarriages at less than 10 weeks. Distinguishing recurrent early pregnancy loss from RPL is important in terms of both prognosis and treatment.

Unexplained recurrent miscarriage is a self-explanatory term indicating that there is no underlying cause for this condition and up to 50% of patients remain without a diagnosis [6]. It is a difficult situation to deal with for the treating clinician and also a frustrating and depressing condition for the couple as majority continue to seek treatments and physicians may try experimental therapies. However, Clifford et al. (1997) showed that women with unexplained RM, and receiving no treatment, have a good prognosis, with a live birth rate up to 75% following referral to a specialized clinic and psychological supportive care [7].

S. Rajaram (✉) • V. Gupta • B. Gupta
Obstetrics and Gynecology, University College of Medical Sciences and GTB Hospital, Delhi, India
e-mail: rajaram.shalini@gmail.com; vasudhamamc@gmail.com

S. Mehta, B. Gupta (eds.), *Recurrent Pregnancy Loss*,
https://doi.org/10.1007/978-981-10-7338-0_12

12.2 Etiology

The most common cause of unexplained RPL is the factor of chance alone. Besides, several endogenous mechanisms, pathologies, and environmental risk factors may contribute to RPL. The endogenous factors include increased maternal age, poor oocyte quality, abnormal sperm morphology and function, poor quality embryos, and nonreceptive endometrium. Environmental factors such as obesity, smoking, alcohol, caffeine, and exposure to certain occupational hazards may increase the chance of RM.

12.2.1 The Factor of Chance

A large number of women suffer from pregnancy losses by chance alone. These women are healthy females who have all normal investigations. They have good prognosis for future pregnancy without any surgical and pharmacological interventions [8]. This is supported by large randomized controlled trials and meta-analysis which have shown no beneficial effect of heparin, albumin, and intravenous immunoglobulin in this group [9, 10]. A number of cohort studies have evaluated the role of supportive care in RPL and have found identical rates of RM and sporadic pregnancy loss (12–25%) in subsequent pregnancy, further strengthening the factor of chance alone [7, 11, 12]. Thus, up to 68% of unexplained RM can be due to chance alone and thus have a favorable outcome with no interventions.

12.2.2 Maternal Age

The incidence of RM due to chance alone also varies with age, with incidence of 0.13%, 0.34%, 1.56%, and 13.3% for ages 20–24, 30–34, 35–39, and 40–44 years, respectively [13]. It has been seen that younger women are more likely to have some underlying cause requiring thorough investigations and further management, while older women may not necessarily benefit from exhaustive investigations and interventions as there could be a factor of chance.

12.2.3 No. of Previous Miscarriages

The high number of miscarriages is less likely due to chance alone [12].

12.2.4 Karyotype of the Products of Conception

In the presence of a normal karyotype, it is less likely to occur as a consequence of chance. In women with RM, the features suggesting a normal karyotype in the products of conceptus are associated with poor prognosis for future pregnancy and a higher number of miscarriages [14, 15]. In contrast, RM occurring due to chance is most commonly associated with sporadic fetal aneuploidy and an abnormal karyotype of the products of conception [4].

12.2.5 Increased Paternal Age

Advanced paternal age is also associated with recurrent miscarriages. The role of sperm remains controversial in recurrent pregnancy loss. Few reported factors are Y chromosome microdeletions, sperm oxidative damage, sperm DNA fragmentation, sperm concentration, morphology, and function [16, 17].

12.2.6 Poor Quality Embryos

Poor quality embryos may have abnormal implantation and chromosomal defects leading to recurrent pregnancy loss [18, 19]. Preimplantation genetic screening and diagnosis may improve the prognosis in this subgroup [20].

12.2.7 Nonreceptive Endometrium

Dysregulation of endometrium at molecular level is a major reason for improper implantation leading to recurrent pregnancy loss.

Recently it has been demonstrated that increased levels of proimplantation cytokines of endometrium in women with recurrent miscarriages lead to superfertility in these women which leads to implantation of poor quality embryos which cause early pregnancy loss [21]. In women with RPL, the endometrial stromal cell migratory activity was similar for high- and low-quality embryos, while in the fertile women, the migratory activity is inhibited in low-quality embryos. These mechanisms that inhibit the migratory activity can serve as a therapeutic target. Also, there is a reduced expression of beta 3 integrins in endometrium of women with RPL.

12.2.8 Systemic Factors

Systemic factors like hypothyroidism, hyperthyroidism [22, 23], insulin resistance, PCOS [24, 25], and immunological reactions like increased uterine natural killer cells are also associated with recurrent pregnancy losses [26].

12.2.9 Environmental Factors

Smoking, alcohol, drug abuse, caffeine, and occupational hazards are also linked with unexplained recurrent pregnancy losses [27].

12.3 Classification of Unexplained RPL

Two types of unexplained recurrent pregnancy loss have been described:

Type 1—It occurs purely by chance. These women are otherwise healthy and carry an excellent prognosis. There is no need of any intervention in these patients, and supportive psychological care (tender loving care) leads to successful pregnancy outcome.

Type 2—It occurs due to an underlying pathology which could not be identified by routine investigations. These women have poor prognosis [8].

It is important to differentiate between patients with type 1 or type 2 miscarriages. Various studies have been done with regard to this. A typical case of type 1 unexplained RM is an older woman (e.g., over 40 years) with three biochemical or early losses, in whom the products of conception of the most recent miscarriage showed aneuploidy. On the other hand, a typical case of type 2 unexplained RM is a young woman (e.g., under 30 years), with four or more losses, all occurring after fetal heart beat had been visualized and in whom the products of conception of the most recent miscarriage showed a normal result [8].

12.4 Markers for Unexplained Pregnancy Loss

Studies have been done to identify potential biomarkers for unexplained RPL.

Maternal serum amyloid A—Ibrahim et al. found that serum amyloid A levels were significantly higher in women with early recurrent pregnancy loss (50.0 μg/mL, interquartile range 26.0–69.0, versus 11.6 μg/mL, interquartile range 6.2–15.5, in controls) [28]. It was found to be an independent indicator of unexplained early pregnancy loss after adjusting for maternal age and gestational age and could represent a novel biomarker for this complication of pregnancy.

Pentraxin 3—Abnormally elevated pentraxin 3 levels indicate the presence of an abnormally exaggerated intrauterine inflammatory or innate immune response that may cause pregnancy failure in women with primary unexplained recurrent pregnancy loss. An increased first-trimester maternal serum levels of pentraxin 3 suggest a significant positive correlation between the numbers of unexplained recurrent pregnancy loss [29].

12.5 Prognosis

Prognosis of women with unexplained recurrent pregnancy loss is excellent because majority occurs by chance in healthy women. Their prognosis is similar to general population [7].

12.6 Treatment

12.6.1 No Pharmacological Treatment

The Royal College of Obstetricians and Gynecologists has recently concluded that unexplained recurrent miscarriages have excellent prognosis without any pharmacological intervention [30].

Studies have shown reduction in rates of pregnancy loss of up to 50% in women who received psychological supportive care in a dedicated clinic, in comparison with patients who either did not return to the clinic or were looked after in a routine antenatal setting. The concept of psychological supportive care/tender loving care (TLC) broadly consists of serial ultrasounds to confirm viability along with access to specialist counseling.

As discussed earlier, the rate of subsequent pregnancy loss is similar to that of general population in this subgroup thereby suggesting that it can be a matter of chance alone. However, it is a positive experience for already stressed women.

12.6.2 Drug Therapy

Aspirin alone, low-molecular-weight heparin, or combination of both does not increase the live birth rate when given in women with unexplained recurrent pregnancy loss and should not be given in non-thrombophilic women [31–33].

A recent retrospective cohort study including 98 subjects with unexplained RPL showed that women receiving luteal HCG support had an increased chance of an ongoing pregnancy compared with those not receiving it (RR = 2.4; 95% CI 1.4–3.6; number need to treat (NNT) = 7; 95% CI 4–18) [34]. There was a significant absolute risk reduction (ARR) of miscarriage in subjects receiving HCG support. However, further randomized controlled trials are required in this field.

Amin et al. did a prospective randomized controlled trial on 80 patients of unexplained recurrent pregnancy loss and found significant increased rate of continuation of pregnancy beyond 20 weeks in patients who were given *N*-acetyl cysteine along with folic acid. Pregnancy is associated with a state of oxidative stress that could initiate and propagate a cascade of changes that may lead to pregnancy wastage. This process of oxidative stress may be suppressed by the antioxidant effect of *N*-acetyl cysteine (NAC) [35].

12.6.3 IVF-Preimplantation Genetic Screening (IVF/PGS) in Unexplained RPL

A recent study in women with unexplained RPL demonstrated that the IVF/PGS strategy had a live birth rate of 53% and a clinical miscarriage rate of 7%, while the live birth rate was 67%, and clinical miscarriage rate was 24% with expectant management. Thus, the former was not a cost-effective approach in management of these women as it was 100-fold more expensive than expectant management [36].

12.6.4 Plasma Exchange

P-incompatibility is one rare but important cause of unexplained RPL. In a case series study, 11 patients with unexplained RPL who had anti-P antibody in their serum were treated by plasma exchange for early antibody removal during their next pregnancies, and all of them progressed to live birth [37].

12.7 Follow-Up

Patients with recurrent miscarriages are often afraid to become pregnant again. These patients require continuous emotional support from family and physician. They should be informed that risk of miscarriage decreases as the pregnancy advances. However, they should also be informed about other abnormal ultrasound findings which can increase the risk of miscarriage like slow or late appearance of cardiac activity and the presence of subchorionic hematomas.

Conclusion

Recurrent pregnancy loss is a frustrating problem for both patients and physician. Important points in management of such patients are frequent communication, education, and emotional support. Epidemiological associations suggest that the majority of older women with unexplained RM do not have any underlying pathology, which would explain the overall good prognosis for this group of women. However, there is another group of women, often younger, who do have a specific underlying pathology that is as yet unidentified, as a cause for their repeated losses. A better understanding of these separate subgroups of women with unexplained RM would lead to different treatment pathways and management strategies.

Key Points

- Unexplained recurrent miscarriage is a self-explanatory term indicating that there is no underlying cause for this condition and up to 50% of patients remain without a diagnosis.
- The most common cause of unexplained RPL is the factor of chance alone constituting the type 1 unexplained RPL group.
- Type 2 group includes women with an underlying pathology which cannot be identified by routine investigations. This includes poor oocyte quality, abnormal sperm morphology and function, poor quality embryos, nonreceptive endometrium, obesity, smoking, alcohol, and exposure to certain occupational hazards.
- Type 1 unexplained RPL has a better prognosis than type 2.
- Psychological supportive care/tender loving care (TLC) is the best treatment for unexplained RPL.
- Benefit of drug therapy is not yet established. Some benefit has been seen with the use of HCG and *N*-acetyl cysteine.

References

1. American Society for Reproductive Medicine. Definitions of infertility and recurrent pregnancy loss. Fertil Steril. 2008;90(Suppl 5):S60.
2. Farquharson RG, Jauniaux E, Exalto N. Updated and revised nomenclature for description of early pregnancy events. Hum Reprod. 2005;20(11):3008–11.
3. Jauniaux E, Farquharson RG, Christiansen OB, Exalto N. Evidence-based guidelines for the investigation and medical treatment of recurrent miscarriage. Hum Reprod. 2006;21:2216–22.
4. Rai R, Regan L. Recurrent miscarriage. Lancet. 2006;368:601–11.
5. Stephenson MD, Awartani KA, Robinson WP. Cytogenetic analysis of miscarriages from couples with recurrent miscarriage: a case-control study. Hum Reprod. 2002;17:446–51.
6. Li TC, Makris M, Tomsu M, Tuckerman E, Laird S. Recurrent miscarriage: aetiology, management and prognosis. Hum Reprod Update. 2002;8:463–81.
7. Clifford K, Rai R, Regan L. Future pregnancy outcome in unexplained recurrent first trimester miscarriage. Hum Reprod. 1997;12:387–9.
8. Saravelos SH, Li TC. Unexplained recurrent miscarriage: how can we explain it? Hum Reprod. 2012;27(7):1882–6.
9. Kaandorp SP, Goddijn M, van der Post JA, et al. Aspirin plus heparin or aspirin alone in women with recurrent miscarriage. N Engl J Med. 2010;362(17):1586–96.
10. Ata B, Tan SL, Shehata F, et al. A systematic review of intravenous immunoglobulin for treatment of unexplained recurrent miscarriage. Fertil Steril. 2011;95(3):1080–5.e1–2.
11. Liddell HS, Pattison NS, Zanderigo A. Recurrent miscarriage—outcome after supportive care in early pregnancy. Aust N Z J Obstet Gynaecol. 1991;31:320–2.
12. Saravelos SH, Regan L. Unexplained recurrent pregnancy loss. Obstet Gynecol Clin North Am. 2014;41(1):157–66.
13. Nybo Andersen AM, Wohlfahrt J, Christens P, Olsen J, Melbye M. Maternal age and fetal loss: population based register linkage study. BMJ. 2000;320:1708–12.
14. Carp H, Toder V, Aviram A, Daniely M, Mashiach S, Barkai G. Karyotype of the abortus in recurrent miscarriage. Fertil Steril. 2001;75:678–82.
15. Ogasawara M, Aoki K, Okada S, Suzumori K. Embryonic karyotype of abortuses in relation to the number of previous miscarriages. Fertil Steril. 2000;73:300–4.
16. Vissenberg R, Goddijn M. Is there a role for assisted reproductive technology in recurrent miscarriage? Semin Reprod Med. 2011;29(6):548–56.
17. Robinson L, Gallos ID, Conner SJ, et al. The effect of sperm DNA fragmentation on miscarriage rates: a systematic review and meta-analysis. Hum Reprod. 2012;27(10):2908–17.
18. Musters AM, Repping S, Korevaar JC, et al. Pregnancy outcome after preimplantation genetic screening or natural conception in couples with unexplained recurrent miscarriage: a systematic review of the best available evidence. Fertil Steril. 2011;95(6):2153–7.e3.
19. Thornhill AR, deDie-Smulders CE, Geraedts JP, et al. ESHRE PGD Consortium 'Best practice guidelines for clinical preimplantation genetic diagnosis (PGD) and preimplantation genetic screening (PGS)'. Hum Reprod. 2005;20(1):35–48.
20. Practice Committee of the American Society for Reproductive Medicine, Practice Committee of the Society for Assisted Reproductive Technology. Preimplantation genetic diagnosis. Fertil Steril. 2006;86(5 Suppl 1):S257–8.
21. Salker M, Teklenburg G, Molokhia M, et al. Natural selection of human embryos: impaired decidualization of endometrium disables embryo-maternal interactions and causes recurrent pregnancy loss. PLoS One. 2010;5(4):e10287.
22. Thangaratinam S, Tan A, Knox E, et al. Association between thyroid autoantibodies and miscarriage and preterm birth: meta-analysis of evidence. BMJ. 2011;342:d2616.
23. Yan J, Sripada S, Saravelos SH, et al. Thyroid peroxidase antibody in women with unexplained recurrent miscarriage: prevalence, prognostic value, and response to empirical thyroxine therapy. Fertil Steril. 2012;98(2):378–82.

24. Smith ML, Schust DJ. Endocrinology and recurrent early pregnancy loss. Semin Reprod Med. 2011;29(6):482–90.
25. Jakubowicz DJ, Iuorno MJ, Jakubowicz S, et al. Effects of metformin on early pregnancy loss in the polycystic ovary syndrome. J Clin Endocrinol Metab. 2002;87(2):524–9.
26. Tang AW, Alfirevic Z, Quenby S. Natural killer cells and pregnancy outcomes in women with recurrent miscarriage and infertility: a systematic review. Hum Reprod. 2011;26(8):1971–80.
27. Saravelos SH, Regan L. The importance of preconception counseling and early pregnancy monitoring. Semin Reprod Med. 2011;29:557–68.
28. Ibrahim MI, Ramy AR, Abdelhamid AS, Ellaithy MI, Omar A, Harara RM, Fathy H, Abolouz AS. Maternal serum amyloid A level as a novel marker of primary unexplained recurrent early pregnancy loss. Int J Gynaecol Obstet. 2017;136(3):298–303.
29. Ibrahim MI, Harb HM, Ellaithy MI, Elkabarity RH, Abdelgwad MH. First trimester assessment of pentraxin-3 levels in women with primary unexplained recurrent pregnancy loss. Eur J Obstet Gynecol Reprod Biol. 2012;165(1):37–41.
30. Royal College of Obstetricians and Gynaecologists. Green top guideline No. 17. The investigation and treatment of couples with recurrent first trimester miscarriage and second trimester miscarriage. RCOG. 2011.
31. Pasquier E, de Saint Martin L, Bohec C, et al. Enoxaparin for prevention of unexplained recurrent miscarriage: a multicenter randomized double blind placebo controlled trial. Blood. 2015;125(14):2200–5.
32. Schleussner E, Kamin G, Seliger G, et al. Low molecular weight heparin for women with unexplained recurrent pregnancy loss: a multicenter trial with a minimization randomization scheme. Ann Intern Med. 2015;162(9):601–9.
33. Jain P, Dhodapkar SB, Daniel M. Combination of aspirin and heparin in unexplained recurrent miscarriages—'Empirical or evidence based'. J Hum Reprod Sci. 2011;4(3):155–6.
34. Fox C, Azores Gococo D, Swart L. Luteal phase HCG support for unexplained pregnancy loss—a low hanging fruit? Reprod Biomed Online. 2016. pii: S1472-6483(16)30693-9.
35. Amin AF, Shaaban OM, Bediaway MA, et al. N-acetyl cysteine for treatment of unexplained recurrent pregnancy loss. Reprod Biomed Online. 2008;17(5):722–6.
36. Murugappan G, Ohno MS, Lathi RB. Cost-effectiveness analysis of preimplantation genetic screening and in vitro fertilization versus expectant management in patients with unexplained recurrent pregnancy loss. Fertil Steril. 2015;103(5):1215–20.
37. Roghaei MA, Jamdar F, Ghaheri A. Application of plasma exchange in patients with history of unexplained recurrent abortion: a case series. Int J Fertil Steril. 2013;7(1):39–42.

Psychological Factors and Stress in RPL

13

Sumita Mehta and Darukshan Anjum

13.1 Introduction

Recurrent miscarriage affects about 1–5% of couples and is unexplained in about 50% of them [1, 2]. Psychological factors and stress are seen to be significant in women with RPL than in those trying to conceive naturally. Brandt and Neilson (1992) found an increased risk for spontaneous abortion in women with a high job demands and low job control [3]. There has been evidence that certain psychological disorders such as anxiety, nervousness, parental conflicts, and negative life events can lead to an increase in medical disorders and impair pregnancy outcomes. A disturbed equilibrium between the immune-endocrine system leads to release of biological mediators which have been implicated in causing miscarriages. Although a cause-effect relation has not been established between stress and RPL, women with RPL exhibit increase in uterine natural killer cells, immune mediators, and oxidative stress which leads to pregnancy loss. Management for recurrent pregnancy loss is a challenge both for woman and for her obstetrician. Successful pregnancy rates have been seen with prenatal care and psychological support by tender love and care.

13.2 Pathophysiology of Stress as a Cause of Recurrent Miscarriage

The role of stress in unexplained recurrent miscarriage has been confirmed from majority of studies which have concentrated on psychological support, and a comparison with the absence of such support found differences in successful pregnancy outcome. These differences have been as varied as 26–84% [4].

S. Mehta (✉) • D. Anjum
Obstetrics and Gynecology, Babu Jagjiwan Ram Memorial Hospital, Delhi, India
e-mail: sumitadr@gmail.com

S. Mehta, B. Gupta (eds.), *Recurrent Pregnancy Loss*,
https://doi.org/10.1007/978-981-10-7338-0_13

The mechanism by which stress leads to pregnancy loss is still not clear. Psychological stress attributes to pregnancy losses by disturbing the equilibrium between the nervous, endocrine, and immune systems.

13.2.1 Stress and Immune Response

Acute and chronic stress has an impact on immune system. Acute stress stimulates the immune system, while chronic stress especially depression downregulates one's immunity. Inflammatory immune response plays a key role in reproductive failure. Cellular immune response mediated by natural killer (NK) and T cells is often dysregulated in recurrent pregnancy loss.

Changes in immune system during stress:

Increased NK cell cytotoxicity: Increased number of NK cells are seen in stress and in peripheral blood of women with recurrent pregnancy loss [5]. Stress elevation of NK activity support a pathophysiological link between NK cells and reproductive failure. NK cells express high levels of β adrenergic receptors, and their adherence to endothelium and migration into blood is affected by catecholamine levels [6].

Hori S et al. found that NK cell activity is positively correlated with woman's self-esteem and negatively correlated with depressive symptoms [7].

Mechanism of action:

- Excessive or inappropriate recruitment of peripheral blood NK cells to the uterus leads to cytotoxic environment in the uterus in which proliferation and differentiation of trophoblast are hampered.
- An altered NK cell cytokine profile modulates the invasive propensity of the trophoblast.
- Uterine NK cells lead to abnormal and inadequate vascular development which in turn leads to oxidative stress and ischemic changes in invading trophoblast.

Alireza Andalib et al. conducted a questionnaire-based study on 45 women with history of RPL and a matched control group [8]. A questionnaire for life events and the Beck Depression Inventory was used to review the sociopsychological events. NK activity was also measured by fresh peripheral blood lymphocytes. They found a positive correlation between depression scores and NK cytotoxicity. Hadinedoushan H et al. did a case control study on 21 patients with RPL within 24 h of last abortion. NK cell cytotoxicity (using flow cytometry) and IL2 and IL10 as well as transforming growth factor B1 were measured. These women had higher NK cytotoxicity compared to controls ($p < 0.045$). Also, the production of IL2 and IL10 was higher in the cases than controls ($p = 0.001$ and 0.002, respectively) [9].

Yamada H et al. prospectively assessed peripheral NK cell activity and subsequent pregnancy activity in 66 pregnant women with a history of RPL. They found that NK activity in women who had a subsequent miscarriage at 6–7 weeks gestational age was significantly higher than the women who had live births later and concluded that high NK cell activity at 6–7 weeks correlates with subsequent miscarriage [5]. Various other studies also gave similar conclusions [10, 11].

Increased decidual release of cytokines: Stress causes an increase in release of pro-inflammatory cytokines. Markert UR et al. found the percentage of degranulated mast cells increased (8% vs. 24%) in the uteri of stressed animals and concluded that mast cells might be the cellular link between the neurotransmitter substance P and increase in decidual TNF alpha release which finally causes the miscarriage [12]. Quack KC et al. studied white blood cells and their activation status in decidua of women with RPL [13]. They found significantly more activated leucocytes and a reduced concentration of CD56+ in decidua of women with RPL as compared to normal age-matched first trimester pregnancies with elective termination procedure. Jasper MJ et al. found reduced levels of IL6 mRNA and IL1 mRNA in endometrial biopsies of women with history of recurrent miscarriages. These interleukins affect the remodeling and angiogenesis in the endometrium and also cause dysregulated trophoblast differentiation and invasion [14].

Cytokines produced by a Th1, namely, TNFα and IFNϒ, mediate abortion by targeting vascular endothelial cells, resulting in ischemic death of the embryo by increased procoagulant activity. There is positive correlation between stress and number of decidua basalis mast cells, CD8+T cells, and TNFα expression [15, 16].

Elevated Th1and Th2 ratio: In pregnancy, a Th1 to Th2 shift has been postulated. Rejection of the trophoblastic cells is selectively inhibited by Th2 cytokines acting unopposed by Th1 cytokines [17].

Kwak-Kim et al. demonstrated significantly higher Th1/Th2 ratios, TNF alpha/IL4, and TNF alpha/IL10 ($p < 0.05$ each) in CD3+/CD8 T helper cells in women with RPL, thereby confirming the dominance of Th1 immune response in peripheral blood lymphocytes in these women [18]. Laird SM et al. reviewed immune cells and molecules in women with RPL and concluded that there is alteration in the ratio of Th1 and Th2 cytokines produced by peripheral blood monocytes and decreased production of pro-inflammatory cytokines such as IL6 in these women [19].

Increased production of mast cell tryptase: Besides the production of inflammatory cytokines, the secretion of decidual mast cell tryptase might imply an additional threat to pregnancy. Mast cell tryptase cleaves proteinase-activated receptor 2 (PAR2) which induces widespread inflammation [20]. A large proportion of primary spinal afferent which express PAR2 has been shown to contain neuropeptide SP. Tryptase directly signals neurons to release these neurotransmitters which induce inflammatory edema which contributes to stress-triggered pro-inflammatory effects of mast cells in human miscarriage deciduas.

13.2.2 Stress and Neurotransmitters

Neurogenic inflammation is caused by neuroimmune linkages due to infection, trauma, or stress. It involves nerves that contain inflammation triggering neuropeptides; the most important are neurotrophin growth factor (NGF) and tachykinin 1 (TAC 1or Subs P). They act by:

- Activation of mast cells and/or other immune cells [21, 22]
- Release of Th1 cytokine TNF alpha

- Upregulation of endothelial ICAM1 (intercellular adhesion molecule) and SELP (Selectin P) and their respective ligands and thereby increasing angiogenesis and mediating the migration of leukocytes [23]

Neurotrophin growth factor: NGF is the first identified member of the family of neurotrophins and plays a critical role in the decidual response to stress. It is a proximal mediator in the complex network of immune rejection seen in stressed women [24–26]. Spontaneous abortion is associated with upregulation of synthesis and aberrant distribution of NGF in placental tissue. It increases ICAM1 in uterine decidua thereby increasing pro-inflammatory and abortogenic cytokines.

Substance P: A number of peptide neurotransmitters in the autonomic and peripheral nerves contain substance P (SP), vasoactive intestinal peptide, enkephalin, and neuropeptide tyrosine. SP-containing nerve fibers are present in human female reproductive organs. SP has a direct effect on vasculature and contracts smooth muscle of airway and gut and is also an immune-modulating peptide [27]. Immunomodulating effects of SP include:

- SP affects the coordination of muscular activity which is important for the transport of sperm and ova in the fallopian tube and also implantation of conceptus.
- SP modulates a variety of immune responses like T-cell proliferation, immunoglobulin synthesis, macrophage activation, mast cell degranulation, and histamine release [28].
- It also induces production of IL-6, IL-1, IFN-ϒ, and TNF-α. Activation of CRH-ACTH-Cortisol cascade is signaled by SP-containing nerve fibers. The interaction between stress neurotransmitters and immune system indicates the close bonds between these systems [29].

13.3 Stress and Hormones

13.3.1 CRH and Glucocorticoids

Hypothalamo-pituitary adrenal ovarian axis gets activated during stress which causes release of CRH (corticotropin-releasing hormone) from hypothalamus. CRH acts on pituitary to release ACTH which further acts on adrenal cortex to release glucocorticoids. Stress is a potent activator of CRH release from the hypothalamus and extra-hypothalamic sites [30]. CRH receptors are found in ovaries, uterus, and placental trophoblast [31]. Cortisol induces estrogen deficiency by suppressing granulosa cell aromatase activity. Estrogen deficiency is seen in anxiety and depression.

Mechanism of action of CRH in causing miscarriage:

- CRH decreases release of GnRH secretion from the hypothalamus and leads to anovulation and interruption of decidualization of endometrium thereby leading to miscarriage.
- Decreases ovarian steroidogenesis leading to ovarian failure [32].

- It induces the release of β endorphins which have a strong impact on immune system [33].
- Increased cortisol causes aging of the trophoblast.
- It also promotes a shift in Th1/Th2 ratio.

Cortisol levels are seen to increase in pregnancy loss; any increase in cortisol in the first 3 weeks of pregnancy is maternal as embryos cannot produce glucocorticoids at 3 weeks. Nepomnaschy et al. concluded that pregnancies exposed to high levels of cortisol were 2.7 times more likely to be unsuccessful than those exposed to normal cortisol levels (95% CI = 1.2–6.2) [34].

13.3.2 Prolactin

The role of prolactin in early pregnancy is controversial. Li W et al. measured serum prolactin levels in 174 women with unexplained RPL [35]. Women who had lower basal prolactin levels were associated with an increased risk of miscarriage in a subsequent pregnancy. Garzia et al. investigated the expression of prolactin, prolactin receptors, and IL 2 at maternofetal interphase. The expression of prolactin was impaired or absent in the villi of women who underwent suction curettage for spontaneous miscarriage as compared to controls (women who had voluntary termination of pregnancy). So, they concluded that prolactin expression is essential for viable pregnancy [36]. But increased levels of prolactin can be detrimental to ongoing pregnancy and can result in miscarriage. The various mechanisms by which hyperprolactinemia causes abortion are:

- Prolactin and growth hormone cause angiogenesis and remodeling of blood vessels [37].
- High prolactin levels in early phase of follicular growth inhibit progesterone secretion and result in luteal phase defects [38, 39].
- Luteal phase defects caused by hyperprolactinemia further reduce LH receptors.
- Prolactin also acts as a cytokine and promotes pro-inflammatory immune responses [40]. It increases the ability of the immune cells to proliferate and produce cytokines such as TNF alpha, IL12, and IL1 beta. This effects results from activation of both intracellular pathways and activation of genes linked to apoptosis and proliferation [41].

Stress that causes an increase in prolactin levels has been recognized since Nicoll first described it in 1960 [42]. Vasopression and peptide histidine isoleucine may be involved in the secretion of prolactin during stress [43]. In a study conducted by Lennartsson AK and Jonsdottir IH, 15 women and 30 men underwent Trier social stress test (TSST). They observed significantly elevated prolactin levels and ACTH levels in response to the stress, but the path of prolactin response did not differ between men and women. However, women had a higher magnitude of increase than men [44].

13.3.3 Progesterone

Progesterone helps during implantation and in maintenance of pregnancy. Progesterone stimulates the production of progesterone-induced blocking factor (PIBF) which induces Th2 cytokine activation in the decidua and thus helps in continuation of pregnancy.

Stress decreases progesterone and hence PIBF. Nepomnaschy et al. in their study on how stress influences reproductive function concluded that stress leads to increase in cortisol levels which cause untimely increases in gonadotrophins and consequently low midluteal progesterone levels and miscarriage [45].

Stephens MA also noted that progesterone levels negatively correlated with ACTH and cortisol in women following TSST in 135 young women. Kajantie et al. also had similar results [46, 47].

13.4 Evidence Supporting Stress in Etiology of Recurrent Miscarriage

The role of stress is unexplained and has been confirmed from two different strategies. Majority of studies have concentrated on psychological support, and a comparison with the absence of such support has found differences in successful pregnancy outcome. These differences have been as varied as 84–26%. The other evidence is in the form of indirect support that stress is an etiological factor in causation of recurrent miscarriages [4].

As early as the 1980s, Stray Pedersen reported an improved pregnancy success rate of 86% in women with recurrent miscarriage who received specific antenatal counseling and psychological support as against 33% observed in women who did not receive such support. None of these women had any abnormal physical factors as a cause for recurrent miscarriage [48].

Neugebauer et al. interviewed 192 women who visited a medical center after spontaneous abortion regarding positive and negative events that had occurred in the past 4–5 months. He concluded that 70% of the women with chromosomally normal losses reported having had one or more negative life events in the months preceding the loss compared with 52% in the women with chromosomally abnormal fetuses (adjusted odds ratio 2.6; 95% CI 1.3–4.6) [49]. Hjollund NH followed a cohort of the first pregnancy planners which included 181 pregnancies of which 32 were subclinical pregnancies [50]. All the women recorded physical strain in a structured diary during early pregnancy. He found that physical strain around the time of implantation was associated with spontaneous miscarriage later. The adjusted risk ratio for women who had higher than average physical strain around day 6 to 9 after the estimated date of ovulation was 2.5 (95% CI 1.3–4.6).

Hamilton BS et al. conducted a case control study in an emergency department, and stress was measured using a life event inventory. They concluded that spontaneous abortion at 11 weeks or greater was seen more in women experiencing more than one life event (adjusted odds ratio 2.9; 95% CI 1.4–6.2) [51].

In another prospective study conducted by Ogasawara M et al., a high depression scale is associated with a high miscarriage rate in women with RPL [52]. In a case control study via a two-stage postal survey of reproductive histories of randomly sampled 603 women, it was found that feeling stressed (including trend with number of stressful or traumatic events) was associated with increased risk of abortion [53].

RCOG guidelines (2011) state that 75% of women with unexplained recurrent pregnancy loss have an excellent prognosis for a successful future pregnancy with supportive care alone. The role of non-pharmacological intervention in the form of tender loving care has a beneficial effect that goes on to show that stress is a causative agent for RPL [54].

Li W et al. investigated the stress status of 45 women with RPL and 50 fertile women and found that women with RPL had significant higher scores on Perceived Stress Scale ($p < 0.05$, adjusted OR 1.13) and lower score on Positive Affect Scale ($p < 0.05$, adjusted OR 1.17) [55]. Various other studies have also shown association between stress and recurrent miscarriages [56, 57].

Contrary to the abovementioned authors, there were studies refuting stress as an etiological factor for recurrent miscarriage.

Fenster et al. examined the relation of work-related psychologic stress to spontaneous abortion in 3953 pregnant women. The psychological stress and social support at work were assessed, and they concluded that overall, stressful work was not associated with an increased risk of spontaneous abortion. But interactions were seen between stressful work and primigravidity ($p = 0.06$), maternal age, and cigarette smoking ($p = 0.02$) [58].

Nelson DB et al. measured stress in women who underwent miscarriage using Perceived Stress Scale, the Prenatal Social Inventory, and the Index of Spousal Abuse. Blood samples of these women were also collected for cortisol and sex hormone levels. They did not find any relation between psychological stress (as calculated by the three stress indices and cortisol levels) and the risk for spontaneous abortion [59]. Mutambudz et al. did a literature review on the psychosocial stress of work on pregnancy outcomes and found that job strain alone was not associated with adverse pregnancy outcomes. Similar results were also reported by Littleton HL et al. [60, 61].

Conclusion

As most of the evidence points toward the role of psychosocial stress in the etiology of recurrent miscarriage, psychological support and reassurance in the form of frequent discussions and sympathetic counseling are crucial to the successful evaluation and treatment of the anxious couple. Pathophysiological changes in response to stress involve neuroendocrine-immune pathways. Lifestyle modification and stress reduction should be emphasized by pointing out a healthy life, free from tobacco and alcohol. Women should be reassured for a successful pregnancy with supportive care.

Key Points

- There has been evidence that negative life events lead to an increase in medical disorders and miscarriages.
- Psychosocial stress attributes to pregnancy loss by disturbing the equilibrium between the neuroendocrine and immune systems.
- Various changes in immune system in response to stress include increase in NK cells, decidual release of pro-inflammatory cytokines, and mast cell tryptase.
- Stress leads to neurogenic inflammation through increase in NGF and Subs P.
- Hypothalamic-pituitary-ovarian axis gets activated by stress leading to increased secretion of CRH, glucocorticoids, and prolactin.
- Psychological support in the form of frequent discussions and sympathetic counseling is crucial to the successful evaluation and treatment of the anxious couple.

References

1. Stephenson M, Kutteh W. Evaluation and management of recurrent miscarriage and early pregnancy loss. Clin Obstet Gynecol. 2007;50(1):132–45.
2. Lee RM, Silver RM. Recurrent pregnancy loss: summary and clinical recommendations. Semin Reprod Med. 2000;18(4):433–40.
3. Brandt LP, Nielson CV. Job stress and adverse outcome of pregnancy: a causal link or recall bias? Am J Epidemiol. 1992;135(3):302–11.
4. Craig M. Stress and recurrent miscarriage. Stress. 2001;4(3):205–13.
5. Yamada H, Kato HE, Kobashi G, et al. High NK cell activity in early pregnancy correlated with subsequent abortion with normal chromosomes in women with recurrent abortion. Am J Reprod Immunol. 2001;46:132–6.
6. Benschop R, Rodriguez-Feuerhahn M, Schedlowski M. Catecholamine induced leukocytosis: early observations, current research, and future directions. Brain Behav Immun. 1996;10:77–91.
7. Hori S, Nakano Y, Furukama TA, Ogasawara M, et al. Psychosocial factors regulating NK cell activity in recent abortions. Am J Reprod Immunol. 2000;44:299–302.
8. Andalib A, Rezaie A, Oreizy F, et al. A study of stress, depression and NK cytotoxic potential in women with recurrent pregnancy abortion. Iran J Allergy Asthma Immunol. 2006;5(1):9–16.
9. Hadinedoushan H, Mirahmadian M, Aflatounian A. Increased NK cell cytotoxicity and IL2 production in recurrent spontaneous abortion. Am J Reprod Immunol. 2007;58(5):409–14.
10. Shakar K, Rosenne E, Loewenthal R, Shakhar G, Carp H, Ben-Eliyahu S. High NK cell activity in recurrent miscarriage: what are we really measuring? Hum Reprod. 2006;21(9):2421–5.
11. Faust Z, Laskarin G, Rukavina D, Szekeres-Bartho J. Progesterone induced blocking factor inhibits degranulation of NK cells. Am J Reprod Immunol. 1999;42:71–5.
12. Markert UR, Arck PC, McBey BA, Manuel J, Croy BA, Marshall JS, et al. Stress triggered abortions are associated with alterations of granulated cells into the decidua. Am J Reprod Immunol. 1997;37(1):94–100.
13. Quack KC, Vassiliadou N, Pudney J, Anderson DJ, Hill JA. Leukocyte activation in the decidua of chromosomally normal and abnormal fetuses from women with recurrent abortions. Hum Reprod. 2001;16(5):949–55.

14. Jasper MJ, Tremellen KP, Robertson SA. Reduced expression of IL6 and IL1 alpha mRNAs in secretory phase endometrium of women with recurrent miscarriage. J Reprod Immunol. 2007;73(1):74–84.
15. Arck PC, Rose M, Hertwig K, Hagen E, Hildebrandt M, Klapp BF. Stress and immune mediators in miscarriage. Hum Reprod. 2001;16:1505–11.
16. Clark DA, Ding JW, Chaouat G, Levy GA. The emerging role of immunoregulation of fibrinogen related procoagulant Fg12 in the success or spontaneous abortion of early pregnancy in mice and humans. Am J Reprod Immunol. 1994;42:71–5.
17. Blois SM, Joachim R, Kandil J, Mrgni R, et al. Depletion of CD8+ cells abolishes the pregnancy protective effect of progesterone substitution with dydrogesterone in mice by altering the Th1/Th2 cytokine profile. J Immunol. 2004;172(10):5893–9.
18. Kwak-Kim JY, Chung-Bang HS, Ng SC, Ntrivalas EI, Mangubat CP, Beaman KD, Beer AE, Gilman-Sachs A. Increased T helper 1 cytokine responses by circulating T cells are present in women with recurrent pregnancy losses and in infertile women with multiple implantation failures after IVF. Hum Reprod. 2003;18(4):767–73.
19. Laird SM, Tuckerman EM, Cork BA, Linjawi S, Blakemore AI, Li TC. A review of immune cells and molecules in women with recurrent miscarriage. Hum Reprod Update. 2003;9(2):163–74.
20. Steinhoff M, Vergonelle N, Young SH, et al. Agonists of proteinase-activated receptor 2 induce inflammation by a neurogenic mechanism. Nat Med. 2000;6:151–8.
21. Black PH. Stress and the inflammatory response: a review of neurogenic inflammation. Brain Behav Immun. 2002;16:622–53.
22. Arck PC, Handjiski B, Peters EM, Peter AS, Hagen E, Fischer A, Klapp BF, Paus R. Stress inhibits hair growth in mice by induction of premature catagen development and deleterious perifollicular inflammatory events via neuropeptide substance P-dependent pathways. Am J Pathol. 2003;162:803.
23. Kappelmayer J, Nagy B Jr, Miszti-Blasius K, Hevessy Z, Setiadi H. The emerging value of SELP as a disease marker. Clin Chem Lab Med. 2004;42:475–86.
24. Tometten M, Blois S, Kuhlmic A, Stretz A, et al. Nerve growth factor translates stress response and subsequent murine abortion via adhesion molecule-dependent pathways. Biol Reprod. 2006;74(4):674–83.
25. Tometten M, Klapp BF, Joachim R, Fest S, et al. Nerve growth factor and it's functional receptor TRKA are upregulated in murine decidual tissue of stress triggered and substance P-mediated abortion. Am J Reprod Immunol. 2004;5(1):86–93.
26. Blois S, Tometten M, Kandil J, Hagen E, Klapp BF, Margni RA, Arck PC. Intercellular adhesion molecule-1/LFA-1 Cross talk is a proximate mediator capable of disrupting immune integration and tolerance mechanism at the feto-maternal interface in murine pregnancies. J Immunol. 2005;174:1820–9.
27. Kowalski ML, Kaliner MA. Neurogenic inflammation, vascular permeability and mast cells. J Immunol. 1988;140:3905–11.
28. Stead RH, Bienestock J. Cellular interactions between the immune and peripheral nervous system: a normal role for mast cells? In: Burger MM, Sordat B, Zinkernagel RM, editors. Cell to cell interaction. Basel: Kargel; 1990. p. 170–87.
29. Donnerer J, Amann R, Skofitsch G, Lembeck F. Substance P afferents regulate ACTH-corticosterone release. Ann N Y Acad Sci. 1991;632:296–30.
30. Rivest S, Rivier C. The role of corticotrophin-releasing hormone and interleukin-1 in the regulation of neurons controlling reproductive functions. Endocr Rev. 1995;16:177–99.
31. Chrousos GP. The hypothalamic-pituitary-adrenal axis and immune mediated inflammation. N Engl J Med. 1995;332:1351–62.
32. Hsueh AJW, Erickson GF. Glucocorticoid inhibition of FSH-mediated estrogen production of cultured rat granulose cells. Steroids. 1983;32:639–43.
33. Petraglia F, Sutton S, Vale W, Plotsky P. Corticotropin releasing factor decreases plasma luteinizing hormone levels in female rats by inhibiting gonadotropin releasing hormone release into hypophysial-portal circulation. Endocrinology. 1987;120:1083–8.

34. Nepomnaschy PA, Welch KB, McConnell DS, Low BS, Strassmann BI, England BG. Cortisol levels and very early pregnancy loss in humans. Proc Natl Acad Sci. 2006;103:3938–42.
35. Li W, Ma N, Laird SM, Ledger WL, Li TC. The relationship between serum prolactin concentration and pregnancy outcome in women with unexplained recurrent miscarriage. J Obstet Gynaecol. 2013;33(3):285–58.
36. Garzia E, Clauser R, Persani L, Borgato S, et al. Prolactin and pro-inflammatory cytokine expression at the feto-maternal interface in first trimester miscarriage. Fertil Steril. 2013;100(1):108–15.
37. Corbacho AM, Martinez De La Escakera G, Clapp C. Role of prolactin, growth hormone and placental lactogen hormone family in angiogenesis. J Endocrinol. 2003;173(2):219.
38. Pluchino N, Drakopoulos P, Wenger JM, Retignat P, et al. Hormonal causes of recurrent pregnancy loss. Hormones. 2014;13(3):314–22.
39. Che H, Fu J, Huang W. Dopamine agonists for preventing future miscarriage in women with idiopathic hyperprolactinemia and recurrent miscarriage history. Cochrane Database Syst Rev. 2016;7:CD008883.
40. Brand JM, Frohn C, Cziupka K, Brockmann C, et al. Prolactin triggers pro-inflammatory immune responses in peripheral immune cells. Eur Cytokine Netw. 2004;15(2):99–104.
41. Fojtikova M, Cerna M, Pavelka K. A review of the effects of prolactin hormone and cytokine on the development and pathogenesis of autoimmune diseases. Vnitr Lek. 2010;56(5):402–13.
42. Nicoll CS, Talwalker PK, Meites J. Initiation of lactation in rats by nonspecific stresses. Am J Physiol. 1960;198:1103–6.
43. Ranabir S, Reetu K. Stress and hormones. Indian J Endocrinol Metab. 2011;15(1):18–22.
44. Lennartsson AK, Jonsdottir IH. Prolactin in response to acute psychosocial stress in healthy men and women. Psychoneuroendocrinology. 2011;36(10):1530–9.
45. Nepomnaschy PA, Welch K, McConnel D, Strassmann LI, England BG. Stress and female reproductive function: a study of daily variations in cortisol, gonadotrophins, and gonadal steroids in a rural Mayan population. Am J Hum Biol. 2004;16(5):523–32.
46. Stephens MA, Mahol PB, McCaul ME, Wand GS. Hypothalamic-pituitary-adrenal axis response to acute psychosocial stress: effects of biological sex and circulating sex hormones. Psychoneuroendocrinology. 2016;66:47–55.
47. Kajantie E, Philips DI. The effects of sex and hormonal status on the physiological response to acute psychological stress. Psychoneuroendocrinology. 2006;31(2):151–78.
48. Stray Pedersen B, Stray Pedersen S. Etiologic factors and subsequent reproductive performance in 195 couples with a prior history of habitual abortion. Am J Obstet Gynecol. 1984;148:140–6.
49. Neugebauer R, Kline J, Stein Z, Shrout P, Warburton D, Susser M. Association of stressful life events with chromosomally normal spontaneous abortion. Am J Epidemiol. 1996;143:588–96.
50. Hjollund NH. Spontaneous abortion and physical strain around implantation: a follow-up of first pregnancy planners. Epidemiology. 2000;11:18–23.
51. Hamilton BS, Ness RB, Grisson AJ, Marcovic N, Bromberger J, CiFellie D. Life events stress and the association with spontaneous abortion in gravid women at an urban emergency department. Health Psychol. 2000;19:510–4.
52. Sugiura-Ogasawara M, Furukawa TA, Nakano Y, Hori S, et al. Depression as a potential causal factor in subsequent miscarriage in recurrent spontaneous aborters. Hum Reprod. 2002;17(10):2580–4.
53. Maconochie N, Doyle P, Prior S, Simmons R. Risk factors for first trimester miscarriage—results from a UK population based case control study. BJOG. 2007;114(2):170–86.
54. Royal College of Obstetricians and Gynecologists. The investigation and treatment of couples with recurrent miscarriage. Guideline No. 17. London: RCOG-UK; 2011.
55. Li W, Newell-Price J, Jones GL, Li TC. Relationship between psychological stress and recurrent miscarriage. Reprod Biomed Online. 2012;25(2):180–9.
56. Legendre G, Gicquel M, Lejeune V, Iraola E, Deffieux X, et al. Psychology and pregnancy loss. J Gynecol Obstet Biol Reprod. 2014;43(10):908–17.

57. Toupet A, Theau A, Goffinet F, Tsatsaris V. Recurrent pregnancy losses: etiological considerations and investigations, the point of view of the obstetrician-gynecologist. Rev Med Interne. 2015;36(3):182–90.
58. Fenster L, Schaefer C, Mathur A, Hiatt RA, et al. Psychologic stress in the workplace and spontaneous abortion. Am J Epidemiol. 1995;142:1176–83.
59. Nelson DB, Grisso JA, Joffe MM, Brensinger C, Shaw L, DAtner E. Does strain influence pregnancy loss. Ann Epidemiol. 2003;13:223–9.
60. Mutambudz M, Meyer JD, Warren N, Reisine S. Effect of psychosocial characteristics of work on pregnancy outcomes: a critical review. Women Health. 2011;51(3):279–97.
61. Littleton HL, Bye K, Buck K, Amacker A. Psychosocial stress during pregnancy and perinatal outcomes: a meta-analytic review. J Psychosom Obstet Gynaecol. 2010;31(14):219–28.

Evidence-Based Clinical and Investigative Workup of RPL Couples

14

Leena Wadhwa and Deepika

Recurrent pregnancy loss (RPL) is defined as two or more failed clinical pregnancies [1]. Recurrent miscarriage is defined as two or more failed pregnancies, which have been documented by either ultrasound or histopathological examination. Evaluation of recurrent pregnancy loss (RPL) can proceed after two or more consecutive clinical pregnancy losses, but it requires a thorough evaluation of couples after three or more pregnancy losses [1, 2].

RPL affects 0.4–1% of couples [3]. This is approximately twice the incidence that would have been expected by chance alone and indicates that an abnormality is likely to be present.

14.1 Clinical Workup of RPL Couples

An evaluation of a case with RPL should always include a complete history, including documentation of previous pregnancies, any pathologic tests that were performed on previous miscarriages, any evidence of chronic or acute infections or diseases, any recent physical or emotional trauma, history of cramping or bleeding with a previous miscarriage, and any previous gynecological surgery or complicating factor. The important clinical points which should be included in history of RPL couples are described below:

14.1.1 Reproductive History

Maternal age and number of previous miscarriages are two independent risk factors for a further miscarriage.

L. Wadhwa (✉) • Deepika
Obstetrics and Gynecology, ESI Post Graduate Institute of Medical Science and Research, Delhi, India
e-mail: drleena_123@yahoo.co.in

S. Mehta, B. Gupta (eds.), *Recurrent Pregnancy Loss*,
https://doi.org/10.1007/978-981-10-7338-0_14

Maternal age: The increase in the risk of miscarriage in advanced age group is due to an increase in chromosomally abnormal conceptus, probably as a result of poor oocyte quality, and a decline in uterine and ovarian function. Advanced paternal age has also been identified as a risk factor for miscarriage. The risk of miscarriage is the highest among couples where the woman is ≥35 years of age and the man ≥40 years of age.

A large prospective study by Regan et al. [4] reported the increase age-related risk of miscarriage in pregnancies as 13% in 12–19 years, 11% in 20–24 years, 12% in 25–29 years, 15% in 30–34 years, 25% in 35–39 years, and 51% in 40–44 years.

No. of previous miscarriages: A woman's obstetric history predicts her future risk of miscarriage. The risk of another miscarriage increases after each subsequent pregnancy loss [5].

After the first pregnancy, the risk of miscarriage is 5–13%; this increases to 14–21% after one miscarriage, 24–29% after two miscarriages, and 31–45% after three miscarriages. Therefore a detailed reproductive history should include age of patient and her partner, as well as detailed history of her prior pregnancies.

14.1.2 Medical Disease

Systemic maternal endocrine disorders such as diabetes mellitus, thyroid disease, PCOS, and hyperprolactinemia have been associated with RPL.

Diabetes mellitus: Women with diabetes who have high hemoglobin A1c levels in the first trimester are at risk of miscarriage and fetal malformation [6].

The points which should be included in history to suggest diabetes are:

Previous history of gestational diabetes mellitus
Previous history of delivery of large baby (>4 kg)
History of congenital malformation in previous pregnancy
Previous traumatic delivery with associated neurological disorder in infant
History of still birth/unexplained neonatal death
History of glycosuria and impaired glucose metabolism

Thyroid disorders: They can lead to RPL and infertility due to anovulation, recurrent abortion, fetal growth restriction, prematurity, still birth, and mental retardation, if left untreated. Antithyroid antibodies have also been linked to recurrent miscarriage and preterm births.

The prevalence of diabetes mellitus and thyroid dysfunction in women who suffer recurrent miscarriage is similar to that reported in the general population. However, well-controlled diabetes mellitus is not a risk factor for recurrent miscarriage nor is treated thyroid dysfunction [7].

Polycystic ovary syndrome (PCOS): It has been linked to an increased risk of miscarriage, but the exact mechanism remains unclear. The increased risk of miscarriage in women with PCOS has been recently attributed to insulin resistance, hyperinsulinemia, and hyperandrogenemia. The prevalence of insulin resistance is increased in women with recurrent miscarriage compared with matched fertile controls. History of weight gain, irregular periods, infertility, hirsutism, or acne is suggestive of PCOS.

PCOS cases should be screened for metabolic syndrome. Risk factors for metabolic syndrome include nonwhite race, sedentary lifestyle, BMI > 25 kg/m^2, age over 40 years, cardiovascular disease, hypertension, insulin resistance, HAIR-AN syndrome, nonalcoholic steatohepatitis, and family history of type 2 diabetes mellitus, gestational diabetes mellitus, or impaired glucose tolerance.

Hyperprolactinemia: Prolactin is the most important hormone involved in the pathophysiology of amenorrhea and/or galactorrhea. Hyperprolactinemia inhibits ovarian steroid synthesis. Thus it results in hypogonadotropic hypogonadism, oligomenorrhea, amenorrhea, anovulation, recurrent pregnancy loss, and many other clinical effects of hypoestrogenism. Prolactin levels should be estimated in all women with galactorrhea, oligomenorrhea, amenorrhea, recurrent pregnancy loss, and infertility.

14.1.3 Anatomical Factors

14.1.3.1 Congenital

Congenital uterine malformations: The reported prevalence of uterine anomalies in recurrent pregnancy loss populations ranges between 1.8 and 37.6% [8]. Incomplete Mullerian fusion or septum is a common cause for uterine malformations. Overall the prevalence of uterine malformations appears to be higher in women with second-trimester miscarriages compared with women who suffer first-trimester miscarriages.

Cervical incompetence: It is a recognized cause of second-trimester pregnancy loss. The diagnosis is usually based on a history of second-trimester pregnancy loss preceded by spontaneous rupture of membranes or painless cervical dilatation.

14.1.3.2 Acquired Factors

These abnormalities include conditions such as intrauterine adhesions, uterine fibroids, and endometrial polyps.

History of any surgical procedure on the cervix mostly midtrimester (conization, forcible dilatation) can cause cervical tear and lead to second-trimester pregnancy losses or preterm deliveries. Therefore history of previous first- or second-trimester pregnancy losses should be mentioned specifically.

14.1.4 Thrombophilia

14.1.4.1 Inherited

History suggestive of inherited thrombophilias includes a detailed family history of thrombosis, recurrent pregnancy loss, still births, or birth defects, and a note of any of these should be taken. The following disorders are included in inherited thrombophilia:

Deficiencies of antithrombin III
Deficiency of protein C/S
Factor v mutation
Prothrombin gene mutation 20210A (PGM)
Dysfibrinogenemia
Hyperhomocysteinemia
MTHFR (methylenetetrahydrofolate reductase) mutation

14.1.4.2 Acquired

Antiphospholipid syndrome: APLA is the only autoimmune condition in which pregnancy loss is part of the diagnostic criteria. Antiphospholipid antibodies (APAs), lupus anticoagulant, anticardiolipin antibodies (ACAs), and anti-B2 glycoprotein-I antibodies are directed against phospholipid-binding plasma proteins.

Antiphospholipid antibodies are present in 15% of women with recurrent pregnancy loss. By comparison, the prevalence of antiphospholipid antibodies in women with a low-risk obstetric history is less than 2%. Antiphospholipid syndrome is the most important treatable cause of recurrent miscarriage.

Criteria for investigative workup for APLA:

(a) Three or more consecutive miscarriages before 10 weeks of gestation
(b) One or more morphologically normal fetal losses after the tenth week of gestation
(c) One or more preterm births before the 34th week of gestation owing to placental disease

It has been hypothesized that thrombophilic disorders cause thrombosis of the utero-placental vasculature (spiral arteries and intervillous space) due to an increased hemostatic response [9]. The subsequent impaired placental perfusion may lead to recurrent pregnancy loss, fetal death, preeclampsia, intrauterine growth restriction, and abruptio placentae.

Considering the above points, a detailed history of prior pregnancies should be taken with respect to any history of high blood pressure record in previous pregnancy, fetal growth restriction or preterm birth, and spontaneous or induced labor (if induced reason for induction). Also, a detailed family history of thrombosis, recurrent pregnancy loss, still births, or birth defects should be taken in evaluation of RPL couples.

14.1.5 Genetic Factors

14.1.5.1 Parental Chromosomal Rearrangements

In approximately 2–5% of couples with recurrent miscarriage, one of the partners carries a balanced structural chromosomal anomaly, and the most common anomaly is balanced reciprocal or Robertsonian translocation [10].

Although carriers of a balanced translocation are usually phenotypically normal, their pregnancies are at increased risk of miscarriage and may result in a live birth with multiple congenital malformations and/or mental disability secondary to an unbalanced chromosomal arrangement.

14.1.5.2 Embryonic Chromosomal Abnormalities

In couples with recurrent pregnancy loss, chromosomal abnormalities of the embryo account for 30–57% of further miscarriages [11]. The risk of pregnancy loss resulting from chromosomal abnormalities of the embryo increases with advancing maternal age. However, it is important to note that as the number of miscarriages increases, the risk of euploid pregnancy loss also increases.

A detailed genetic history should be included in clinical workup of RPL couples. There should be history of previous cytogenetic results to determine any numeric chromosome abnormality [6].

Pedigree charts are useful in genetic studies. These are commonly used in family to track genetic disease and calculate the probability of child having that disorder.

14.1.6 Infective Agents

The presence of bacterial vaginosis in the first trimester of pregnancy has been reported as a risk factor for second-trimester miscarriage and preterm delivery [12], but the evidence for an association with first-trimester miscarriage is inconsistent. A randomized placebo-controlled trial [13] reported that treatment of bacterial vaginosis early in the second trimester with oral clindamycin significantly reduces the incidence of second-trimester pregnancy loss and preterm birth in the general population. History suggestive of post-abortion or postpartum fever (direct infection of the uterus, fetus, or placenta), prolonged foul-smelling or abnormal discharge per vaginum (endometritis), and sexually transmitted disease should be taken.

14.1.7 Lifestyle, Environmental, and Occupational Factors

History of exposure to smoking, alcohol, and caffeine along with sedentary lifestyle are important risk factors for pregnancy losses.

History of occupational and environmental exposure to organic solvents, medications, ionizing radiation, and toxins as they could possibly have a role in RPL should also be elicited.

14.2 Examination

A complete examination is a must so as to identify any previously undiagnosed systemic disorder. A general physical examination should be performed to detect signs of metabolic illness including PCOS, diabetes, hyperandrogenism, and thyroid or prolactin disorders. The points to be noted are:

Height, weight, and blood pressure: BMI (kg/m^2) may be abnormal in diabetics and in thyroid dysfunction
Thyroid swelling
Evidence of galactorrhea as seen in hyperprolactinemia
Skin texture
Clinical features of hyperandrogenemia such as hirsutism, acne, and acanthosis nigricans
Pedal edema
Pelvic examination: A per speculum and a bimanual pelvic examination to identify local infection, uterine size and shape, torn cervix, or a grossly short cervix and any gross uterine anomaly.

14.3 Recommended Investigations of Couples with RPL

Assessment of RPL focuses on screening for genetic factors and antiphospholipid syndrome, assessment of uterine anatomy, hormonal and metabolic factors, and lifestyle variables. These may include:

Screening for medical disease (diabetes, thyroid, prolactin disorders, and PCOS). Thyroid function should be assessed in women known to have a history of thyroid disease or with the clinical manifestations thereof. The American Thyroid Association recommends measuring serum thyroid-stimulating hormone in pregnant women in the following cases [14]:

- Symptomatic for thyroid disease
- From an area known with iodine insufficiency
- Family or personal history of thyroid disease
- Presence of thyroid peroxidase antibodies
- Type 1 diabetes
- History of preterm delivery or miscarriage
- History of head or neck radiation
- Morbid obesity
- Infertility

Screening of asymptomatic women for subclinical thyroid disease is controversial. However, certain authors recommend measurement of thyroid peroxidase antibodies in patients with RPL or preterm birth, where no other cause can be identified [15].

Investigations for PCOS include:

Lipid profile, glucose tolerance test, fasting insulin, serum LH/FSH ratio, and serum DHEAS level
Serum prolactin level
Blood sugar level and HbA1c level in suspected insulin resistance

14.3.1 Screening for Thrombophilia

14.3.1.1 Inherited

Testing for inherited thrombophilia in women with a history of unexplained RPL is controversial [9]. Screening should be done for factor V Leiden and prothrombin gene mutation (G2010A), as well as antithrombin III, protein C, and protein S deficiency [1] in cases with suspicious family history and personal or family history of venous thromboembolic events. Screening with fasting homocysteine levels or methylenetetrahydrofolate reductase mutation analyses is not recommended routinely [1]. A meta-analysis [16] from 31 retrospective studies reported that association between thrombophilia and late pregnancy loss has been consistently stronger than for early pregnancy loss. It also reported a strong association between second-trimester miscarriage and inherited thrombophilias: factor V Leiden, factor II (prothrombin) gene mutation, and protein S deficiency.

14.3.1.2 Acquired Antiphospholipid Syndrome

Antiphospholipid syndrome refers to the association between antiphospholipid antibodies, lupus anticoagulant, anticardiolipin antibodies, and anti-B2 glycoprotein-I antibodies and adverse pregnancy outcome or vascular thrombosis.

All women with RPL should be screened for antiphospholipid syndrome before the next pregnancy [17]. The workup includes testing for anticardiolipin IgG and IgM, lupus anticoagulant (LA) IgG and IgM, anti-B2 glycoprotein 1 IgG, and IgM antibodies. The tests should be done twice, 6–8 weeks apart, to rule out a false-positive result. The diagnosis of antiphospholipid syndrome requires at least two positive results for either lupus anticoagulant or anticardiolipin IgG or IgM antibodies. Women with one positive test result and a second negative test result should have a third test to confirm the diagnosis. False-positive results may be due to infection, suboptimal methods of sample collection and preparation, and lack of standardization of laboratory testing.

14.3.2 Anatomical Factors

All women with recurrent first-trimester miscarriages or with one or more second-trimester pregnancy loss should have a pelvic ultrasound scan to assess the uterine anatomy [1]. Thereafter, if uterine anomalies are suspected, hysterosalpingography can be done, and diagnosis can be confirmed using three-dimensional pelvic ultrasound. 3D USG has a sensitivity of 99.27 and 100% specificity to diagnose uterine anomalies. Other diagnostic modalities are hysteroscopy, laparoscopy or sonohysterography (it provides information on the internal contour of the uterus), and magnetic resonance imaging (MRI). MRI is seldom indicated because it is expensive, and its specificity and sensitivity varies between 33–100% and 29–100%, respectively.

Laparohysteroscopy is seen as the gold standard for the diagnosis of intrauterine anomalies, and most abnormalities can also be treated during the procedure; it has 100% sensitivity and specificity [18].

14.3.3 Karyotyping

14.3.3.1 Karyotyping of Products of Conception

Cytogenetic analysis should be performed on the products of conception of third and subsequent consecutive miscarriages. Structural chromosomal rearrangements in the fetus may be inherited or sporadic and are an indication for parental karyotyping. The most common inborn parental chromosomal abnormality that leads to recurrent abortion are balanced translocations. The live offspring will either be carrier of monosomy or trisomy for translocated chromosomal DNA. Trisomies (e.g., trisomy 13, 18, and 21) have better prognosis and survival than monosomies. Mosaicism along with insertions, deletions, and single-gene defect can also contribute to recurrent pregnancy loss.

The role of preimplantation genetic diagnosis (PGD) with IVF has been reviewed, and it has not been found to be cost-effective in the management of RPL [19]. In patients with RPL, the spontaneous birth rate is still 50%; with PGD the miscarriage rate may be decreased, but only 33% of women become pregnant after each PGD/IVF cycle.

14.3.3.2 Parental Peripheral Blood Karyotyping

Parental peripheral blood karyotyping of both partners should be performed in couples with recurrent miscarriage where testing of products of conception reports an unbalanced structural chromosomal abnormality.

14.4 Recommended Guidelines for Investigative Protocol of Couples with RPL

14.4.1 Royal College of Obstetricians and Gynecologists (RCOG) Guidelines

RCOG guidelines were first published in 1998, updated in 2003, and most recently updated in 2011. These guidelines recommend fetal karyotyping, 3D ultrasound, hydrosonography/hysteroscopy for uterine abnormalities, and antiphospholipid testing [20].

Parental karyotyping is no longer recommended except in the presence of unbalanced chromosomal abnormality in the products of conception. Moreover, assessment of thyroid function, antithyroid antibodies, alloimmune testing, and immunotherapy and assessment of TORCH and other infective agents are also not recommended. There is no role of assessment of bacterial vaginosis (BV) and progesterone and HCG supplementation. These guidelines suggest that there may be association of factor V Leiden deficiency or other hereditary thrombophilia with the second-trimester pregnancy loss but not with the first-trimester loss.

14.4.2 American Society of Reproductive Medicine (ASRM) Guidelines

These guidelines have replaced the American College of Obstetricians and Gynecologists (ACOG) guidelines.

They clearly warrant the investigation after two recurrent pregnancy losses. Unlike RCOG, ASRM clearly suggests that management can be tailored depending on the needs of individual patient, available resources, and limitations of particular institution or type of practice [21].

In contrast to RCOG guidelines, ASRM recommends parental karyotyping, and prenatal diagnosis should be offered if one of the patients is having chromosomal abnormality. It also recommends karyotyping of the abortus. Uterine cavity assessment should be done, and septum should be resected if present, for second-trimester loss. Screening of antiphospholipid antibodies is recommended with treatment with aspirin and unfractionated heparin rather than low molecular weight heparin. These guidelines recommend against screening for antithyroid antibodies and infective agents like chlamydia, mycoplasma or BV, alloimmune testing, parental leucocyte immunization, or intravenous immunoglobulin (IVIg).

14.4.3 European Society of Human Reproduction and Embryology (ESHRE) Guidelines [22]

These were published in 2006, and recently updated in Nov 2017. The diagnosis of RPL could be considered after the loss of two or more pregnancies. Ectopic and molar pregnancies are not included in RPL.

These guidelines discuss the investigations of cause and treatment interventions separately and don't figure level of evidence for its recommendation unlike RCOG. It recommends testing of blood sugar levels, thyroid testing, testing of antiphospholipid antibodies (LAC and ACL), parental karyotyping, and uterine cavity assessment by pelvic ultrasound or hysterosalpingography. Laparoscopy and hysteroscopy are categorized under "advanced investigations," but the "group of patients" whom to subject to these advanced investigations has not been mentioned. A new category of investigations under "framework of clinical trial" includes fetal karyotyping, natural killer (NK) cell testing, luteal phase endometrial biopsy, and homocysteine levels [22].

Table 14.1 Comparison between ESHRE, RCOG, and ASRM guidelines

Investigation/ treatment option	ESHRE (2017) [22]	RCOG (2011) [20]	ASRM (2012) [21]
Karyotyping			
Parental	R	NR	R
Fetal	Trials needed	R	R
Assessment of uterine cavity	R	R	IE
Resection of uterine septum	–	IE	Should be considered
Antiphospholipid assessment (ACA and LAC)	R	R	R
Infective agents			
TORCH	NR	NR	NR
Bacterial vaginosis	–	IE	NR
Thyroid function tests	R	–	R
Glucose challenge test	R	–	–
Prolactin estimation	–	–	R
Investigation of luteal phase defect	IE	–	NR
Hereditary thrombophilias	Recommended as advanced investigation	Recommended for midtrimester losses	NR
Alloimmune testing	IE	NR	NR
Immunotherapy	IE; RCTs needed for IVIg and third-party leucocytes; no proven effect of paternal leucocyte injection	NR	NR

RCOG Royal College of Obstetricians and Gynecologists, *ESHRE* European Society of Human Reproduction and Embryology, *APS* antiphospholipid syndrome, *RCT* randomized controlled trial, *IVIg* intravenous immunoglobulin, *TORCH* toxoplasma, rubella, cytomegalovirus, herpes, and others, *ACA* anticardiolipin antibody, *LAC* lupus anticoagulant, *R* recommended, *NR* not recommended, *IE* insufficient evidence

Table 14.1 shows the comparison between the three guidelines. Complete dependability on these guidelines will leave the clinicians in quandary, regarding which investigations to be done and what treatment to be offered. Thus there is a need to follow a tailored approach depending on the patient's clinical profile.

Conclusion

Evaluation of RPL can proceed after two or more consecutive clinical pregnancy losses. The evaluation of any couple with RPL should include a complete history, including their age, obstetric, gynecological, medical, surgical, genetic, social, and family history, as well as a physical examination. A detailed history of the previous losses is essential, including the gestational age. There should be focus on screening for hormonal and metabolic factors, antiphospholipid syndrome, assessment of uterine and cervix anatomical factors, and lifestyle variables.

Key Points

- A clinical evaluation of a case with RPL should include a complete history, including details of previous pregnancies, medical history and family history. A detailed systemic examination is required with along with assessment of BMI, thyroid, pedal edema, abdominal and pelvic examination.
- Assessment of RPL focuses on screening for genetic factors and antiphospholipid syndrome, assessment of uterine anatomy, hormonal and metabolic factors including diabetes, thyroid dysfunction.
- All women should undergo evaluation of anatomic factors by HSG, 3D ultrasound. Lapro-hysteroscopy is the gold standard in diagnosis.
- There is no uniform recommendation for screening for inherited thrombophilias, infective screen, antithyroid antibodies and karyotyping.

References

1. Practice Committee of the American Society for Reproductive Medicine. Definitions of infertility and recurrent pregnancy loss. Fertil Steril. 2008;89:1603.
2. Regan L, Backos M, Rai R. The investigation and treatment of couples with recurrent first-trimester and second-trimester miscarriage. RCOG Green-top Guideline No. 17. April 2010. Accessed 1 April 2011.
3. Salat-Baroux J. Recurrent spontaneous abortions. Reprod Nutr Dev. 1988;28:1555–68.
4. Regan L, Braude PR, Trembath PL. Influence of past reproductive performance on risk of spontaneous abortion. BMJ. 1989;299:541–5.
5. Stirrat GM. Recurrent miscarriage. Lancet. 1990;336(8716):673–5. http://dx.doi.org/10.1016/0140-6736(90)92159-F.
6. Hanson U, Persson B, Thunell S. Relationship between haemoglobin A1C in early type 1 (insulin-dependent) diabetic pregnancy and the occurrence of spontaneous abortion and fetal malformation in Sweden. Diabetologia. 1990;33:100–4.
7. Abalovich M, Gutierrez S, Alcaraz G, Maccallini G, Garcia A, Levalle O. Overt and subclinical hypothyroidism complicating pregnancy. Thyroid. 2002;12:63–8.
8. Grimbizis GF, Camus M, Tarlatzis BC, Bontis JN, Devroey P. Clinical implications of uterine malformations and hysteroscopic treatment results. Hum Reprod Update. 2001;7:161–74.
9. Lockwood C, Wendel G, Committee on Practice Bulletins—Obstetrics. Practice bulletin no. 124: inherited thrombophilias in pregnancy. Obstet Gynecol. 2011;118:730–40.
10. de Braekeleer M, Dao TN. Cytogenetic studies in couples experiencing repeated pregnancy losses. Hum Reprod. 1990;5:519–28.
11. Stephenson MD, Awartani KA, Robinson WP. Cytogenetic analysis of miscarriages from couples with recurrent miscarriage: a case-control study. Hum Reprod. 2002;17:446–51.
12. Leitich H, Kiss H. Asymptomatic bacterial vaginosis and intermediate flora as risk factors for adverse pregnancy outcome. Best Pract Res Clin Obstet Gynaecol. 2007;21:375–90.
13. Ugwumadu A, Manyonda I, Reid F, Hay P. Effect of early oral clindamycin on late miscarriage and preterm delivery in asymptomatic women with abnormal vaginal flora and bacterial vaginosis: a randomised controlled trial. Lancet. 2003;361:983–8.

14. Stagnaro-Green A, Abalovich M, Alexander E, et al. Guidelines of the American Thyroid Association for the diagnosis and management of thyroid disease during pregnancy and post-partum. Thyroid. 2011;21(10):1081–125. http://dx.doi.org/10.1089%2Fthy.2011.0087.
15. Alexander EK. Thyroid autoantibodies and pregnancy risk. Nat Rev Endocrinol. 2011;7(9):501–2.
16. Rey E, Kahn SR, David M, Shrier I. Thrombophilic disorders and fetal loss: a meta-analysis. Lancet. 2003;361:901–8.
17. Out HJ, Kooijman CD, Bruinse HW, Derksen RH. Histopathological findings in placentae from patients with intra-uterine fetal death and anti-phospholipid antibodies. Eur J Obstet Gynecol Reprod Biol. 1991;41:179–86.
18. Homer HA, Li TC, Cooke ID. The septate uterus: a review of management and reproductive outcome. Fertil Steril. 2000;73(1):1–14.
19. Christiansen O, Nybo Andersen A, Bosch E, Daya S, Delves PJ, Thomas V. Evidence-based investigations and treatments of recurrent pregnancy loss. Fertil Steril. 2005;83(4):821–39.
20. The investigation and treatment of couples with recurrent first trimester and second trimester miscarriage. Greentop guideline no. 17, Aprill 2011.
21. Jauniaux E, Farquharson RG, Christiansen OB, Exalto N. Evidence based guidelines for the investigation and medical treatment of recurrent miscarriage. Hum Reprod. 2006;21: 2216–22.
22. https://www.eshre.eu/Guidelines/Guidelines/Recurrent Pregnancy loss. Nov 2017.

Evidence Based Management in Recurrent Pregnancy Loss

15

Rashmi

Recurrent pregnancy loss (RPL) is defined as three pregnancy losses before the 20th week of gestation and excludes ectopic, molar, and biochemical pregnancies. The American Society of Reproductive Medicine (ASRM) recommends clinical evaluation following two first-trimester pregnancy losses [1]. RPL has been associated with factors related to genetics; age; anatomic, immunological, congenital, and acquired thrombophilias; errors of metabolism; hormonal imbalance; infections; sperm parameters; and lifestyle issues. But still despite a thorough evaluation, 50% of cases of RPL will remain unexplained (Fig. 15.1).

Evaluation and treatment are generally started after two consecutive miscarriages, more so if the couple have had infertility treatment or when the woman is older than 35 years of age.

RPL evaluation includes a complete history and diagnostic evaluation for all possible causes enumerated in Table 15.1. There is paucity of level one evidence in literature regarding the investigations to establish etiology and therapeutic interventions. The evidence-based treatment available will be discussed in this chapter.

15.1 Genetic Factors

Miscarriages due to chromosomal abnormalities either structural or numerical are seen in 30–57% of cases, most common being aneuploidy [2]. Autosomal trisomy is commonest and present in approximately 50% of chromosomally abnormal

Rashmi
Obstetrics and Gynecology, University College of Medical Sciences and GTB Hospital, Delhi, India
e-mail: rashmi.malik2011@gmail.com

S. Mehta, B. Gupta (eds.), *Recurrent Pregnancy Loss*,
https://doi.org/10.1007/978-981-10-7338-0_15

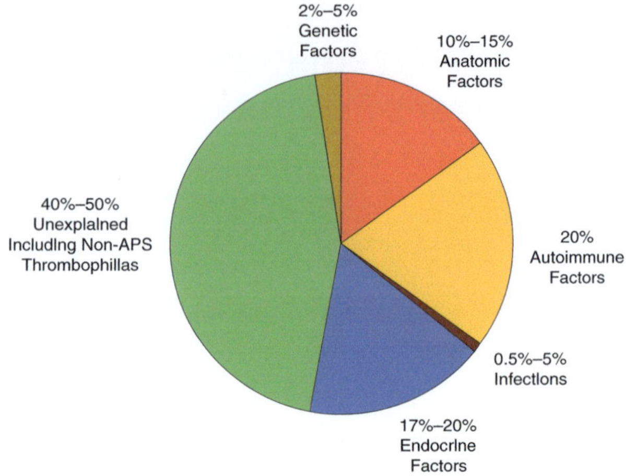

Fig. 15.1 Etiology of recurrent pregnancy loss

APS Antiphospholipid syndrome

Table 15.1 Definitions of pregnancy and RPL

Pregnancy	Pregnancy is confirmed by ultrasonography or histopathologic examination
Clinical miscarriage	When the pregnancy loss occurs before the 20th week of gestation
RPL: classic definition	Three pregnancy losses before the 20th week of gestation; it does not include ectopic, molar, and biochemical pregnancies
RPL: evaluation indicated according to ASRM	Clinical evaluation may proceed when a patient comes with history of two first-trimester pregnancy losses
Primary RPL	RPL in a patient who has never had a live birth
Secondary RPL	RPL in a patient who has had at least one live birth

abortuses. In cases of RPL with parental chromosomal abnormality, the options may include preimplantation genetic diagnosis (PGD) and in vitro fertilization (IVF) and gamete donation. In cases of RPL with recurrent aneuploidy, the option may include preimplantation genetic screening (PGS) and IVF.

15.1.1 Preimplantation Genetic Testing

Women with translocation errors should be offered IVF and prenatal genetic testing. There is lack of evidence supporting PGS in RPL as prospective trials comparing placebo with IVF-PGD are lacking [3]. Only several case series have been published which have shown lesser miscarriages and shorter time to successful pregnancy but have not considered the emotional and financial cost of a failed cycle [3, 4].

IVF with PGD is an expensive option and has not been found to be cost-effective in management of RPL [5].

The only large intent-to-treat study in carriers of translocations was carried out by Scriven and colleagues [6]. They concluded that PGS is beneficial for patients with a high risk of unbalanced viable offspring but not so for couples with lower-risk translocations. Such conceive more quickly without PGS and have a high rate of healthy offspring with spontaneous conception.

Though assisted reproduction provides genetic screening to patients who have an increased risk of aneuploidy, the evidence is limited [7, 8]. Pregnancy rates are better when embryo biopsy is done at the blastocyst stage, as opposed to the cleavage stage, and using 23 chromosome microarrays has further improved the rates [9, 10]. Preimplantation genetic screening as a treatment of recurrent miscarriage is still not recommended due to lack of evidence (Evidence level II).

15.1.2 Donor Gametes

Genetic conditions that always cause embryonic aneuploidy are helped by using donor gametes.

15.2 Anatomic Causes of RPL

Congenital and acquired uterine anomalies are found in 10–15% of women with RPL compared with 7% of all reproductive-aged women [10]. Of these uterine anomalies, intrauterine adhesions and uterine fibroids or polyps are the commonest.

15.2.1 Congenital Uterine Anomalies

A review of several studies found that congenital uterine anomalies are present in 4.3% of normal population (range 2.75–16.7%) and in 12.6% (range 1.5–37.6%) of patients with RPL [11]. A high rate of miscarriage occurred in patients with septate ($n = 5499$, 44.3% loss), bicornuate ($n = 5627$, 36.0% loss), and arcuate ($n = 5241$, 25.7% loss) uteri.

At present, there is no prospective study evaluating the efficacy of uterine surgery. In a case-control study by Sugiura-Ogasawara et al., surgical resection of uterine septums showed beneficial effects ($n = 5366$, live birth rate 83.2%, range 77.4–90.9%) [12].

Limited evidence shows that almost normal pregnancy outcomes are seen in patients undergoing hysteroscopic septum resection. They have a term delivery in approximately 75% and live birth rates in about 85% [13]. Sixty percent of women who do not undergo septal resection also have a successful pregnancy in 78%. Therefore, more evidence is needed to recommend metroplasty in these women [12] (Evidence level II).

15.2.2 Acquired Uterine Abnormalities

Surgical intervention in patients with RPL with acquired uterine abnormalities, such as adhesions, polyps, retained products of conception, and fibroids, is debated. Only fibroids that distort the uterine cavity, such as the ones located in the cavity and intramural fibroids with an intracavitary component, result in infertility and recurrent miscarriage. The role of myomectomy in smaller leiomyomas is unclear.

Excessive curettage of endometrium or genital tuberculosis leads to intrauterine adhesions (Asherman's syndrome) thus impairing implantation. There are no randomized controlled trials showing that surgical intervention decreases the subsequent miscarriage rate; however, the consensus is that hysteroscopic correction of these defects is helpful because of the potential impact on subsequent fertility, miscarriage, and pregnancy outcomes.

15.2.3 Cervical Incompetence

Cervical incompetence commonly causes pregnancy loss in the second trimester. Uterine abnormalities such as septate or bicornuate uterus are causative in causing incompetence of cervix. It may also be acquired following conization, loop electrosurgical excision procedures, obstetric injury, and over-dilatation of the cervix during termination of pregnancy. There are no diagnostic tests to confirm cervical insufficiency. Cervical incompetence is treated with expectant management, cervical cerclage, and/or progestogen therapy.

According to a meta-analysis of four trials, cerclage in women with a history of previous preterm birth and a short cervix helps in continuation of pregnancy [14, 15] (Evidence level 1). The American College of Obstetricians and Gynecologists (ACOG) and Royal College of Obstetricians and Gynecologists (RCOG) recommend that cerclage should be offered to women if their cervical length is less than 2.5 cm on ultrasound before 24 weeks gestation. This is more pertinent if such women have a history of one or more spontaneous midtrimester losses or preterm births [16, 17]. Women with history of three or more previous preterm births and/or second-trimester losses should also undergo cerclage.

The CERVO trial showed no added benefit of cervical occlusion to cerclage [18]. Evidence supports emergency cerclage as compared to bed rest [19] (Evidence level III). Shirodkar technique for ultrasound-indicated cerclage is better compared to the McDonald cerclage in singleton pregnancies (Evidence level III) [20]. However, vaginal progesterone and mechanical pessary are equally effective when short cervix is detected on midtrimester scan (Evidence level II) [21]. Cervical length is not very accurate predictor of preterm delivery [22].

15.3 Endocrinologic Causes of RPL

Endocrine factors may contribute to 8–12% of recurrent pregnancy loss and so an evaluation for endocrine disorders should form part of workup of women with RPL.

15.3.1 Thyroid Disorders

The cutoff for normal upper limit of TSH in pregnancy is still unclear, but the aim should be to maintain baseline TSH < 2.5 mU/L [1, 23]. In early pregnancy, requirement of thyroid hormone is higher [1, 24]. Women with raised TPO antibodies with raised TSH should be given levothyroxine. However, observation suggests that empirical thyroxine therapy in TPO Ab-positive women with normal TSH does not improve outcome status [25]. The randomized controlled trial, thyroid antibodies and levothyroxine study (TABLET), is ongoing, and the primary objective is to study the pregnancy and neonatal outcomes with levothyroxine treatment in women positive for thyroid peroxidase antibody (TPO) and normal thyroid function tests (http://www.controlled-trials.com/ISRCTN15948785/). The trial results will be available in 2018. Thus, in the absence of good evidence, thyroxine treatment is not recommended in women if they are positive for thyroid antibody, but the thyroid function tests are normal (Evidence level III).

15.3.2 Diabetes Mellitus

Poorly controlled diabetes is associated with pregnancy loss, and blood sugar should be properly controlled with insulin and/or oral hypoglycemic drugs like metformin and glyburide. Increase in early pregnancy loss and congenital malformations is well correlated to high-glycosylated hemoglobin (HbA1C) values (>8%) [24]. In women with well-controlled diabetes mellitus, there is no increased risk of miscarriage.

15.3.3 Hyperprolactinemia

Hyperprolactinemia causes changes in hypothalamic-pituitary-ovarian axis, thereby impairing follicle formation, abnormal maturation of oocyte, and short luteal phase. A randomized trial demonstrated improvement in pregnancy outcomes after prolactin levels fell down to normal following treatment with dopamine agonist [26].

15.3.4 Luteal Phase Deficiency

Luteal phase deficiency (LPD) is defined as endometrial development unsuitable for embryonic implantation due to decreased progesterone levels due to corpus luteum insufficiency. The use of histologic and/or biochemical testing for diagnosis is unreliable and not reproducible (Evidence level III) [27]. Therefore assessment for luteal phase defect in women with RPL is not advocated.

15.3.5 Empirical Progesterone Supplementation

Progesterone supplementation is usually given empirically in cases of RPL for not only to correct any undiagnosed luteal phase defect but also due to immunomodulatory role of the progesterone.

A Cochrane review of four small trials showed that women who received progesterone had a significantly lower risk of miscarriages than those who received placebo or no treatment [28]. A more recent double-blind, placebo-controlled, randomized trial of oral dydrogesterone also showed that progesterone was helpful in reducing subsequent miscarriage [29]. Rates of live births were not assessed in any of these trials. According to a large, randomized, placebo-controlled trial (Progesterone in Recurrent Miscarriages [PROMISE]), progesterone therapy in the first trimester of pregnancy does not significantly increase live births among women with a history of unexplained recurrent miscarriages [30]. In this study progesterone treatment was initiated after pregnancy confirmation, and so it is difficult to say whether progesterone supplementation could be more effective if given before pregnancy is confirmed, i.e., in the luteal phase.

The types of progesterone supplements vary; but in general, intramuscular injections and vaginal suppositories are the most widely used. Oral progesterone is ineffective at increasing uterine progesterone levels. Recommendations differ on the timing of empirical progesterone supplement. Traditionally, progesterone administration was given after ovulation in the luteal phase.

Although evidence demonstrating benefit is not very clear, progesterone supplementation is advisable as there is no harm following treatment. With the PROMISE trial's results, routine use of progesterone in early pregnancy in cases of RPL doesn't seem beneficial (Evidence level II). Routine use of progesterone is not recommended and is entirely based on clinician's discretion (Evidence level III).

15.3.6 PCO, Elevated LH, and Insulin Resistance

Mechanisms of RPL include hypersecretion of basal LH and insulin resistance [31, 32]. The role of metformin for treatment in RPL is not clear. Some studies have shown that metformin may reduce insulin levels, thus reducing the risk of miscarriage by restoring normal hemostasis [33]. In women with RPL and associated PCOS, metformin treatment is not advocated (Evidence level III).

15.3.7 Diminished Ovarian Reserve

Miscarriages are increased in women with an increased level of follicle-stimulating hormone (FSH), a low anti-Mullerian hormone (AMH), and a diminished antral follicle count. Although these conditions cannot be treated, their presence should be followed up with appropriate counseling.

15.4 Immune Factors in RPL

Immune factors implicated as cause of RPL can be either autoimmune or alloimmune.

15.4.1 Autoimmune Factors: Antiphospholipid Antibody Syndrome (APS)

The treatment of documented APS consists of low-dose aspirin (usually 75 mg daily) preconceptionally and heparin (usually 5000 units by subcutaneous injection twice a day) beginning with a positive pregnancy test, reducing miscarriage rates by 54% [34, 35]. Aspirin or low-molecular-weight heparin alone has not been found much useful [36].

Glucocorticoids can be used in secondary APS with underlying connective tissue disorder. Obstetric outcomes in APS have not shown to improve and may be associated with an increased risk of gestational hypertension and gestational diabetes after addition of prednisone [35].

Multiple large randomized trials examining the use of heparin and/or aspirin in women with RPL not meeting strict criteria for APS have shown no difference in clinical outcomes [37]. Therefore, the use of heparin and aspirin should be limited to only women who have met both the clinical and laboratory criteria for APS.

15.4.2 Alloimmune Factors (Immunotherapy)

Although immunological mechanisms have been implicated as an important cause of RPL, there is no evidence for routine testing for immunological causes of recurrent miscarriages, and testing for peripheral blood natural killer (NK) cells and cytokine tests is not done (Evidence level I).

Treatments designed to develop immune tolerance, such as paternal white blood cell immunization (also known as lymphocyte immunization therapy), donor leukocytes, and trophoblast membranes, have not been shown to be effective at decreasing the risk of miscarriage and also do not increase the live birth rate [38]. Randomized controlled trials using intravenous immunoglobulin (IvIG) have shown them to be ineffective [37, 39, 40]. Further sub-analyses revealed increase in the rates of live birth in secondary recurrent miscarriage with IvIG [41]. Complications with IvIG include immunological side effects and risk of transmitting infections like cytomegalovirus. Investigations and treatment for immunological causes should be only in research context [39, 40] (Evidence level II).

15.4.3 Hereditary Thrombophilias

Screening for inherited thrombophilias may be justified in patients with either a personal history of thrombosis or a first-degree relative who is a high risk for thrombophilia and recurrent miscarriage [1]. Unlike APS, the role of low molecular weight heparin for treatment of thrombophilia-related RPL is not very clear due to lack of good-quality studies, and treatment is only recommended to prevent thromboembolism [41, 42] (Evidence level I).

15.4.4 Hyperhomocysteinemia and MTHFR Mutation

Testing for MTHFR mutation is routinely recommended [39] (Evidence level II). The use of high-dose folic acid (5 mg) and vitamin B12 (0.5 mg once daily) for treatment of recurrent miscarriage is not recommended, although they help reduce levels of homocysteine (Evidence level III).

15.5 Microbiologic Factors as a Cause of RPL

Routine screening for infectious agents in patients with RPL is not recommended [1]. The use of empirical antibiotics in patients with asymptomatic RPL is not supported by randomized prospective studies [1].

There is no need to test for TORCH group of infections when investigating recurrent miscarriage (Evidence level II) except syphilis which needs to be treated before next pregnancy.

Bacterial vaginosis (BV) is an important risk factor for preterm delivery and late miscarriages, and screening for BV is recommended in women at high risk for the same [41]. Oral clindamycin early in the second trimester is recommended for treatment (Evidence II).

15.6 Male Factor

Association between sperm DNA defragmentation and recurrent miscarriage is not significant, and tests are not recommended in clinical practice outside research settings (Evidence level II) [40].

A semen analysis and/or referral to a urologist may be informative in couples taking longer than expected to conceive, but no sperm testing should be considered for routine evaluation for a couple with RPL [1].

15.7 Environmental and Psychological Factors

Association between stress, environmental toxins, and addictions has not been shown to be significant [43]. RPL is extraordinarily impactful on a patient's emotional well-being, and awareness of the psychological needs of these patients is important. The grief and sense of loss for these couples can manifest itself in all aspects of personal and work life and may impact success with future pregnancies. Lifestyle modification by improvements in diet, exercise, abstinence from drugs, and stress reduction improve pregnancy outcomes (Evidence level III).

15.8 Unexplained Recurrent Miscarriage

In the absence of any cause for repeated miscarriages, unproven therapies, especially if they are invasive and expensive, should not be undertaken. Reassurance and emotional support are the most effective in such cases.

15.8.1 Tender Loving Care and Lifestyle Advice

The strategy of emotional support and reassurance works well in unexplained cases as even no treatment shows a good prognosis in 60–80% cases (Evidence level III) [1]. Some small prospective studies have shown a positive influence in patients with RPL with the use of tender loving care (TLC) defined as psychological support with weekly medical and ultrasound [44].

15.8.2 Drug Therapy

There is no role of aspirin in unexplained RPL [45] (Evidence level II). As mentioned earlier, after the PROMISE trial, there seems to be no role of progesterone in cases of RPL (Evidence level II). Further evidence is required whether progesterone started in luteal phase is helpful (Evidence level III). The role of LMWH is only established in APS, and its use in other clinical situations of preventing RPL is not recommended (Evidence level II). Evidence also fails to support the use of hCG for preventing miscarriages (Evidence level II) [46]. The evidence to recommend the use of steroids, IV immunoglobulins, or intralipid for unexplained recurrent miscarriage is weak (Evidence level III).

Table 15.2 Diagnosis and management of RPL

Etiology	Diagnostic evaluation	Therapy
Genetic	Parental karyotyping POC karyotyping	Genetic counseling Donor gamete, PGD/PGS
Anatomic	2D USG Hysterosalpingography Hysteroscopy Sonohysterography Transvaginal 3D ultrasound MRI	Resection of septum Myomectomy Adhesions lysis
Endocrinologic	Progesterone (midluteal) TSH Serum prolactin Glycosylated HbA1c	Progesterone Supplement thyroxine Bromocriptine/cabergoline Metformin
Immunologic	Lupus anticoagulant Anticardiolipin antibodies Anti B2 glycoprotein	Aspirin + heparin
Psychologic	Interview and counseling	Support group
Iatrogenic	Obesity, addiction to smoking, alcohol, exposure to chemicals	Eliminate consumption Eliminate exposure

POC products of conception; *PGD/PGS* preimplantation diagnosis/screening, *TSH* thyroid-stimulating hormone, *USG* ultrasonography

Table 15.2 summarizes the evidence-based investigative workup of cases of RPL, and recommendations by various societies are compared in Table 15.3.

To conclude, treatment for recurrent miscarriage is still an obstetrician's dilemma as there is lack of randomized studies and multicenter trials, and treatment strategies are still based on expert opinions (Table 15.4).

Key Points

- Couples with unexplained recurrent miscarriage have a high chance of a successful outcome with empathic care and support and no medical treatment.
- The role of surgical correction of uterine anomaly is not well established in improving pregnancy outcomes.
- Antiphospholipid syndrome is successfully treated with aspirin and heparin; however, the role in inherited thrombophilia is not well established.
- Routine chromosomal analysis of products of conception is not recommended in resource poor settings although it may yield useful prognostic information.
- Balanced translocations are seen in 2–4% patients and is of limited clinical relevance.
- Role for immunotherapy is limited. Role of metformin, hCG, and progesterone therapy is also unclear.

Table 15.3 Evidence-based workup of couples with recurrent pregnancy loss

Genetic counseling and screening
– All patients should undergo genetic counseling and karyotyping of products of conception – Amniocentesis: all women of advanced maternal age – Parental karyotyping: This is done when karyotyping of the abortus is abnormal or in men with family history of genetic abnormalities
ACAs (IgG and IgM) and lupus anticoagulant
– Should be done in all women, before the next pregnancy. At least two readings 6–8 weeks apart should be undertaken
Mullerian anomalies
– Pelvic ultrasound and hysteroscopy should be done in all patients – Treatment is according to the anomaly detected
Screening for infection
– Universal screening for syphilis and bacterial vaginosis in women with risk of preterm delivery and late recurrent miscarriage
TSH, fasting glucose/HbA1c
– Routine screening is recommended in all women with RPL

ACAs anticardiolipin antibodies, *TSH* thyroid-stimulating hormone, *HbA1c* glycosylated hemoglobin

Table 15.4 Comparison of three protocols for investigations and treatment of RPL

Investigation or treatment	RCOG protocol [5]	ASRM protocol [1]	ESHRE protocol
Parental karyotyping	Not recommended	Recommended	Recommended
Fetal karyotyping	Recommended	Recommended	Trial required
Uterine cavity assessment	Recommended	Insufficient evidence	Recommended
Resection of septum	Insufficient evidence	Should be considered	–
APS assessment (ACA and LA)	Recommended	Recommended	Recommended
APS treatment with aspirin and heparin	Recommended	Recommended	Insufficient evidence
Luteal phase investigation	–	Not recommended	Insufficient evidence trials required
Progesterone supplementation	Insufficient evidence	Insufficient evidence	Insufficient evidence more RCTs required
hCG supplementation	Insufficient evidence	–	–
Bacterial vaginosis	Insufficient evidence	Not recommended	–
Hereditary thrombophilias	Recommended for second-trimester losses	Not recommended	Recommended as advanced investigation
Anticoagulants for hereditary thrombophilias	Insufficient evidence	–	Insufficient evidence
Thyroid function	–	Recommended	Recommended

(continued)

Table 15.4 (continued)

Investigation or treatment	RCOG protocol [5]	ASRM protocol [1]	ESHRE protocol
Glucose challenge test	–	–	Recommended
Prolactin estimation	–	Recommended	–
TORCH	Not recommended	Not recommended	Not recommended
Alloimmune testing	Not recommended	Not recommended	Insufficient evidence
Immunotherapy	Not recommended	Not recommended	Insufficient evidence. RCT required for IVIg and third-party leucocyte. PLI no proven effect
Tender loving care	Insufficient evidence	Recommended	Recommended
Diet, smoking, alcohol	–	–	Recommended
Folic acid for hyperhomocysteinemia	–	–	Insufficient evidence
Vitamin supplementation	–	–	Not recommended
Steroids	Not recommended	Not recommended	Not recommended

Note: *RCOG* Royal College of Obstetricians, *ASRM* American Society of Reproductive Medicine, *ESHRE* European Society of Human Reproduction and Embryology, *APS* antiphospholipid syndrome, *RCT* randomized controlled trial, *IVIg* intravenous immunoglobulin G

References

1. Practice Committee Opinion of the American Society of Reproductive Medicine. Evaluation and treatment of recurrent pregnancy loss: a committee opinion. Fertil Steril. 2012;98:1103–11.
2. Regan L, Backos M, Rai R. The investigation and treatment of couples with recurrent first-trimester and second-trimester miscarriage. RCOG Green-top Guideline No. 17. April 2010. http://www.rcog.org.uk/files/rcog-corp/GTG17recurrentmiscarriage.pdf.
3. Fischer J, Colls P, Escudero T, et al. Preimplantation genetic diagnosis (PGD) improves pregnancy outcome for translocation carriers with a history of recurrent losses. Fertil Steril. 2010;94:283–9.
4. Lim CK, Jun JH, Min DM, et al. Efficacy and clinical outcome of preimplantation genetic diagnosis using FISH for couples of reciprocal and Robertsonian translocations: the Korean experience. Prenat Diagn. 2004;24:556–61.
5. Christiansen OB, Nybo Andersen AM, Bosch E, Daya S, Delves PJ, Hviid TV, et al. Evidence-based investigations and treatments of recurrent pregnancy loss. Fertil Steril. 2005;83:821–39.
6. Scriven PN, Flinter FA, Khalaf Y, et al. Benefits and drawbacks of preimplantation genetic diagnosis (PGD) for reciprocal translocations: lessons from a prospective cohort study. Eur J Hum Genet. 2013;21:1035–41.
7. Mastenbroek S, Twisk M, van Echten-Arends J, et al. In vitro fertilization with preimplantation genetic screening. N Engl J Med. 2007;357:9–17.
8. Practice Committee of Society for Assisted Reproductive Technology, Practice Committee of American Society for Reproductive Medicine. Preimplantation genetic testing: a Practice Committee opinion. Fertil Steril. 2008;90:S136–43.
9. Forman EJ, Tao X, Ferry KM, et al. Single embryo transfer with comprehensive chromosome screening results in improved ongoing pregnancy rates and decreased miscarriage rates. Hum Reprod. 2012;27:1217–22.

10. Acien P, Acien M, Sanchez-Ferrer M. Complex malformations of the female genital tract. New types and revision of classification. Hum Reprod. 2004;19:2377–84.
11. Grimbizis GF, Camus M, Tarlatzis BC, et al. Clinical implications of uterine malformations and hysteroscopic treatment results. Hum Reprod Update. 2001;7:161–74.
12. Sugiura-Ogasawara M, Ozaki Y, Katano K, Suzumori N, Mizutani E. Uterine anomaly and recurrent pregnancy loss. Semin Reprod Med. 2011;29:514–21.
13. Shahine L, Lathi R. Recurrent pregnancy loss: evaluation and treatment. Obstet Gynecol Clin North Am. 2015;42:117–34.
14. Berghella V, Odibo AO, To MS, Rust OA, Althuisius SM. Cerclage for short cervix on ultrasonography: meta-analysis of trials using individual patient-level data. Obstet Gynecol. 2005;106:181–9.
15. Owen J, Hankins G, Iams JD, Berghella V, Sheffield JS, Perez-Delboy A, et al. Multicenter randomized trial of cerclage for preterm birth prevention in high-risk women with shortened midtrimester cervical length. Am J Obstet Gynecol. 2009;201:375.e1–8.
16. American College of Obstetrics and Gynecologist. ACOG practice bulletin No 142. Cerclage for the management of cervical insufficiency. Obstet Gynecol. 2014;123(2 Pt 1):372–9.
17. Royal College of Obstetricians & Gynecologists. Green Top Guidelines No 60. Cervical cerclage. https://www.rcog.org.uk/en/guidelines-research-services/guidelines/gtg60.
18. Brix N, Secher NJ, McCormack CD, Helmig RB, Hein M, Weber T, et al. Randomised trial of cervical cerclage, with and without occlusion, for the prevention of preterm birth in women suspected for cervical insufficiency. BJOG. 2013;120:613–20.
19. Namouz S, Porat S, Okun N, Windrim R, Farine D. Emergency cerclage: literature review. Obstet Gynecol Surv. 2013;68:379–88.
20. Hume H, Rebarber A, Saltzman DH, Roman AS, Fox NS. Ultrasound-indicated cerclage: Shirodkar vs. McDonald. J Matern Fetal Neonatal Med. 2012;25:2690–2.
21. Conde-Agudelo A, Romero R, Nicolaides K, Chaiworapongsa T, O'Brien JM, Cetingoz E, et al. Vaginal progesterone vs. cervical cerclage for the prevention of preterm birth in women with a sonographic short cervix, previous preterm birth, and singleton gestation: a systematic review and indirect comparison metaanalysis. Am J Obstet Gynecol. 2013;208:42.e1–8.
22. Melamed N, Hiersch L, Domniz N, Maresky A, Bardin R, Yogev Y. Predictive value of cervical length in women with threatened preterm labor. Obstet Gynecol. 2013;122:1279–87.
23. Groot LD, Abalovich M, Alexander EK, et al. Management of thyroid dysfunction during pregnancy and postpartum: an Endocrine Society clinical practice guideline. J Clin Endocrinol Metab. 2012;97:2543–65.
24. Greene MF, Hare JW, Cloherty JP, et al. First-trimester hemoglobin A1 and risk for major malformation and spontaneous abortion in diabetic pregnancy. Teratology. 1989;39:225–31.
25. Yan J, Sripada S, Saravelos SH, Chen ZJ, Egner W, Li TC. Thyroid peroxidase antibody in women with unexplained recurrent miscarriage: prevalence, prognostic value, and response to empirical thyroxine therapy. Fertil Steril. 2012;98:378–82.
26. Hirahara F, Andoh N, Sawai K, Hirabuki T, Uemura T, Minaguchi H. Hyperprolactinemic recurrent miscarriage and results of randomized bromocriptine treatment trials. Fertil Steril. 1998;70:246–52.
27. Murray MJ, Meyer WR, Zaino RJ, et al. A critical analysis of the accuracy, reproducibility, and clinical utility of histologic endometrial dating in fertile women. Fertil Steril. 2004;81:1333–43.
28. Haas DM, Ramsey PS. Progestogen for preventing miscarriage. Cochrane Database Syst Rev. 2013;(10):CD003511.
29. Kumar A, Begum N, Prasad S, Aggarwal S, Sharma S. Oral dydrogesterone treatment during early pregnancy to prevent recurrent pregnancy loss and its role in modulation of cytokine production: a double-blind, randomized, parallel, placebo-controlled trial. Fertil Steril. 2014;102(5):1357.e3–63.e3.
30. Coomarasamy A, Williams H, Truchanowicz E, Seed PT, et al. A randomized trial of progesterone in women with recurrent miscarriages. N Engl J Med. 2015;373:2141–8.

31. Rai R, Backos M, Rushworth F, Regan L. Polycystic ovaries and recurrent miscarriage: a reappraisal. Hum Reprod. 2000;15:612–5. [PubMed: 10686206].
32. Li ZL, Xiang HF, Cheng LH, Cao YX, Wei ZL, Liu C, et al. Association between recurrent miscarriages and insulin resistance: a meta analysis. Zhonghua Fu Chan Ke Za Zhi. 2012;47:915–9.
33. Carrington B, Sacks G, Regan L. Recurrent miscarriage: pathophysiology and outcome. Curr Opin Obstet Gynecol. 2005;17:591–7.
34. de Jong PG, Kaandorp S, Di Nisio M, et al. Aspirin and/or heparin for women with unexplained recurrent miscarriage with or without inherited thrombophilia. Cochrane Database Syst Rev. 2014;(7):CD004734.
35. Lockshin MD, Druzin ML, Qamar T. Prednisone does not prevent recurrent fetal death in women with antiphospholipid antibody. Am J Obstet Gynecol. 1989;160:439–43.
36. Ziakis PD, Pavlou M, Voulgarelis M. Heparin treatment in antiphospholipid syndrome with recurrent pregnancy loss. A systematic review and meta-analysis. Obstet Gynecol. 2010;115:1256–62.
37. Hutton B, Sharma R, Fergusson D, et al. Use of intravenous immunoglobulin for treatment of recurrent miscarriage: a systematic review. BJOG. 2007;114:134–42.
38. Porter TF, LaCoursiere Y, Scott JR. Immunotherapy for recurrent miscarriage. Cochrane Database Syst Rev. 2006;(2):CD000112.
39. Creus M, Deulofeu R, Peñarrubia J, Carmona F, Balasch J. Plasma homocysteine and vitamin B12 serum levels, red blood cell folate concentrations, C677T methylenetetrahydrofolate reductase gene mutation and risk of recurrent miscarriage: a case-control study in Spain. Clin Chem Lab Med. 2013;51:693–9.
40. Zini A. Are sperm chromatin and DNA defects relevant in the clinic? Syst Biol Reprod Med. 2011;57:78–85.
41. Leitich H, Kiss H. Asymptomatic bacterial vaginosis and intermediate flora as risk factors for adverse pregnancy outcome. Best Pract Res Clin Obstet Gynaecol. 2007;21:375–90.
42. Kaandorp S, Di Nisio M, Goddijn M, Middeldorp S. Aspirin or anticoagulants for treating recurrent miscarriage in women without antiphospholipid syndrome. Cochrane Database Syst Rev. 2009;(1):CD004734.
43. Niekerk EC, Siebert I, Kruger TF. An evidence based approach to recurrent pregnancy loss. S Afr J Obstet Gynaecol. 2013;19(3):61–5.
44. Stray-Pedersen B, Stray-Pedersen S. Etiologic factors and subsequent reproductive performance in 195 couples with a prior history of habitual abortion. Am J Obstet Gynecol. 1984;148:140–6.
45. Kaandorp SP, Goddijn M, van der Post JA, Hutten BA, Verhoeve HR, Hamulyák K, et al. Aspirin plus heparin or aspirin alone in women with recurrent miscarriage. N Engl J Med. 2010;362:1586–96.
46. Morley LC, Simpson N, Tang T. Human chorionic gonadotrophin (hCG) for preventing miscarriage. Cochrane Database Syst Rev. 2013;(1):CD008611.

Part III

Beyond Convention

16 Establishing a One-Stop Recurrent Pregnancy Loss Clinic

Pooja Sikka

16.1 Introduction

Recurrent pregnancy loss (RPL) is associated with significant psychological grief, hopelessness, and anxiety in a couple. These keep on increasing further as the number of miscarriages increase. The couple obviously seeks an explanation for the miscarriages. Expectations from the doctor are thus very high, especially in those with no identifiable cause. Hence part from comprehensive evaluation, emphasis should also be on compassionate care [1–4]. A lot of time is required for counseling which should be sympathetic, scientific, and evidence based.

In a routine obstetrics and gynecology clinic, there is a mix of patients, and the attending doctor deals with all kinds of problems. Moreover, in public hospitals there is a huge rush of patients with a low doctor to patient ratio. After waiting in long queues for her interaction with the doctor, the woman is sometimes only handed over a long list of investigations at the initial visit, and the average time per patient is not more than 10–15 min. When she comes back, she meets a new doctor who does not have any clue about her history. This can further aggravate fear, anger, depression, and guilt in these women. The situation can sometimes become difficult to manage.

An exclusive, dedicated team for this vulnerable group of women is thus needed. An outpatient clinic with reproductive gynecologists specialized in evidence-based RPL care can be established to provide a focused treatment to the couple. The clinic apart from doctors should also have a team of nurses, ultrasound technologists, and counselors. Medical students, resident doctors, and student technologists may also be involved. This clinic should be a one-stop recurrent pregnancy loss clinic where at one time and one place the examination,

P. Sikka
Department of Obstetrics and Gynaecology, Postgraduate Institute of Medical Education and Research, Chandigarh, India
e-mail: drpoojasikka@yahoo.com

S. Mehta, B. Gupta (eds.), *Recurrent Pregnancy Loss*,
https://doi.org/10.1007/978-981-10-7338-0_16

evaluation, and treatment can be provided to the couple. A recurrent miscarriage clinic should be organized in such a way that individual care from one doctor is provided to the couple and a clear roadmap is provided regarding further evaluation and treatment [5]. Working in the clinic, the doctor and his team should try to establish underlying risk factors or cause for recurrent pregnancy loss in the couple as quickly as possible.

16.2 Logistic Requirements

16.2.1 The "Care" Team

Comprehensive management of patients with RPL requires teamwork with close coordination between different caregivers. The team should comprise of the following members:

1. *Consultant gynecologists* who have special interest in the field can come together in the establishment of clinic. RPL care should be provided by only one doctor per couple.
2. *Paramedical staff and nurses* to assist the doctors during examination and procedures. It is important that all staff dealing with RPL couples should be trained in emotional aspects of pregnancy loss.
3. *Geneticist* for genetic counseling in the setting of abnormal karyotype in one of the parents or of the aborted fetus or embryo can help affected parents in deciding the further plan.
4. *Counselors* are essential for emotional support of both the patient and her partner. Depression and feelings of hopelessness can persist for a long time after pregnancy loss. Counselors can provide empathetic support themselves and can also arrange participation of the couples in support groups. Counselors may pick up signs of depression in the couple. Consultation by a psychiatrist should be advised in patients with significant anxiety and depression.
5. *Administrative staff* is required to coordinate management and provide a contact point for the patient.
6. *Lab technicians* for investigative workup.

16.2.2 Location

Patients with RPL may be upset if they see women with normal pregnancies and small children while waiting in the clinic. Thus the RPL clinic should not be located close to the antenatal clinic. Instead, it can be a part of the gynecology outpatient clinic. At least two rooms are required, one room for history taking and performing physical examination and another for counselors. Counselors should ideally be provided with a separate room for privacy. A separate area for performing transvaginal examination should be maintained.

16.2.3 Record Keeping

Good record keeping is essential. History, examination, and sonographic findings should be documented and secured. A standardized protocol for workup should be used. In this way, all patients will be asked same standard basic questions, and chance of missing an important finding will be low.

16.2.4 Laboratory Services

Laboratory services form the backbone of the workup of RPL patients and should ideally be provided under a single roof. Access to a basic facility is needed where hematological, biochemical, and microbiological workup can be carried out. Multidisciplinary support will be provided by other departments such as clinical genetics, pathology, endocrinology, internal medicine, radiology, and hematology.

The basic set up of the clinic has been shown in Fig. 16.1.

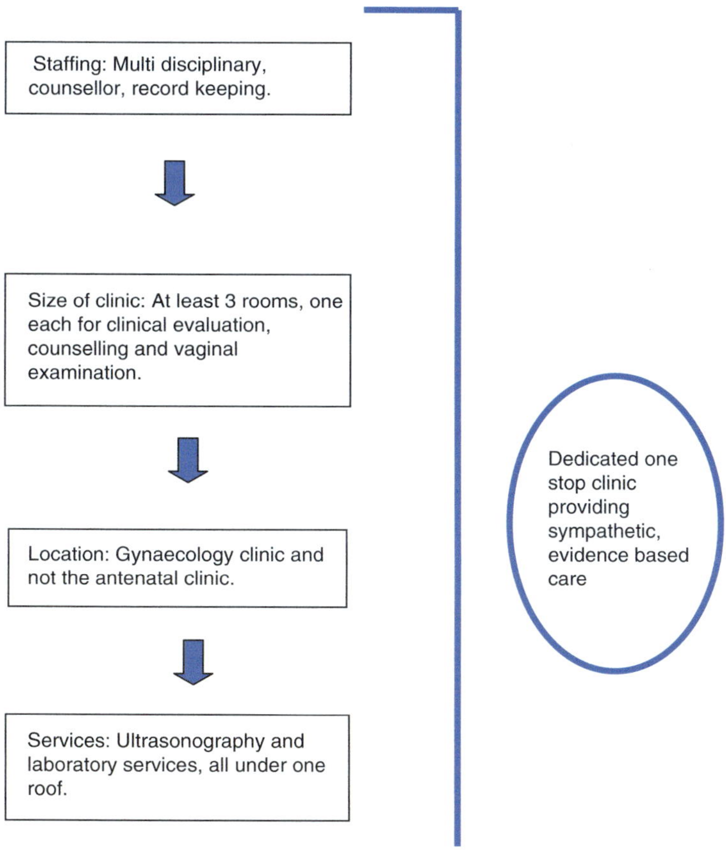

Fig. 16.1 Basic setup of recurrent pregnancy loss clinic

16.3 Who Should Be Referred to the RPL Clinic?

Women with recurrent pregnancy loss represent a very heterogeneous population. In some of them, RPL is attributable to chance alone, while in others there is a genuine cause which cannot be identified by basic investigations. The traditional definition of RPL includes those couples with three or more spontaneous, consecutive pregnancy losses. The American Society of Reproductive Medicine has defined it as a distinct disorder characterized by two or more failed clinical pregnancies [6]. Ideally, a woman with three or more recurrent pregnancy losses should be referred to the RPL clinic. However, clinical evaluation may proceed following two first-trimester pregnancy losses also, especially when the woman is older than 35 years of age or when the couple had difficulty in conceiving [7, 8].

16.4 RPL Clinic Protocol

What constitutes a complete evaluation is still not clearly defined. Clinicians often do not adhere to clinical guidelines regarding RPL. There are wide variations in the investigation and treatment protocols even today. Past studies have focused on endocrine and immunological causes of RPL. Recent research is focused on spermatozoa, embryonic, and endometrial causes behind RPL [9, 10]. Out of desperation, patients and the doctors try to overdiagnose and overtreat. The management of each patient should be individualized according to the medical history and the presence or absence of risk factors.

The following protocol may be followed in the RPL clinic:

First visit: Patients referred to this clinic with RPL will normally have had a first consultation with a gynecologist or an obstetrician. Occasionally, it may be a self-referral by the couple. At their first visit to the RPL clinic, a detailed history with regard to prior miscarriages and medical, social, obstetric, and family factors should be taken. A standardized protocol should be used for documentation of the history and examination findings. Participation of both the partners should be encouraged. Decision to perform diagnostic tests will depend largely on individual history and examination findings. The couple should be reassured that all risk factors for RPL would be explored. However, all couples need not go through all diagnostic tests. Diagnostic tests should not be performed just to reassure the woman that something is being done and should be tailored according to the clinical findings. Both partners should be made aware of the workup before they leave the clinic. The further plan should be discussed in detail.

Subsequent visits: The results of the diagnostic tests should be discussed. Treatment options should be explained. At the second visit, the couple should be seen by a counselor. Contact details of the counselor should preferably be provided to the patient. This relieves anxiety, enforces faith of the patient, and also facilitates any emergency care if required. Couples need not make many visits to the clinic. Two to three visits are enough for making a future plan for the couple.

If the couple achieves pregnancy, the RPL clinic should arrange an ultrasound scanning and discuss the future plan for the pregnancy. The woman should then directly be booked in the antenatal clinic or high-risk pregnancy clinic. In case the pregnancy ends up in a missed abortion, facility for medical method of termination of pregnancy or a surgical evacuation should be available.

Conclusion

To conclude, couples with recurrent pregnancy loss need dedicated and supportive clinical care. They need a doctor who is accessible, listens to them, has knowledge of their obstetric history, and gives them information about their recurrent losses. Tender loving care and health advice are one of the main treatments of RPL. Thus all women who present with recurrent pregnancy loss should have access to a specialized one-stop clinic where they can be guided by one doctor. Establishment of dedicated clinics will increase the understanding of pathophysiology of recurrent pregnancy loss, enhance research work in this field, and would result in a more favorable and successful outcome for the couples.

Key Points

- An exclusive, one-stop, dedicated clinic and team is required for management of couples with RPL where diagnosis, investigations, and treatment can be provided at the same place.
- The team should consist of a specialized doctor, nurses, geneticist, ultrasonologist, counselors, and laboratory support staff.
- RPL clinic should not be located close to the antenatal clinic and can be a part of the gynecology outpatient clinic.
- Woman with three or more recurrent pregnancy losses or older woman (>35 years of age) with history of infertility after two first-trimester pregnancy losses should be referred to an RPL clinic.

References

1. Royal College of Obstetricians and Gynaecologists. Green top guideline No. 17. The investigation and treatment of couples with recurrent first trimester miscarriage and second trimester miscarriage. RCOG. 2011.
2. American College of Obstetricians and Gynecologists. ACOG practice bulletin. Management of recurrent pregnancy loss. Number 24, February 2001. (Replaces Technical Bulletin Number 212, September 1995). American College of Obstetricians and Gynecologists. Int J Gynaecol Obstet. 2002;78:179–90.
3. Musters AM, Koot YE, van den Boogaard NM, et al. Supportive care for women with recurrent miscarriage: a survey to quantify women's preferences. Hum Reprod. 2013;28:398–405.
4. Liddell HS, Pattison NS, Zanderigo A. Recurrent miscarriage—outcome after supportive care in early pregnancy. Aust N Z J Obstet Gynaecol. 1991;31:320–2.
5. Habayeb OM, Konje JC. The one-stop recurrent miscarriage clinic: an evaluation of its effectiveness and outcome. Hum Reprod. 2004;19:2952–8.
6. Practice Committee of the American Society for Reproductive Medicine. Evaluation and treatment of recurrent pregnancy loss: a committee opinion. Fertil Steril. 2012;98:1103–11.

7. Committee on Gynecologic Practice of American College of Obstetricians and Gynecologists; Practice Committee of American Society for Reproductive Medicine. Age-related fertility decline: a committee opinion. Fertil Steril. 2008;90(5 Suppl):S154–5.
8. Practice Committee of the American Society for Reproductive Medicine. Aging and infertility in women. Fertil Steril. 2006;86(5 Suppl 1):S248–52.
9. Smith ML, Schust DJ. Endocrinology and recurrent early pregnancy loss. Semin Reprod Med. 2011;29:482–90.
10. Cumming DC, Honoré LH, Scott JZ, Williams KP. The late luteal phase in infertile women: comparison of simultaneous endometrial biopsy and progesterone levels. Fertil Steril. 1985;43:715–9.

Role of Imaging

17

Vaishali Upadhyaya

17.1 Introduction

Recurrent pregnancy loss (RPL), defined as three consecutive pregnancy losses occurring before 20 weeks from the last menstrual period, is a cause of physical and emotional stress for affected women [1]. As the risk of further pregnancy loss increases after each such event, diagnostic evaluation becomes important. If the cause of RPL can be ascertained and subsequently treated, if possible, such patients may be able to carry and deliver safely and need not relive the entire traumatic experience.

Anatomic abnormalities which are responsible for RPL in about 10–15% cases include congenital uterine anomalies, intrauterine adhesions, submucosal fibroids or large intramural fibroids, and endometrial polyps [1]. Cervical incompetence can be considered among the acquired causes, though it causes pregnancy loss in the second trimester.

The imaging modalities used for diagnosis and radiological features of each of these abnormalities will be described in this chapter.

17.2 Imaging Modalities

17.2.1 Hysterosalpingography (HSG)

It is the primary screening modality used to evaluate patients with RPL. Water-soluble contrast medium such as Urografin (diatrizoate meglumine) is instilled into the uterine cavity through a catheter placed in the cervical canal after which radiographs are taken which show early uterine filling, completely distended uterus and

V. Upadhyaya
Department of Radiodiagnosis, Vivekananda Polyclinic and Institute of Medical Sciences, Ramkrishna Mission Sewashram, Lucknow, India
e-mal: vshali77@yahoo.co.in

S. Mehta, B. Gupta (eds.), *Recurrent Pregnancy Loss*,
https://doi.org/10.1007/978-981-10-7338-0_17

fallopian tubes, and intraperitoneal spillage of contrast. The procedure is performed during days 7–12 of the menstrual cycle, and the patient is asked to abstain from intercourse till the day of the examination. Image analysis is facilitated by proliferative thin endometrium. Prior to the procedure, it is important to rule out pregnancy and acute pelvic infection as these are absolute contraindications. Complications of the procedure include bleeding, pain, and infection. Other rare complications include a reaction to the contrast material, uterine perforation, and radiation exposure of an early pregnancy [2].

17.2.2 Ultrasound (US)

Two-dimensional (2D) transvaginal sonography (TVS) is a widely available low-cost imaging modality for evaluation of the uterus and adnexa. It is noninvasive and there is no radiation exposure during the procedure. It provides good-quality images of pelvic lesions with the use of high-frequency transducers. Problems which are encountered in transabdominal scanning (TAS) such as evaluation of obese women, those unable to fill their bladder, or retroverted uterus are overcome by TVS [3].

An US examination can also be supplemented by color Doppler to assess the vascularity of any detected pathology. The recent development of three-dimensional (3D) sonography has further enhanced the diagnostic capability of sonography. 3D sonography provides a coronal image of the uterus and enables assessment of the endometrium, myometrium as well as superior serosal aspect of the uterus. Thus, 3D sonography is superior to 2D imaging with the added advantage of not being operator dependent [4, 5]. It also is noninvasive and allows complete assessment of uterine morphology. Uterine dimensions can be measured, thus evaluating the likely success of any surgical intervention.

Sonohysterography (SHG) is sometimes performed in patients with RPL. Here, sterile saline is instilled into the endometrial cavity under transvaginal sonographic guidance. This enables good visualization of the endometrium and can help differentiate between endometrial and myometrial lesions. Patency of the fallopian tubes can also be assessed [6]. The procedure is carried out between fourth and tenth day of the menstrual cycle. This ensures the presence of a thin endometrium which facilitates diagnosis. A pre-procedure TVS is done to assess uterine size, cervical orientation, any obvious mass lesion, or evidence of active pelvic infection in which case the examination may have to be delayed. To ensure a successful examination, a comforting environment, counseling of the patient, use of warmed speculum and saline, gradual saline infusion, and pre-procedure nonsteroidal anti-inflammatory drug (NSAID) are useful measures [6].

17.2.3 Magnetic Resonance Imaging (MRI)

It is an excellent imaging modality for evaluation of the uterus and adnexa which can accurately characterize Mullerian duct anomalies and other abnormalities detected on US or HSG and help to decide appropriate management [7]. Its advantages include high contrast resolution, multiplanar imaging, noninvasive nature, and absence of exposure to ionizing radiation. These reasons have made it increasingly popular and greatly decreased the need for a computed tomography (CT) scan which requires intravenous contrast and exposes patients to ionizing radiation.

A combination of T1-weighted and T2-weighted sequences in axial plane and T2-weighted sequence in coronal and sagittal planes is usually performed for pelvic MRI. A coronal T2-weighted sequence to cover the lower abdomen especially the kidneys is indicated in uterovaginal anomalies. Fat suppression and gadolinium-based contrast that enhanced T1-weighted sequence may be acquired whenever indicated [8]. However, gadolinium-based contrast media are nephrotoxic, and the patient's renal profile needs to be assessed before contrast administration. In patients with cardiac pacemakers, cerebral aneurysm clips, cochlear implants, or ferromagnetic foreign bodies in the eye globe, MRI is contraindicated as the strong external magnetic field may induce their movement and harm the patient.

Patient should fast for about 3–6 h before the procedure. She can empty her bladder about 1–2 h before the examination. A full bladder is not required as wall contraction can lead to motion artifacts [8]. Anti-spasmodics may be given to improve image quality. In females of reproductive age, the uterus shows intermediate signal intensity in T1-weighted images. T2-weighted images nicely delineate its zonal anatomy. The innermost endometrium appears bright or hyperintense. The middle junctional zone which is the innermost layer of the myometrium appears dark or hypointense. The outer myometrium shows intermediate signal intensity. The cervix shows a central hyperintense zone due to cervical epithelium and mucus and an outer hypointense zone due to fibrous stroma [9].

A comparison of MRI with 3D ultrasound is shown in Table 17.1.

17.3 Ultrasound Findings in Early Pregnancy Loss

When a patient with suspected pregnancy loss comes for an US, it is important for the sonologist to diagnose the miscarriage and also characterize it as either complete, incomplete, or delayed. Terms such as trophoblastic bleeding, anembryonic sac, and blighted ovum are discouraged, and they should not be used while reporting the scan. Miscarriage is considered complete on US when endometrial thickness is <15 mm and there is no evidence of retained products. It is incomplete when there is a heterogeneous lesion within the endometrial cavity. In cases of delayed miscarriage, the diameter of the gestational sac is 20 mm or more without a fetal pole/yolk sac, or the fetal pole measures more than 6 mm without cardiac activity (Fig. 17.1). Pregnancy loss can also be classified as early or late. In early pregnancy loss, there is either an empty gestational sac or fetus <12 weeks without cardiac activity. In late pregnancy loss, loss of fetal cardiac activity occurs after 12 weeks [10, 11].

Besides the size of the gestational sac, other supportive signs of pregnancy loss include deformed contour of the gestational sac, poor echogenicity of the

Table 17.1 Comparison of MRI and 3D ultrasound in etiology of RPL

Modality	Advantages	Limitations	Sensitivity/specificity
MRI	– No radiation exposure – No use of iodinated contrast – Noninvasive – Both external fundal contour and the uterine cavity can be assessed – Can differentiate between septate and bicornuate uteri – Can assess length and thickness of the uterine septum – Can simultaneously assess renal anomalies – Enables detection of cervical and vaginal septa – Can differentiate between short subseptate and arcuate uteri – Can detect small uterine remnants	Not suitable for claustrophobic patients Cannot be done if patient has a pacemaker or other contraindications for MRI May miss rare anomalies Distortion of image anatomy by large fibroids	Sensitivity of 77–100% Specificity of 33–100% PPV of 83–100% NPV of 25–100% (Mullerian duct anomalies)
3D US	– No radiation exposure – Low cost – Less time-consuming – Better tolerated (no claustrophobia) – Iodinated contrast media not required – Noninvasive – Can show external fundal contour as well as the uterine cavity – Can differentiate between septate and bicornuate uteri – Can assess length and thickness of the uterine septum – Can simultaneously assess renal anomalies	Poor resolution in very obese patients Limited ability to detect small uterine remnants Difficulty in recognition of intermediate forms of bicornuate and septate uteri May miss rare anomalies Distortion of image anatomy by large fibroids	Sensitivity of 86.6–100% Specificity of 96.9–100% PPV of 99.3–100% NPV of 54.4–100% (Mullerian duct anomalies)

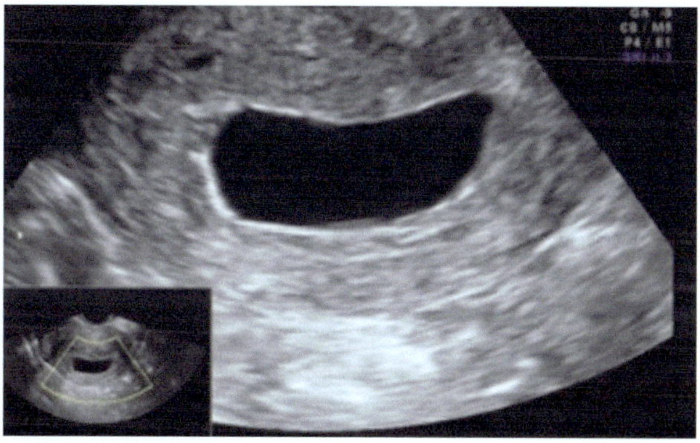

Fig. 17.1 US image in a case of early miscarriage showing a large gestational sac without a fetal pole or yolk sac (Image Courtesy—Dr. Manju (Handa) Virmani, New Delhi)

trophoblast, <2 mm thickness of the trophoblastic reaction, and an abnormal low position of the gestational sac [3].

Some other sonographic findings are suggestive of a poor outcome of the pregnancy. These include embryonic bradycardia (FHR <80 beats/min with CRL <5 mm, FHR <100 beats/min with CRL 5–9 mm, and FHR <110 beats/min with CRL 10–15 mm), cardiac arrhythmia, mean diameter of the gestation sac <5 mm greater than the CRL at 5.5–9 weeks gestation age, very small or abnormally large yolk sac, calcified yolk sac, subchorionic hematoma, and disproportionately large amniotic sac [3, 12].

Doppler evaluation can show high-pressure blood flow in the decidual spiral arteries with RI (resistivity index) >0.55. This is associated with increased flow in the intervillous space with detachment of immature villi and miscarriage. Women with RPL also have increased PI (pulsatility index) of the uterine artery [13, 14].

17.4 Ultrasound Markers of Aneuploidy

There is also need to emphasize the importance of assessing the previous imaging records of patients with RPL. It is possible that there may be signs of aneuploidy in the fetus prior to miscarriage. In that case, the management of the patient will be different, and she is likely to be advised serum biochemical screening and karyotyping.

The commonest aneuploidy is trisomy 21 or Down syndrome. The sonographic marker used for its detection is nuchal translucency (NT). This is an anechoic fluid collection in the subcutaneous plane behind the neck of the fetus (Figs. 17.2 and 17.3). It occurs due to mesenchymal edema associated with improper lymphatic development. NT is thickened if its value is more than 95% for CRL. There is a 35% risk of chromosomal anomaly if NT is more than 3 mm in the first trimester [15]. A thickened NT is also seen in trisomy 18 and 13. Fetuses with thickened NT show increased risk for congenital anomalies such as cardiac defects, diaphragmatic hernia, abdominal wall defects, and body stalk anomalies. For proper measurement of the NT, the fetus should be in midsagittal plane and should occupy majority of the

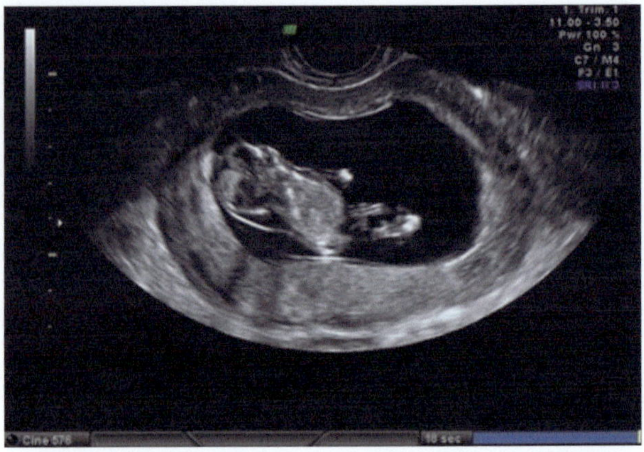

Fig. 17.2 US image of a fetus with thickened nuchal translucency (Image Courtesy—Dr. Manju (Handa) Virmani, New Delhi)

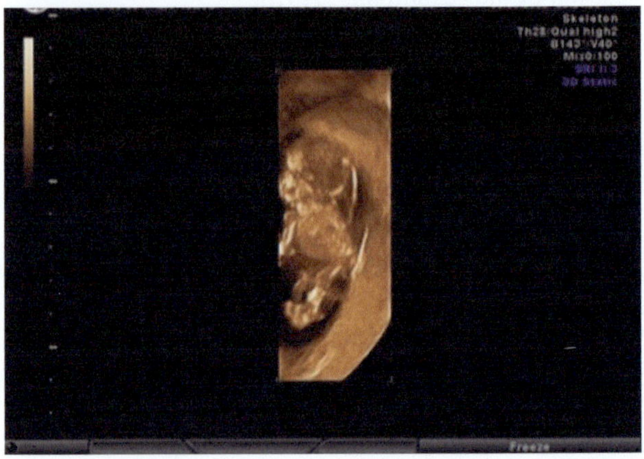

Fig. 17.3 3D US image of another fetus with thickened nuchal translucency (Image Courtesy—Dr. Manju (Handa) Virmani, New Delhi)

image with the head in neutral position. The tip of nose should be seen in profile. The measurement is made perpendicular to the long axis of the fetus and is repeated thrice. The largest of the three values is then recorded [3].

Other markers for aneuploidies in the first trimester include cystic hygroma which is a multiseptate fluid collection behind the fetal neck and upper back (Fig. 17.4), flattened facies, reversal of blood flow in the ductus venosus, and tricuspid regurgitation.

Sonographic markers in the second trimester for detection of aneuploidies include thickened nuchal fold, absence of fetal nasal bone, echogenic bowel, echogenic intracardiac focus, mild pyelectasis, and short humeral length. All these markers have been variably associated with trisomy 21. The nuchal fold is measured in an axial section of the fetal head which includes the thalami, cerebellar hemispheres, cisterna magna, and occipital bone. It extends from the occipital bone till the skin surface, and a finding of 5 mm or more is considered abnormal. Bowel is considered echogenic if its appearance is similar to the adjacent bone. In mild pyelectasis, the anteroposterior diameter of the renal pelvis is 4 mm or more [3].

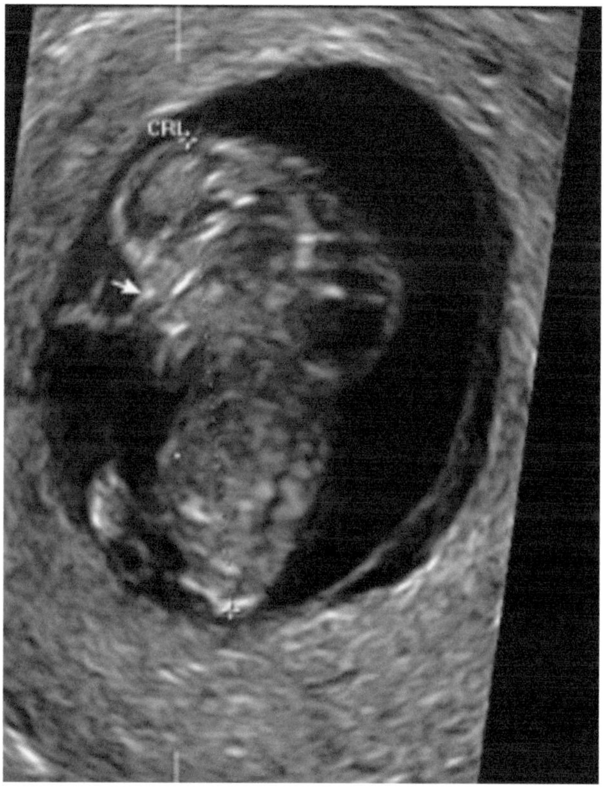

Fig. 17.4 US image of a fetus with a cystic hygroma seen as a multiseptate collection behind the fetal neck (Image Courtesy—Dr. Manju (Handa) Virmani, New Delhi)

17.5 Imaging Findings in Etiology of RPL

17.5.1 Congenital Uterine Anomalies

Detection and characterization of Mullerian duct anomalies (MDAs) are of immense importance in women with RPL. Nearly 15% of women with RPL have such anomalies [16].

A classification given by the American Society of Reproductive Medicine divides MDAs into class I–VII. Uterine hypoplasia and agenesis are seen in class I. Class II includes unicornuate uterus, class III is uterus didelphys, class IV is bicornuate uterus, class V is septate uterus, class VI is arcuate uterus, and class VII is diethylstilbestrol-related anomalies [17].

Among these uterine anomalies, the septate, bicornuate, and unicornuate uteri are associated with increased risk of midtrimester pregnancy loss. The arcuate uterus is associated with increased risk of miscarriage in the second trimester [18–20]. Proposed factors for miscarriage in patients with uterine anomalies include implantation on the septum which has a different composition and vascularity than the rest of the uterine walls and differences in uterine vasculature [21].

Although HSG findings can besuggestive of MDAs, it cannot differentiate between the different types. An important limitation is that the external uterine contour cannot be assessed. A review of many studies by Saravelos et al. showed that HSG had a sensitivity of 78%, specificity of 90%, positive predictive value (PPV) of 83%, negative predictive value (NPV) of 91%, and accuracy of 86% in the diagnosis of congenital uterine anomalies when compared with hysteroscopy [22]. 2D US has a sensitivity of less than 60% although specificity is nearly 100%. Hence, both HSG and 2D US can be useful only for screening of these anomalies [22, 23].

3D US and MRI are the preferred modalities for diagnosis and characterization of MDAs. They allow assessment of external uterine contour as well as associated renal anomalies. 3D US has a reported accuracy of about 90–92%, and MRI has a very high accuracy of about 100% for characterization of MDAs [7, 23]. 3D US has a sensitivity of 86.6–100%, specificity of 96.9–100%, PPV of 99.3–100%, and NPV of 54.4–100% for the diagnosis of Mullerian duct anomalies [5, 24, 25]. MRI has a sensitivity of 77–100%, specificity of 33–100%, PPV of 83–100%, and NPV of 25–100% for the diagnosis of Mullerian duct anomalies [25–27].

MRI scores over 3D US in the depiction of septal and vaginal anomalies as well as uterine remnants. Despite this, MRI has some limitations which occur due to lack of a combined clinical and radiological classification of the anomalies, failure to identify rare anomalies, distortion of uterine anatomy by fibroids, and misinterpretation of cervical mucosal fold as a septum [28]. Some patients may be claustrophobic and may need sedation. In some others, there may be contraindications to MRI. Here, 3D US is the best alternative. It is cheaper and widely available, provides images of high resolution, and is not operator dependent [28]. The scan time is also shorter and there is no exposure to ionizing radiation.

17.5.1.1 Septate Uterus

This is the commonest anomaly in patients with RPL having a reported prevalence of 6.1% [21]. Differentiating a septate uterus from a bicornuate uterus by imaging is important as management of these patients is different [29].

If the external fundal contour is normal, it suggests a septate uterus, whereas in a bicornuate uterus, there is a cleft in the external fundal contour. Initial imaging by HSG can be helpful, but it has a diagnostic accuracy of only 55% in differentiating between a septate and bicornuate uterus. In a septate uterus, the angle of divergence between the two uterine cavities is less than or equal to 75° (Fig. 17.5a, b). When this angle is more than 105°, a bicornuate uterus is likely. In case the angle is between 75° and 105°, further imaging studies are required to establish the diagnosis [30].

2D US is not very helpful in differentiating between septate and bicornuate uteri, but 3D US can help establish the diagnosis as it enables visualization of the external fundal contour in the coronal plane (Figs. 17.6 and 17.7). The dimensions of the septum and cavity volume can also be calculated [31]. The fundal contour is normally either convex, flat, or has a subtle concavity. The upper muscular part of the septum shows similar echogenicity as the rest of the myometrium but inferiorly appears hypoechoic due to fibrous composition.

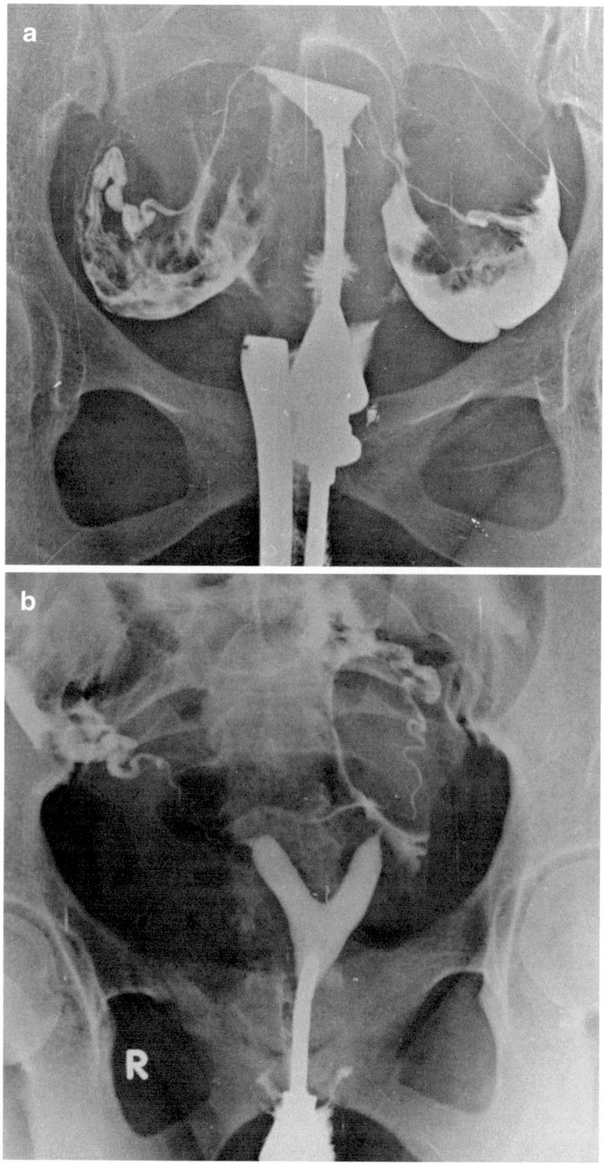

Fig. 17.5 (**a**) HSG image of a normal uterus with an inverted triangle appearance. The tubes are patent with bilateral free peritoneal spillage of contrast. (**b**) HSG image of a septate uterus (partial). The angle of divergence between the two uterine cavities is less than 75°

In the coronal plane, an interostial line can be drawn. If the apex of the fundal contour is more than 5 mm above this line, it suggests a septate uterus. In a bicornuate or didelphys uterus, the apex of the fundal contour is below this line or less than 5 mm above it [29].

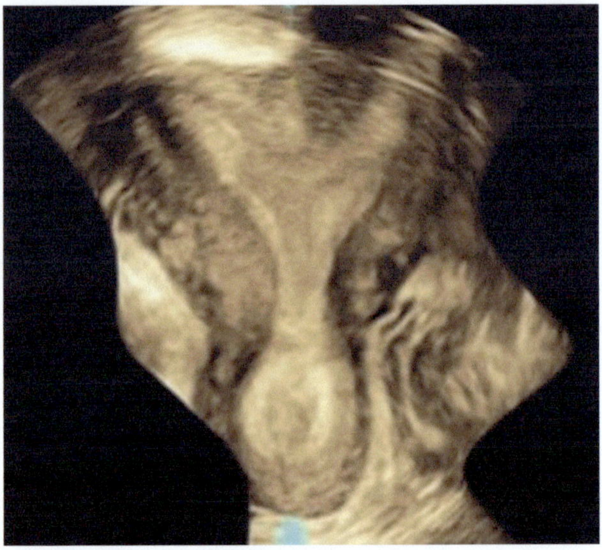

Fig. 17.6 3D US image of a septate uterus showing normal external fundal contour (Image Courtesy—Dr. Manju (Handa) Virmani, New Delhi)

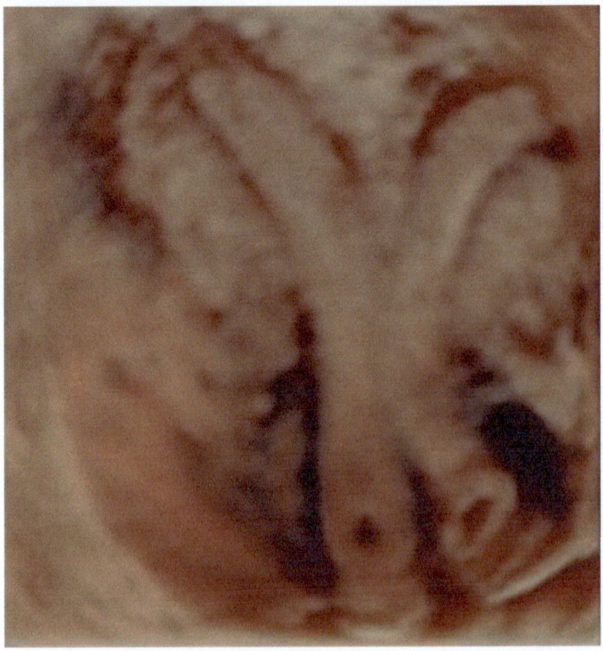

Fig. 17.7 3D US image of a septate uterus. (complete) where the septum is extending till the external os (Image Courtesy—Dr. Manju (Handa) Virmani, New Delhi)

MR imaging in the coronal plane nicely delineates the septate uterus and enables assessment of the extent and nature of the septum (Fig. 17.8a, b). A muscular septum appears thick with signal intensity similar to rest of myometrium in T2-weighted images, whereas a fibrous septum appears thin with hypointense signal in T2-weighted images [7]. An advantage of MRI over 3D US is that it can also identify vaginal septa. These appear hypointense as compared to the vaginal walls [31].

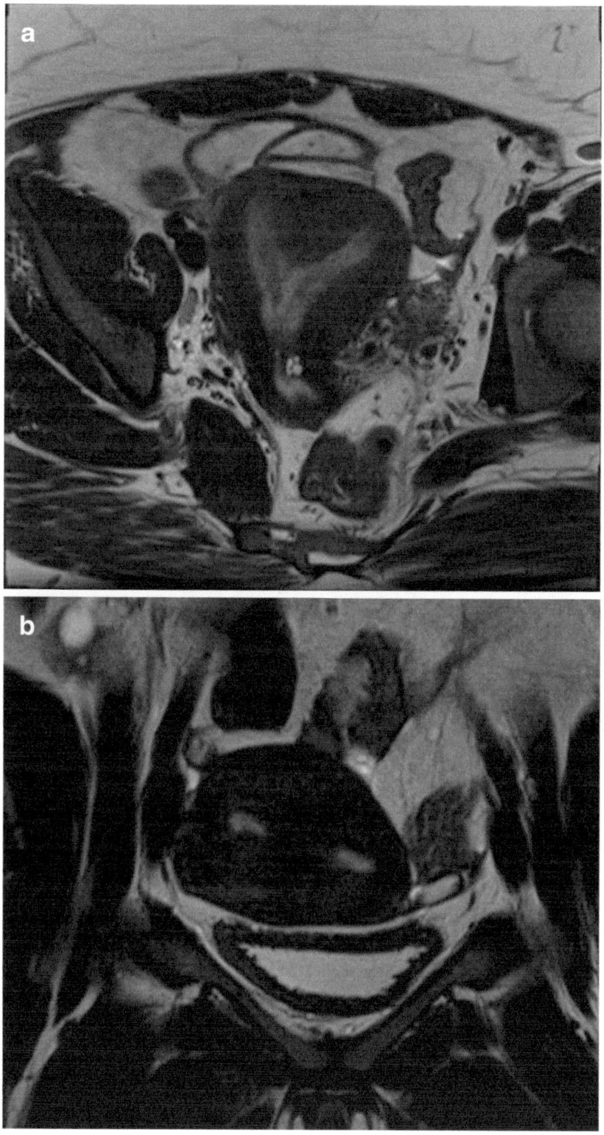

Fig. 17.8 (**a**) and (**b**) Axial and Coronal T2-weighted MR images showing a uterine septum (partial). The external fundal contour is normal

17.5.1.2 Bicornuate Uterus

HSG shows two symmetric fusiform uterine horns, each with its own fallopian tube. If the angle of divergence between them is more than 105°, it suggests a bicornuate uterus [30] (Fig. 17.9). 3D US can show a deep fundal cleft with divergent uterine horns (Fig. 17.10). The optimal time to demonstrate the separate uterine cavities is when the endometrium appears echogenic during the secretory phase of the menstrual cycle [23]. The diagnosis may be difficult when the uterus is extremely

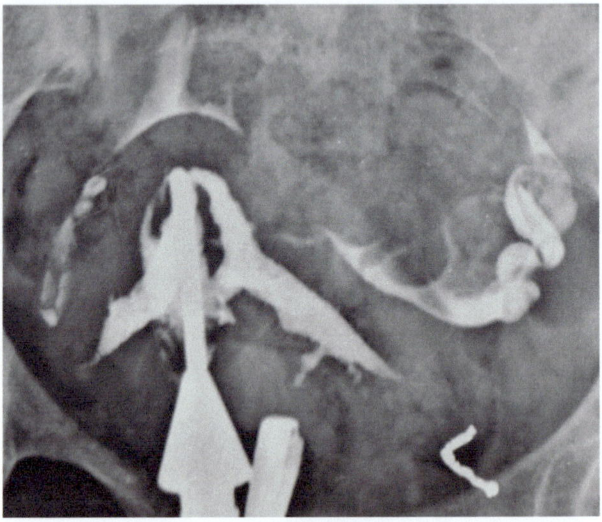

Fig. 17.9 HSG image of a bicornuate unicollis uterus where the angle of divergence between the two uterine cavities is more than 105°

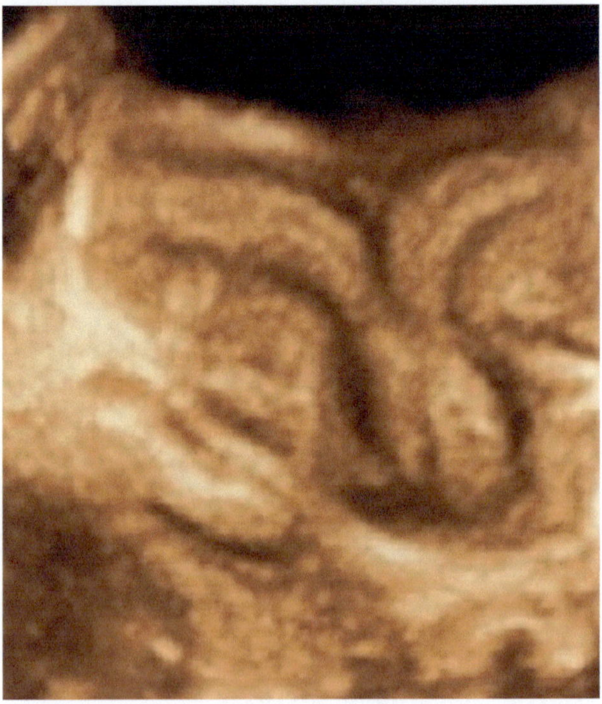

Fig. 17.10 3D US image of a bicornuate bicollis uterus with a deep fundal cleft and divergent uterine horns (Image Courtesy—Dr. Manju (Handa) Virmani, New Delhi)

anteflexed or retroflexed and uterine contour is deformed by fibroids. MR imaging in the coronal plane clearly shows the fundal cleft which is at least 1.0 cm in depth. Normal zonal anatomy and endometrial-to-myometrial ratio are seen in each of the horns [29]. (Fig. 17.11).

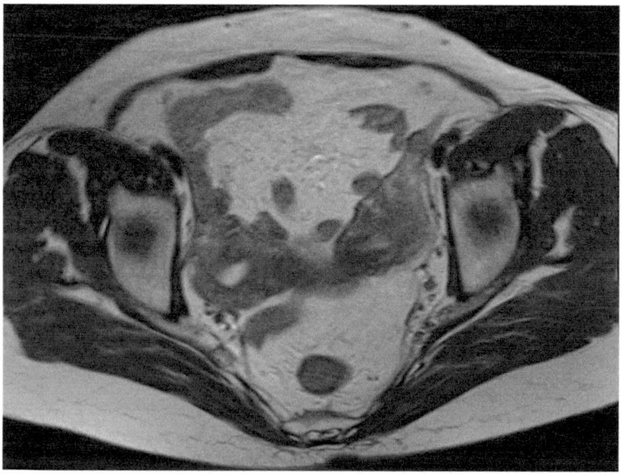

Fig. 17.11 Axial T2-weighted MR image of a bicornuate uterus with divergent uterine horns and each with normal zonal anatomy

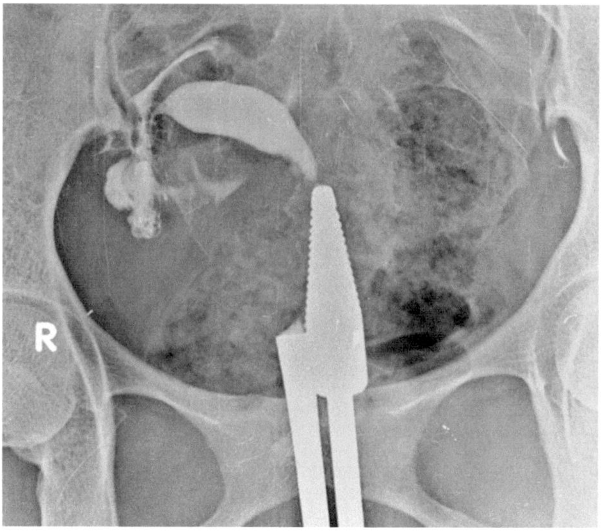

Fig. 17.12 HSG image of a unicornuate uterus with a single laterally deviated uterine horn and single fallopian tube

17.5.1.3 Unicornuate Uterus

This occurs when one Mullerian duct shows normal development, but the other fails to elongate. Renal anomalies associated with a unicornuate uterus include renal agenesis, ectopic kidney, horseshoe kidney, or dysplastic kidney [29].

On HSG, unicornuate uterus appears as a laterally deviated single uterine horn with single fallopian tube (Fig. 17.12). 3D US and MRI also easily demonstrate the unicornuate uterus (Figs. 17.13 and 17.14). Sometimes, there may be an associated rudimentary horn with or without a communicating cavity. It is in detection of the rudimentary uterine horn as well as visualization of endometrium and zonal anatomy within it where MRI scores over US [7, 23]. It is difficult to identify the rudimentary horn with US where it may look like a pelvic mass or cervix [29].

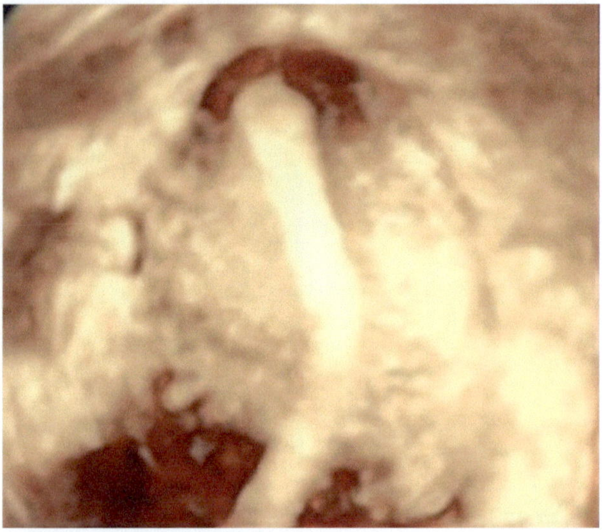

Fig. 17.13 3D US image showing a unicornuate uterus (Image Courtesy—Dr. Manju (Handa) Virmani, New Delhi)

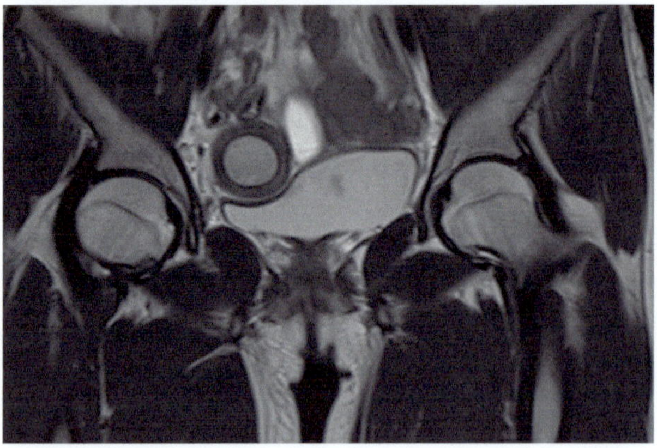

Fig. 17.14 Coronal T2-weighted MR image showing a unicornuate uterus with collection in uterine cavity

17.5.1.4 Arcuate Uterus

Here, both the Mullerian ducts have fused and septal reabsorption is nearly complete. It is considered by some as a normal variant. HSG shows a single uterine cavity with a smooth broad-based indentation at the fundus [7] (Fig. 17.15). 3D US shows a normal external uterine contour with a broad-based myometrial prominence at the fundus (Fig. 17.16). MRI also demonstrates the normal external contour of the uterus and the prominent soft tissue at fundus which shows signal intensity same as rest of myometrium [23] (Fig. 17.17).

17.5.2 Acquired Uterine Anomalies

These include adhesions in the uterine cavity, leiomyomas or fibroids, and endometrial polyps. There is a wide variation in the frequency of acquired anomalies in

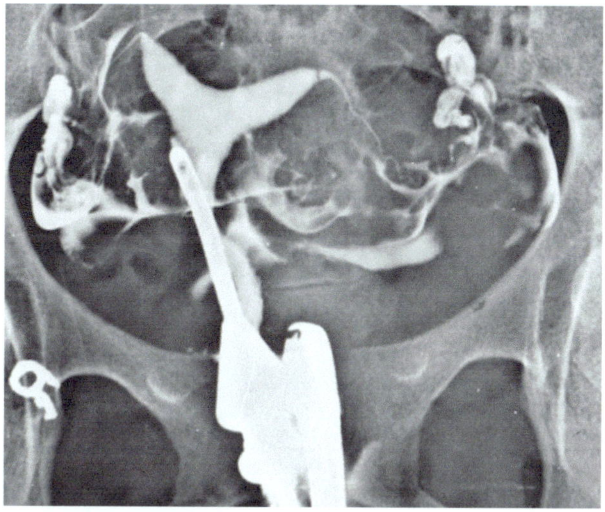

Fig. 17.15 HSG image of an arcuate uterus showing a single uterine cavity with a broad-based indentation at the fundus

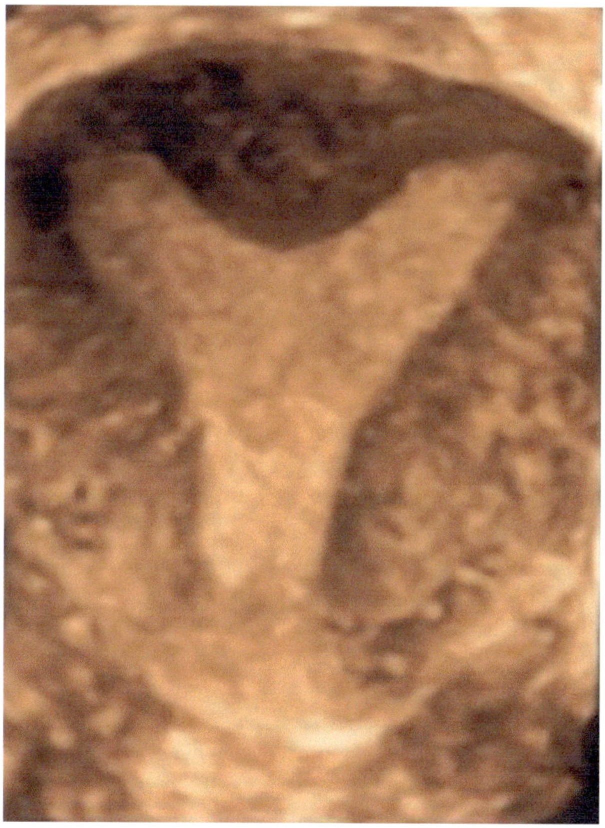

Fig. 17.16 3D US image of an arcuate uterus (Image Courtesy—Dr. Manju (Handa) Virmani, New Delhi)

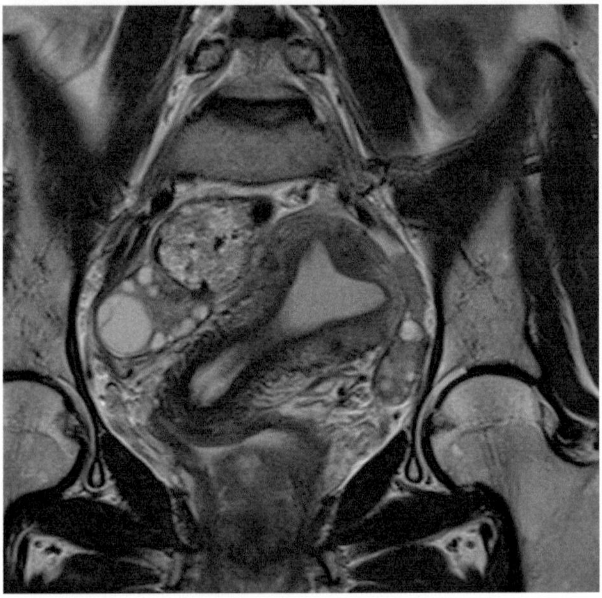

Fig. 17.17 Coronal T2-weighted MR image showing an arcuate uterus which is deviated to left side

women with RPL ranging from 1 to 33% with an average of about 12%. The reason for this variation is the lack of clear-cut diagnostic criteria [21].

17.5.2.1 Intrauterine Adhesions

They occur in about 5.5% of women with RPL [21]. When these adhesions partially or totally cause obliteration of the uterine cavity, this is known as Asherman's syndrome. This syndrome clinically presents with infertility, RPL, menstrual abnormalities, and pelvic pain [32]. Various classifications have been proposed to assess disease severity based on degree of cavity obliteration, thickness of the adhesions, menstrual pattern of the patient, and patency of the tubal ostia, but there is lack of clarity in their usage [32, 33].

Findings on HSG include multiple irregular filling defects, such as small and distorted cavity [2, 7]. However, HSG has a high false-positive rate and overestimates disease severity in patients who have adhesions only in the lower uterine segment [32].

2D transvaginal US is not very useful to detect adhesions as they get compressed in the uterine cavity. However, if saline hysterography (SHG) is carried out, adhesions can be seen as echogenic bands traversing the uterine cavity. These bands may be thin or thick and may be associated with scarring of the endometrium [34]. 3D transvaginal US enables visualization of the adhesions and accurately grades their extent and degree of obliteration of the uterine cavity (Fig. 17.18). A study by Knopman and Copperman revealed a sensitivity of 66.7% for HSG and 100% for 3D US in grading the intrauterine adhesions [35].

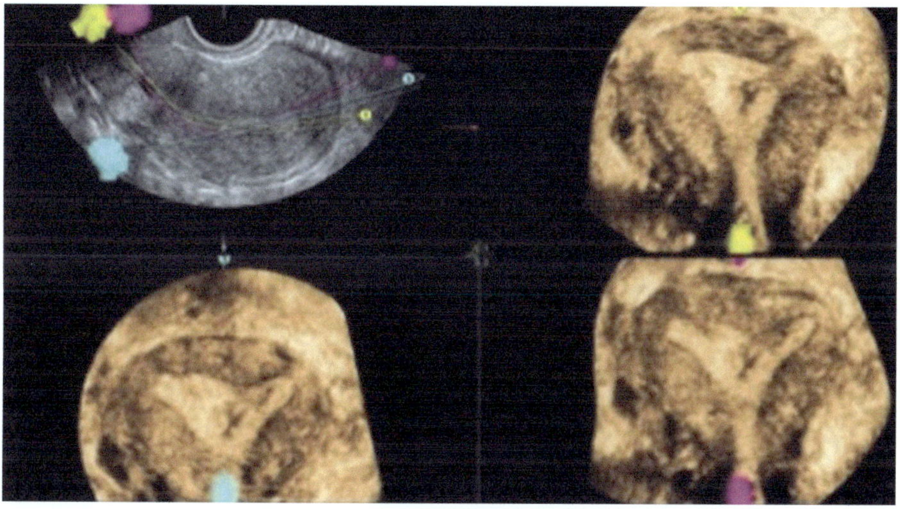

Fig. 17.18 3D US image showing intrauterine adhesions. The uterine cavity is not obliterated (Image Courtesy—Dr. Manju (Handa) Virmani, New Delhi)

MRI is not yet commonly used for evaluation of intrauterine adhesions. It may provide additional information to that obtained from HSG or US [36].

17.5.2.2 Leiomyomas/Fibroids

Submucosal fibroids and large intramural fibroids (>5 cm) are the ones associated with RPL [1, 37]. Submucosal fibroids are seen in about 4.5% of women with RPL [21]. Factors which lead to miscarriage include implantation over the surface of a submucous fibroid, location close to placenta, irregular myometrial contractions due to abnormal myocytes, and unfavorable effect of the fibroid on the endometrium [21, 37, 38].

On HSG, submucosal lesions are seen as filling defects in the initial phase after instillation of contrast into the uterine cavity. Large intramural lesions can deform the uterine cavity [2].

Leiomyomas are well visualized on transvaginal US. They appear as well-defined hypoechoic solid mass lesions or may appear heterogeneous with interspersed calcific foci. They can have a whorled appearance and associated acoustic shadowing. Cystic areas may be seen if the lesion has undergone degeneration [7, 39]. 3D US nicely delineates these lesions and their relationship to the uterine cavity (Fig. 17.19). On SHG, even the volume of a submucosal lesion projecting into the endometrial cavity can be assessed [34]. Limitations of US include its operator dependence and difficulty in assessment of an enlarged uterus when the field of view is limited.

MRI is considered the imaging modality of choice for evaluation of leiomyomas. It can detect the lesions and classify them accurately according to their location. It can assess the relationship of the leiomyoma to the endometrial cavity and the zonal anatomy (Figs. 17.20 and 17.21). Thus, it facilitates surgical planning and enables optimal patient management [40]. Non-degenerated leiomyomas are seen as well-defined

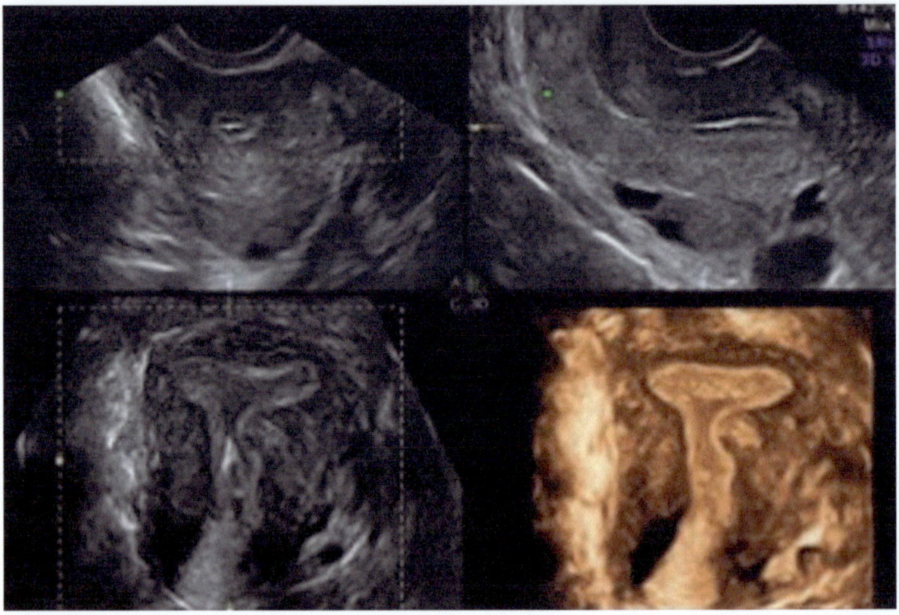

Fig. 17.19 3D US image of a small submucous fibroid along the left lateral wall (Image Courtesy—Dr. Manju (Handa) Virmani, New Delhi)

Fig. 17.20 Coronal T2-weighted fat-suppressed image showing a hypointense submucous fibroid with a whorled appearance

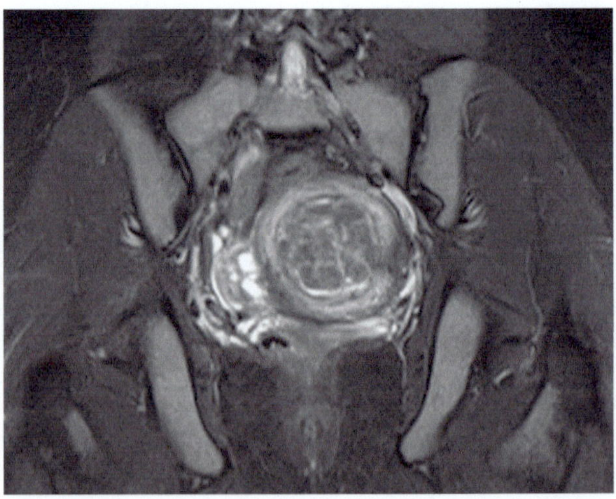

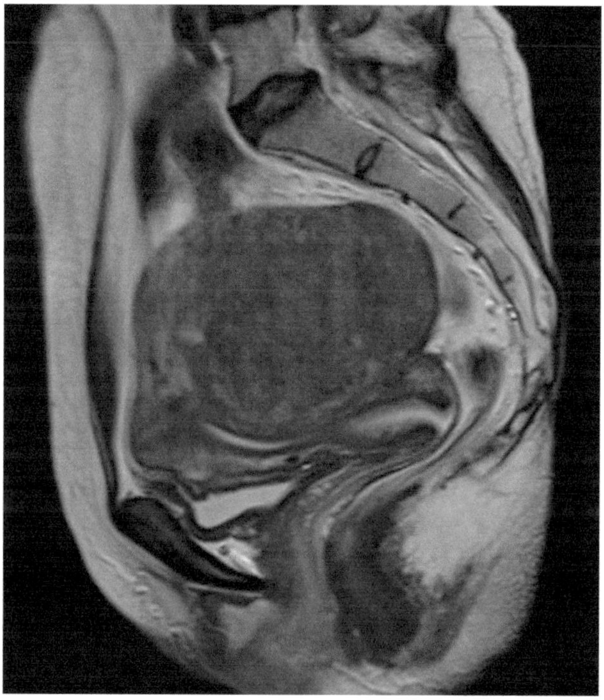

Fig. 17.21 Sagittal T2-weighted MR image of a large posterior wall uterine fibroid which is compressing the uterine cavity (Image Courtesy—Dr. Karthik Ganesan, Mumbai)

homogeneous hypointense mass lesions in T2-weighted images as compared to normal myometrium. They appear more conspicuous with contrast as they enhance less than the normal myometrium. Cellular leiomyomas have brighter signal intensity in T2-weighted images and enhance with contrast. Degenerated lesions can show high T2 signal intensity due to cystic areas or myxoid changes [8, 40].

17.5.2.3 Endometrial Polyps

Polyps are the least common of the acquired causes of RPL and are seen in about 2.4% of cases [21].

At HSG, polyps are seen as well-defined filling defects in the initial phase of contrast instillation into the uterine cavity (Fig. 17.22). At transvaginal US, polyps usually appear as small homogeneous hyperechoic mass lesions within the endometrial cavity (Fig. 17.23). Color Doppler can show the central vascular stalk. SHG helps differentiate polyps from endometrial hyperplasia where there is generalized endometrial thickening and also from submucosal leiomyomas where it enables visualization of the elevated echogenic endometrium [41].

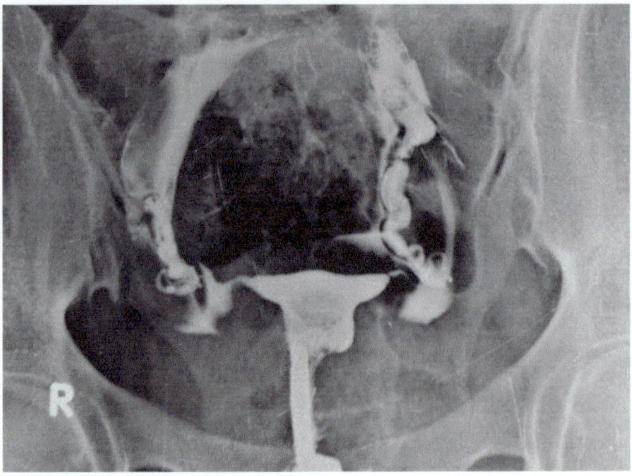

Fig. 17.22 HSG image of a well-defined filling defect in the uterine cavity due to a polyp

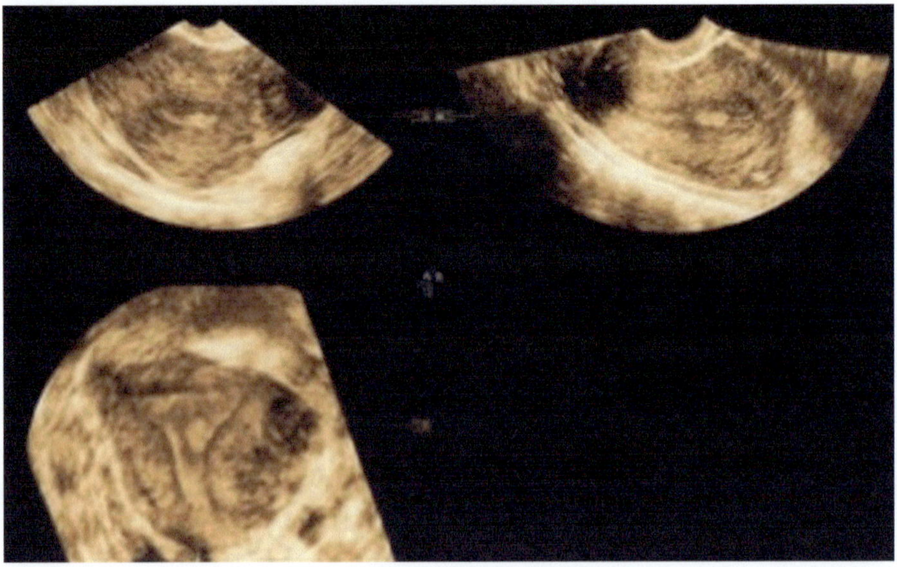

Fig. 17.23 3D US image showing a small endometrial polyp (Image Courtesy—Dr. Manju (Handa) Virmani, New Delhi)

At MRI, polyps are intracavitary mass lesions which show intermediate signal intensity in T1-weighted images and appear heterogeneously hyperintense in T2-weighted images (Fig. 17.24). It is difficult to identify small lesions which merge with the adjacent endometrium. Other findings include presence of a T2 hypointense fibrous core in the mass and intralesional cysts. Polyps can show homogeneous enhancement with contrast or heterogeneous enhancement due to presence of cysts [42].

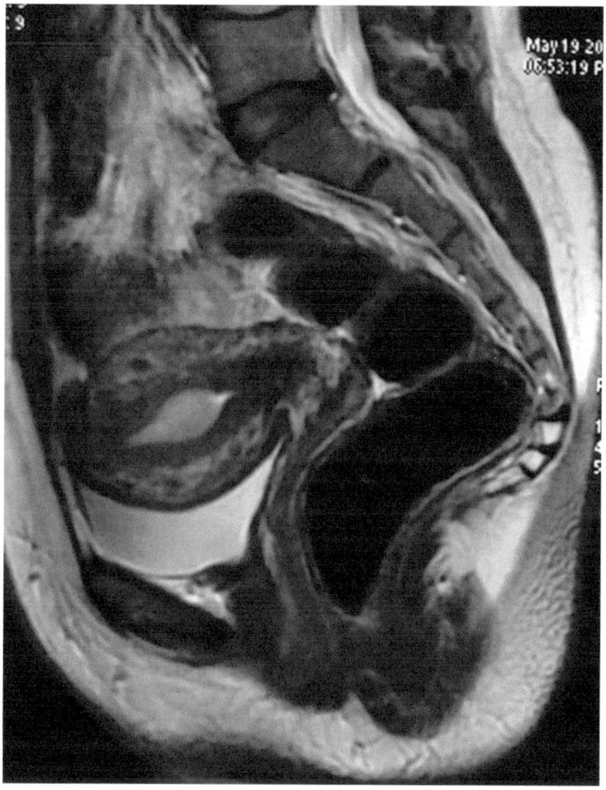

Fig. 17.24 Sagittal T2-weighted MR image showing a hyperintense lesion in the uterine cavity which is a polyp

17.5.2.4 Cervical Incompetence

This causes cervical dilatation without uterine activity leading to pregnancy loss in the second trimester. For cervical evaluation, transvaginal sonography is the modality of choice. A probe with frequency of 5 MHz or more is used for the scan. Findings on TVS include shortest cervical length < 25 mm at 24–28 weeks gestation age, cervical funneling which implies dilatation of the internal os, >5 mm shortening of cervical length after application of transfundal pressure for 15 s, debris in the amniotic fluid, and progressive shortening of the cervix on serial scans [3].

Conclusion

A sound knowledge of the various causes of RPL and their radiological features can help the radiologist choose the appropriate imaging modality, establish the diagnosis, and facilitate patient management. Usually a preliminary HSG or 2D US can be followed by 3D US or pelvic MRI to identify the cause of RPL, delineate its extent, and decide treatment strategy.

Key Points

- Causes of RPL include congenital uterine anomalies, intrauterine adhesions, submucosal fibroids or large intramural fibroids, and endometrial polyps.
- Preliminary imaging is by HSG and 2D US, but these need to be supplemented by 3D US or MRI to establish the correct diagnosis and decide treatment strategy.
- The chief advantages of both 3D US and MRI are that they are noninvasive, do not entail radiation exposure, and generate high-resolution images of both the uterine cavity as well as external fundal contour.

References

1. Ford HB, Schust DJ. Recurrent pregnancy loss: etiology, diagnosis and therapy. Rev Obstet Gynecol. 2009;2(2):76–83.
2. Simpson Jr WL, Beitia LG, Mester J. Hysterosalpingography: a reemerging study. Radiographics. 2006;26:419–31.
3. Salem S. Gynecology. In: Rumack CM, Wilson SR, Charboneau JW, Levine D, editors. Diagnostic ultrasound. Philadelphia: Elsevier Mosby; 2011. p. 547–612.
4. Bocca SM, Abuhamad AZ. Use of 3-dimensional Sonography to assess uterine anomalies. J Ultrasound Med. 2013;32:1–6.
5. Moini A, Mohammadi S, Hosseini R, Eslami B, Ahmadi F. Accuracy of 3-dimensional sonography for diagnosis and classification of congenital uterine anomalies. J Ultrasound Med. 2013;32:923–7.
6. Allison SJ, Horrow MM, Kim HY, Lev-Toaff AS. Saline-infused sonohysterography: tips for achieving greater success. Radiographics. 2011;31:1991–2004.
7. Steinkeler JA, Woodfield CA, Lazarus E, Hillstrom MM. Female infertility: a systematic approach to radiologic imaging and diagnosis. Radiographics. 2009;29:1353–70.
8. Forstner R, Kinkel K. Female pelvis. In: Haaga JR, Dogra VS, Forsting M, Gilkeson RC, Ha HK, Sundaram M, editors. CT and MRI of the whole body. Philadelphia: Elsevier Mosby; 2009. p. 2075–129.
9. Hricak H. MRI of the female pelvis: a review. AJR. 1986;146:1115–22.
10. Jauniaux E, Jones J, Burton GJ. The role of ultrasound imaging in diagnosing and investigating early pregnancy failure. Ultrasound Obstet Gynecol. 2005;25:613–24.
11. Royal College of Obstetricians and Gynaecologists. The management of early pregnancy loss. Guideline No. 25. London: RCOG; 2006.
12. Doubilet PM, Benson CB. Embryonic heart rate in the early first trimester: what rate is normal ? J Ultrasound Med. 1995;14:431–4.
13. Jaffe R, Dorgan A, Abramowicz JS. Color Doppler imaging of the uteroplacental circulation in the first trimester: value in predicting pregnancy failure or complication. AJR Am J Roentgenol. 1995;164:1255–8.
14. Nakatsuka M, Habara T, Noguchi S, et al. Impaired uterine arterial blood flow in pregnant women with recurrent pregnancy loss. J Ultrasound Med. 2003;22:27–31.
15. Nicolaides KH, Azar G, Byrne D, et al. Fetal nuchal translucency: ultrasound screening for chromosomal defects in first trimester of pregnancy. BMJ. 1992;304:867–9.
16. Devi Wold AS, Pham N, Arici A. Anatomic factors in recurrent pregnancy loss. Semin Reprod Med. 2006;24(1):25–32.
17. The American Fertility Society classifications of adnexal adhesions, distal tubal occlusion, tubal occlusion secondary to tubal ligation, tubal pregnancies, Mullerian anomalies and intrauterine adhesions. Fertil Steril. 1988;49(6):944–55.

18. Woelfer B, Salim R, Banerjee S, Elson J, Regan L, Jurkovic D. Reproductive outcomes in women with congenital uterine anomalies detected by three-dimensional ultrasound screening. Obstet Gynecol. 2001;98:1099–103.
19. Chan YY, Jayaprakasan K, Tan A, Thornton JG, Coomarasamy A, Raine-Fenning NJ. Reproductive outcomes in women with congenital uterine anomalies: a systematic review. Ultrasound Obstet Gynecol. 2011;38:371–82.
20. Jayaprakasan K, Chan YY, Sur S, Deb S, Clewes JS, Raine-Fenning NJ. Prevalence of uterine anomalies and their impact on early pregnancy in women conceiving after assisted reproduction treatment. Ultrasound Obstet Gynecol. 2011;37:727–32.
21. Jaslow CR. Uterine factors. Obstet Gynecol Clin N Am. 2014;41:57–86.
22. Saravelos SH, Cocksedge KA, Li T-C. Prevalence and diagnosis of congenital uterine anomalies in women with reproductive failure: a critical appraisal. Hum Reprod Update. 2008;14(5):415–29.
23. Behr SC, Courtier JL, Qayyum A. Imaging of Mullerian duct anomalies. Radiographics. 2012;32:E233–50.
24. Wu MH, Hsu CC, Huang KE. Detection of congenital Mullerian duct anomalies using three-dimensional ultrasound. J Clin Ultrasound. 1997;25:487–92.
25. Deutch TD, Bocca S, Oehninger S, Stadtmauer L, Abuhamad AZ. Magnetic resonance imaging versus three-dimensional transvaginal ultrasound for the diagnosis of Mullerian anomalies. Fertil Steril. 2006;86:S308.
26. Letterie GS, Haggerty M, Lindee G. A comparison of pelvic ultrasound and magnetic resonance imaging as diagnostic studies for Mullerian tract abnormalities. Int J Fertil Menopausal Stud. 1995;40:34–8.
27. Carrington BM, Hricak H, Nuruddin RN, Secaf E, Laros RK Jr, Hill EC. Mullerian duct anomalies: MR imaging evaluation. Radiology. 1990;176:715–20.
28. Mueller GC, Hussain HK, Smith YR, Quint EH, Carlos RC, Johnson TD, et al. Mullerian duct anomalies: comparison of MRI diagnosis and clinical diagnosis. AJR. 2007;189:1294–302.
29. Troiano RN, McCarthy SM. Mullerian duct anomalies: imaging and clinical issues. Radiology. 2004;233:19–34.
30. Reuter KL, Daly DC, Cohen SM. Septate versus bicornuate uteri: errors in imaging diagnosis. Radiology. 1989;172:749–52.
31. Bermejo C, Ten PM, Cantarero R, Diaz D, Pedregosa JP, Barron E, et al. Three-dimensional ultrasound in the diagnosis of Mullerian duct anomalies and concordance with magnetic resonance imaging. Ultrasound Obstet Gynecol. 2010;35:593–601.
32. Fischer C, Copperman A. Use of three dimensional ultrasound imaging in evaluation of Asherman's syndrome. In: Minin O, editor. Ultrasound imaging—medical applications. InTech. https://doi.org/10.5772/16533.
33. I-Ferne T, Robertson M. The role of imaging in the investigation of Asherman's syndrome. AJUM. 2011;14(3):15–8.
34. O'Neill MJ. Sonohysterography. Radiol Clin N Am. 2003;41:781–97.
35. Knopman J, Copperman AB. Value of 3D ultrasound in the management of suspected Asherman's syndrome. J Reprod Med. 2007;52(11):1016–22.
36. Letterie GS, Haggerty MF. Magnetic resonance imaging of intrauterine synechiae. Gynecol Obstet Investig. 1994;37(1):66–8.
37. Bajekal N, Li TC. Fibroids, infertility and pregnancy wastage. Hum Reprod Update. 2000;6(6):614–20.
38. AAGL: Advancing Minimally Invasive Gynecology Worldwide. AAGL practice report: practice guidelines for the diagnosis and management of submucous leiomyomas. J Minim Invasive Gynecol. 2012;19(2):152–71. https://doi.org/10.1016/j.jmig.2011.09.005.
39. Sue W, Scott-Barrett S. Radiological appearances of uterine fibroids. Indian J Radiol Imaging. 2009;19(3):222–31.
40. Murase E, Siegelman ES, Outwater EK, Perez-Jaffe LA, Tureck RW. Uterine leiomyomas: histopathologic features, MR imaging findings, differential diagnosis, and treatment. Radiographics. 1999;19:1179–97.

41. Jorizzo JR, Chen MYM, Riccio GJ. Endometrial polyps: sonohysterographic evaluation. AJR. 2001;176:617–21.
42. Grasel RP, Outwater EK, Siegelman ES, Capuzzi D, Parker L, Hussain SM. Endometrial polyps: MR imaging features and distinction from endometrial carcinoma. Radiology. 2000;214:47–52.

Fetal Autopsy and Placental Examination as a Complimentary Tool

18

Priyanka Gogoi

18.1 Introduction

Miscarriage, one of the commonest complications of pregnancy, is the spontaneous loss of a pregnancy before the fetus has reached viability. The term therefore includes all pregnancy losses from the time of conception until 24 weeks of gestation. Recurrent pregnancy loss (RPL), also referred to as *recurrent miscarriage* or *habitual abortion*, is defined as the loss of three or more consecutive pregnancies and affects 1% of couples trying to conceive [1]. It has been suggested that RPL is a distinct clinical entity having different etiopathological mechanisms than spontaneous abortions and needs to be addressed separately. At present, studies evaluating the etiology of RPL have focused on factors related to epidemiology including maternal age and number of previous miscarriages [2, 3], advanced paternal age [4], lifestyle issues [5–11], antiphospholipid antibody syndrome [12, 13], genetics [14–19], congenital uterine malformations and cervical weakness [20–23], endocrine disorders [24–33], immunology [34–37], infections [38–42], and inherited thrombophilic defects [43–47]. Based on these studies, recommendations regarding evaluation and management of RPL have been published [48–50]. However, there is no clear consensus about the causes of RPL as most studies of pregnancy loss are based on sporadic miscarriages and not RPL. Regardless of the numerous causes and treatment options, RPL is emotionally devastating with enormous psychological implications for the patient. Estimating the risk for a subsequent fetal loss and the identification of a treatable etiology for the disorder form the cornerstone on which the management of RPL is based. However a definitive diagnosis is possible in only 50% of cases, and significant number of RPL remains unexplained despite intensive

P. Gogoi, M.D. (Pathology)
Department of Pathology, University College of Medical Sciences and Guru Teg Bahadur Hospital, Delhi, India
e-mail: drpriyankagogoi@gmail.com

S. Mehta, B. Gupta (eds.), *Recurrent Pregnancy Loss*,
https://doi.org/10.1007/978-981-10-7338-0_18

investigations of probable causes [51, 52]. The autopsy of the fetus as well the placental examination can help by providing additional information beyond that achieved by conventionally recommended investigations.

18.2 The Value of Placental Examination and Fetal Autopsy in the Causes of RPL

Fetal growth and development are regulated in a very complex manner and critically hinge on the growth and development of the placenta. This unique organ of fetal origin has been indicated to predict not only the outcome of a pregnancy but also the long-term health of the baby. At various stages during fetal development, the placenta performs a remarkable range of functions until the fetal organs become functional. Acknowledging this key role of the placenta, its many histologic and pathologic variants, and its complicated derivation, the relevance of a meticulous examination and alterations viewed by the pathologist cannot be overlooked. Thus, it can be anticipated that an objective, thorough, well-documented analysis of the products of conception would be a valuable source of data both about the mechanisms and the causes of RPL.

18.2.1 Histopathological Examination of Products of Conception in RPL

Products of conception are one of the most common specimens submitted for histopathological examination as an integral and routine component of the management of patients with pregnancy failure. Such an examination aims to document the presence of an intrauterine pregnancy and to exclude gestational trophoblastic diseases. Furthermore, histopathological examination of products of conception at times elucidates the pathogenic mechanisms of the underlying cause of pregnancy failure, particularly in the setting of RPL or detecting unexpected fetal pathology. Based on the period of gestation at which it occurs, abortions are divided into two significantly different groups, early (up to 12 weeks) and late (>12 weeks).While chromosomal abnormalities are associated with early spontaneous abortions generally, placental and maternal factors are responsible for most late abortions.

There is a paucity of data regarding the importance of routine histopathological examination of products of conception in the setting of RPL. Studies based on routine histopathological examination of products of conception in RPL demonstrate that in the majority of cases it serves to simply confirm an intrauterine gestation. Several histopathological classification systems based on several criteria including the morphology of the conceptus, the presence and absence of an embryo or fetus, the state of preservation of the conceptus, and the placental morphology have been described to elucidate the etiology of the abortion or to establish the timing of the teratological insult [53–55]. However such classification systems are cumbersome for routine use and subject to interobserver variations. These histopathological systems have largely been replaced by sensitive methods including karyotyping for detection of fetal aneuploidy and serial sonography for timing of intrauterine death.

18.2.2 Role of Routine Histopathological Examination in Specific Clinicopathological Conditions Associated with RPL

18.2.2.1 Chromosomal Abnormalities

Demonstrable chromosomal anomalies of the embryo account for 30–57% of further miscarriages in patients of RPL [49]. Trisomies are the most frequent cytogenetic abnormality detected followed by triploidy and monosomy X [49]. Gross assessment of the products of conception may reveal abnormality in the contents of the chorionic cavity, if the contents are identified. An abnormally large amniotic sac often prematurely fused to the chorion may be present in some cases. Anomalies in the embryo, either generalized or localized developmental defects, point to a high probability of a chromosomal anomaly. On the other hand, a normal well-developed embryo suggests the possibility of a maternal cause of abortion, although 20–25% of morphologically normal embryo with chromosomal anomalies, particularly triploidy, are known to occur. In early spontaneous abortions, the gross morphology may at times be helpful in suggesting the possibility of a chromosomal anomaly as the chorionic cavity and its contents are identifiable. However in the fragmented tissues of curetted specimen, gross assessment of the embryo and/or placenta is, at best, suboptimal. Microscopically, various nonspecific dysmorphic features have been described in the villi of abortions with abnormal karyotypes. These features, including villous enlargement with myxoid stroma, irregular villous outlines, multiple trophoblastic invaginations, and individual trophoblastic cells in the villous stroma though common and prominent in karyotypically abnormal abortions, are also in abortions with normal karyotype. Hence, in the present scenario, the accurate identification of chromosomal anomalies either fetal or of parental origin is best accomplished by genetic evaluation of villous stroma and trophoblast and by techniques such as karyotyping.

Hydatidiform moles (HM) have been implicated as a cause of recurrent abortions in a minority of patients ranging from 1 to 2% following a molar pregnancy [56–60] to as high as 23% for women with two consecutive molar pregnancies [61]. HM is also associated with a significant increased risk of developing gestational trophoblastic neoplasia (GTN), ranging from 1 to 15% for partial mole (PM) and complete mole (CM), respectively [61]. The absence of fetal tissue in high-resolution ultrasound and abnormally high hCG level early in pregnancy clinches the diagnosis of a complete molar pregnancy and poses little problem from the third month of pregnancy onward with 80% of cases diagnosed [62–65]. By contrast, the ultrasound diagnosis of partial mole is less accurate, and around 70% of those cases will be missed by routine ultrasound examination [64]. Histologically, HM is characterized by hydropic swelling of the placental villi, hyperplasia of villous trophoblast, and absent, or abnormal, fetal development, and morphological examination of the products of conception reliably demonstrates this condition [66] (Fig. 18.1). Classical villous histological criteria supplemented by adding features of the materno-embryonic interface greatly increase the sensitivity and specificity of routine microscopic examination [67]. The diagnosis of a molar pregnancy assumes significance as the patient would require surveillance both for recurrence in future pregnancies and for detection of persistent gestational trophoblastic neoplasia. Ploidy analysis by flow cytometry allows further categorization of molar specimens [68, 69]. Analysis of molar DNA on a routine basis can be done using newer molecular biology techniques such as fluorescent in situ hybridization (FISH) which are easier, faster, and cheaper than cell culture [69–74]. These techniques are now well established, can be performed on paraffin-embedded tissues, and are becoming increasingly available. A combination of histopathology, FISH, and DNA analysis of the microsatellites serves to accurately diagnose and classify HM.

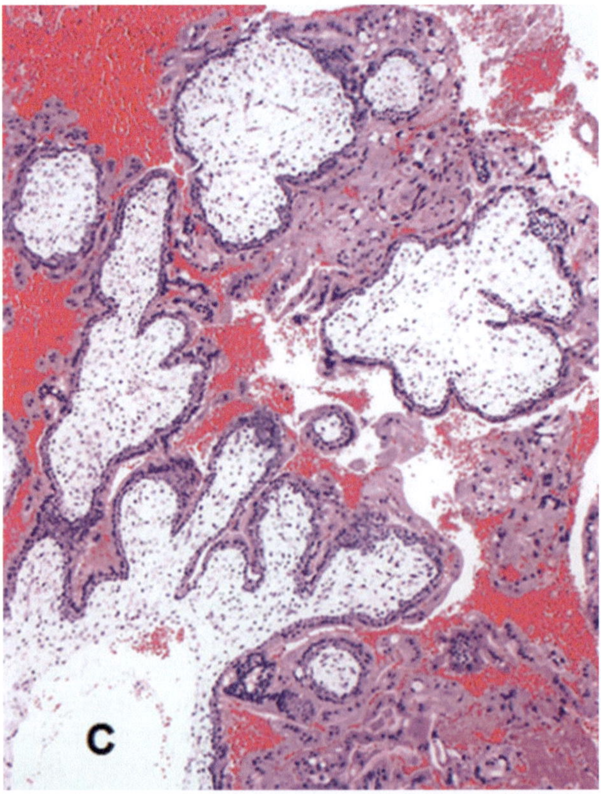

Fig. 18.1 Early complete hydatidiform mole. Villi have extensive stromal edema with central cisterns (C). The periphery of the villi expands into bulbous projections with more prominent stromal cells. There is a large amount of proliferative trophoblast in this field (Courtesy of Dr. B. Ronnett) (Reproduced with permission from Kurman R.J, Ellenson L. H and Ronnett B.M (Eds.) Blaustein's Pathology of the Female Genital Tract. 6th edn. Springer, New York)

Rarely, women with recurrent HM include patients with familial recurrent hydatidiform mole (FRHM), a rare autosomal recessive condition characterized by recurrent, usually complete molar pregnancies of biparental rather than androgenetic origin [75]. It has been shown that mutations in genes, NLRP7 and KHDC3L, account for 75 and 5% of cases of FRHM, respectively [76, 77]. Diagnosis of this condition is by genotyping of the CM.

Chronic histiocytic intervillositis (CHI) is a histopathologically recognizable cause of recurrent spontaneous abortion, characterized by the presence of an intervillous infiltrate of mononuclear cells of maternal origin, usually associated with villous and intervillous fibrin deposition and focal villitis along with placental insufficiency and poor perinatal outcome [79–82] (Fig. 18.2). Immunohistochemically, the chronic inflammation of CHI is composed predominantly of monocytes/macrophages with scattered T-lymphocytes [78]. In their study on CHI associated with recurrent miscarriage, Boyd and Redline showed that approximately 42% of patients with CHI had recurrent spontaneous abortions [80]. This has a bearing on the future reproductive management of these patients. However this condition is relatively rare and has been reported in only around 6/10,000 placentas analyzed in the second and third trimester [80] and in 4.4% of first trimester miscarriages with normal karyotype [79].

Antiphospholipid antibody (aPL) syndrome is one of the most important treatable causes of RPL with a prevalence rate of 15% in women with recurrent abortions [12, 83]. However the role of histopathological examination of products of conception in this condition in the setting of recurrent abortions has not been extensively studied. The primary placental pathology described in the placentas of patients with antiphospholipid antibody syndrome is chronic uteroplacental

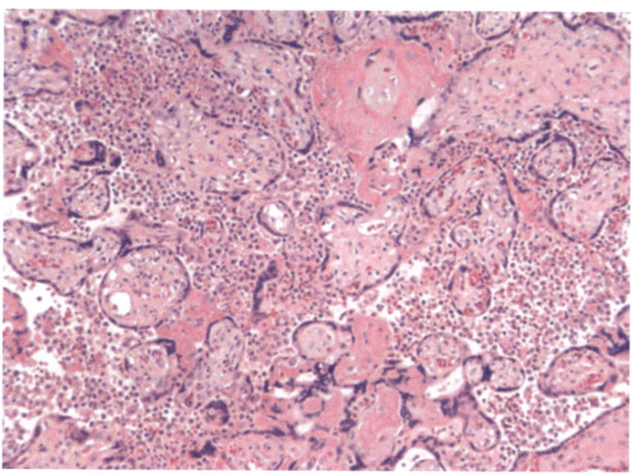

Fig. 18.2 Chronic histiocytic intervillositis. There is diffuse infiltration of the intervillous space by monocyte macrophages (Reproduced with permission from Kurman R.J, Ellenson L. H and Ronnett B.M (Eds.) Blaustein's Pathology of the Female Genital Tract. 6th edn. Springer, New York)

vasculopathy, specifically placental infarction, besides intervillous thrombosis and perivillous fibrin deposition [84–89] (Figs. 18.3 and 18.4). However other studies show that the prevalence of placental infarction is similar in RPL, regardless of the status of antiphospholipid antibodies [90]. Hence morphology alone though suggesting possible mechanism of fetal loss is not helpful in the diagnosis of aPL syndrome and does not provide additional help in the management of these patients.

18.2.2.2 Thrombophilic Disorders

The association of thrombophilias including factor V Leiden, activated protein C resistance, and prothrombin G20210A mutation with recurrent fetal loss is well

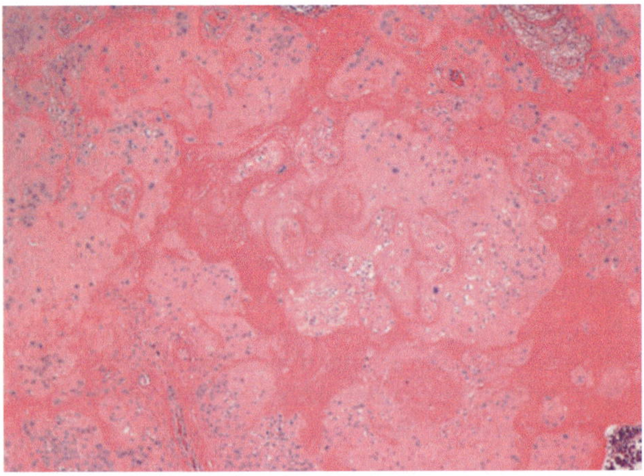

Fig. 18.3 Massive perivillous fibrin deposition (MFD). Villi are separated by and enmeshed in dense perivillous fibrinoid containing intermediate trophoblast (Reproduced with permission from Kurman R.J, Ellenson L. H and Ronnett B.M (Eds.) Blaustein's Pathology of the Female Genital Tract. 6th edn. Springer, New York)

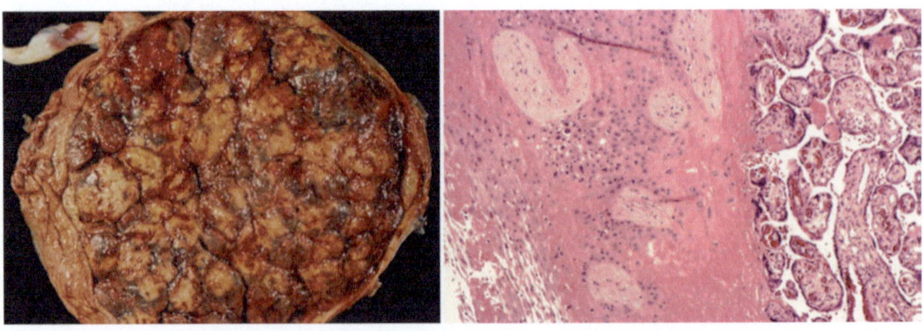

Fig. 18.4 Maternal floor infarct (MFI). The maternal surface is diffusely discolored and firm (left). The basal villi are entrapped in fibrinoid (right) (Reproduced with permission from Kurman R.J, Ellenson L. H and Ronnett B.M (Eds.) Blaustein's Pathology of the Female Genital Tract. 6th edn. Springer, New York)

established. While factor V Leiden has been found to have a stronger association with late recurrent fetal loss, activated protein C resistance and prothrombin G20210A mutation have an association with first trimester recurrent fetal loss [43]. There is no specific placental lesion unique to or specific for maternal thrombophilia. Excessive thrombosis of the placental vessels, placental infarction, and secondary uteroplacental insufficiency has been observed in the placentas of thrombophilic women with fetal loss [91] (Figs. 18.3, 18.4, 18.5, and 18.6) and has been proposed to be a common underlying mechanism of fetal loss in these patients. On the contrary, the absence of placental thrombosis has also been observed in women with thrombophilia and adverse pregnancy outcome [92], thereby

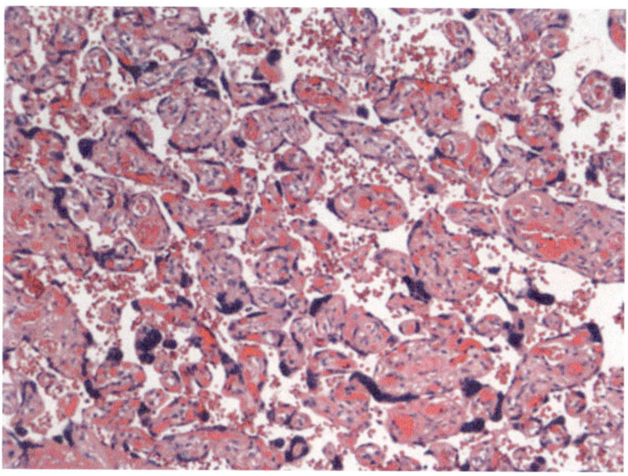

Fig. 18.5 Maternal underperfusion. Increased syncytial knots. Syncytiotrophoblastic nuclei clustered in the distal villi (Reproduced with permission from Kurman R.J, Ellenson L. H and Ronnett B.M (Eds.) Blaustein's Pathology of the Female Genital Tract. 6th edn. Springer, New York)

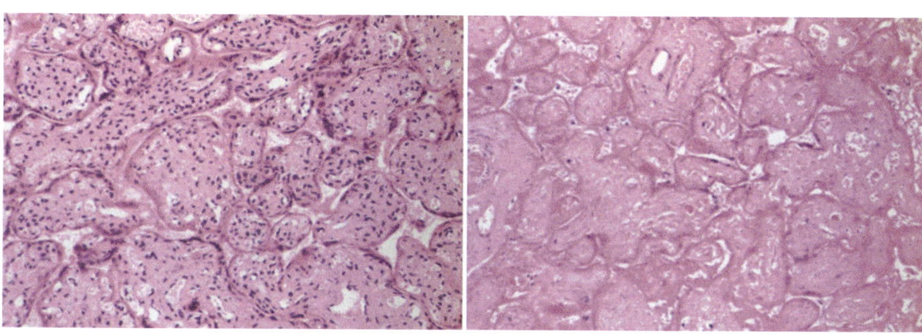

Fig. 18.6 Maternal underperfusion. Infarcts. The intervillous space is collapsed with necrotic villi undergoing progressive necrosis eventuating in ghost-like villous remnants (Reproduced with permission from Kurman R.J, Ellenson L. H and Ronnett B.M (Eds.) Blaustein's Pathology of the Female Genital Tract. 6th edn. Springer, New York)

suggesting the role of other pathophysiological pathways in fetal loss in thrombophilias. Thrombophilic factors have been suggested to prevent implantation by damage to decidual or chorionic vessels or impairing trophoblast invasiveness, similar to the mechanism described in antiphospholipid antibody syndrome [93]. As such, the histomorphological finding of placental thrombosis alone neither is specific for diagnosing thrombophilias nor does it distinguishes spontaneous from recurrent abortions. The role of histopathological examination in these patients would be to suggest screening of all patients of RPL with placental thrombosis for the presence of both acquired and inherited thrombophilias with coagulation studies.

18.2.2.3 Beyond Routine Histomorphology

An additional sampling technique, placental bed biopsies from some but not all patients with miscarriages have demonstrated defects in hemochorial placentation [94–96]. This defect is characterized by the presence of a thinner and fragmented trophoblast shell, and impaired early trophoblastic invasion is also associated with premature intervillous space blood flow with subsequent oxidative damage. In patients with a history of RPL who had miscarriage, defective placentation was observed in only a subset of patients, while placentation was normal in others [96]. Other authors have us found interactions between fetal trophoblast and maternal uNK cells to influence placentation in human pregnancy [97, 98]. Immunohistochemistry, immunoblotting, and in vitro studies have showed a significant relation between abnormal trophoblast invasion resulting in recurrent miscarriage and impaired expression of molecules such as kisspeptins and STMN1 [99, 100]. Research-based techniques attempting to investigate the possible etiology of RPL have been used by several authors. Experimental in vitro studies concentrating on the anchorage pattern in the developing placenta in normal and abnormal pregnancies suggest disturbed anchorage leading to instability and defective invasion of maternal vessels by the extravillous cytotrophoblast [101]. Other studies have used sera of women with recurrent spontaneous abortions in inhibition assay of trophoblast adhesion to endothelial cells [102].

Cinar O. et al. used comparative immunofluorescent tissue labeling of decidual tissue for evaluation of the existence and distribution of decidual apoptosis in normal pregnancies and miscarriages and found significantly higher number of apoptotic cells preferentially localized to sites of origin of decidualization in patients with RPL [103].

There is a growing body of evidence suggesting an immunological basis in the pathogenesis of RPL. Various subsets of immune effectors including T cells, NK cells, monocytes, or DCs and cytokines and chemokines secreted by these cells influence implantation and early trophoblast invasion by altering the maternofetal immunologic tolerance balance. Several studies have postulated that a fine balance exists between factors promoting immune tolerance and rejection at the maternal-fetal interface, and any alteration in this would negatively affect pregnancy outcome.

Some authors have attempted to supplement routine morphology with immunohistochemistry techniques. Routinely collected and processed histopathological specimens of products of conceptus were used for studying infiltrating cells, usually leukocyte subpopulations and their activation status in decidua of women with a history of RPL [104–110]. Other authors have used techniques such as flow cytometry, Western blotting, and RT-PCR for demonstration of a proinflammatory bias in the deciduas of these patients [111–119]. Though providing a basis for possible immunological pathogenesis of pregnancy losses, these markers are currently not recommended for routine use and are unlikely to affect clinical management. However further work aimed at characterizing and manipulating the infiltrating cell population in the decidua in patients with RPL appears promising in terms of possible therapeutic intervention in these patients.

Recently, there has been much focus on the miRNA expression profiles in villus or decidua from patients with a history RPL [120–122]. Differentially expressed miRNAs in this setting were predicted to target a large number of genes involved in various cellular functions, including proliferation, differentiation, and migration. These miRNAs may have the potential to serve as diagnostic and prognostic biomarkers with clinical utility and facilitate the development of new strategies for targeted therapy against RPL.

Conclusion

The role of routine histopathological examination of evacuated products of conception in determining the etiology of RPL has generated a lot of debate and controversy. The limited amount of material available as well as the fragmented nature of the specimens submitted makes the morphological study particularly challenging. While not recommended as a part of routine workup of a patient of RPL currently, it cannot be denied that such an exercise allows identification of important etiology in few cases while giving direction for further diagnostic workup in others. However in the majority of cases the morphological examination alone is unlikely to alter clinical management. An optimized protocol for the histopathological evaluation of products of conceptus in RPL, supplemented with use of newer advanced techniques including immunohistochemistry, FISH, PCR, and microarray profiling, is the need of the hour to extract maximum diagnostic yield from these specimens. This would in turn require a very close collaboration between multiple disciplines including obstetricians, geneticists, and pathologist.

References

1. Stirrat GM. Recurrent miscarriage. Lancet. 1990;336(8716):673–5.
2. Nybo Anderson AM, Wohlfahrt J, Christens P, Olsen J, Melbye M. Maternal age and fetal loss: population based register linkage study. BMJ. 2000;320:1708–12.
3. Regan L, Braude PR, Trembath PL. Influence of past reproductive performance on risk of spontaneous abortion. BMJ. 1989;299:541–5.
4. de la Rochebrochard E, Thonneau P. Paternal age and maternal age are risk factors for miscarriage; results of a multicentre European study. Hum Reprod. 2002;17:1649–56.
5. Lindbohm ML, Sallmén M, Taskinen H. Effects of exposure to environmental tobacco smoke on reproductive health. Scand J Work Environ Health. 2002;28(Suppl 2):84–96.

6. Rasch V. Cigarette, alcohol, and caffeine consumption: risk factors for spontaneous abortion. Acta Obstet Gynecol Scand. 2003;82:182–8.
7. Peck JD, Leviton A, Cowan LD. A review of the epidemiologic evidence concerning the reproductive health effects of caffeine consumption: a 2000–2009 update. Food Chem Toxicol. 2010;48:2549–76.
8. Kesmodel U, Wisborg K, Olsen SF, Henriksen TB, Secher NJ. Moderate alcohol intake in pregnancy and the risk of spontaneous abortion. Alcohol Alcohol. 2002;37:87–92.
9. Marcus M, McChesney R, Golden A, Landrigan P. Video display terminals and miscarriage. J Am Med Womens Assoc. 2000;55:84–8, 105.
10. Shuhaiber S, Koren G. Occupational exposure to inhaled anaesthetic. Is it a concern for pregnant women? Can Fam Physician. 2000;46:2391–2.
11. McGregor DG. Occupational exposure to trace concentrations of waste anesthetic gases. Mayo Clin Proc. 2000;75:273–7.
12. Rai RS, Regan L, Clifford K, Pickering W, Dave M, Mackie I, et al. Antiphospholipid antibodies and beta-2-glycoprotein-I in 500 women with recurrent miscarriage: results of a comprehensive screening approach. Hum Reprod. 1995;10:2001–5.
13. Rai RS, Clifford K, Cohen H, Regan L. High prospective fetal loss rate in untreated pregnancies of women with recurrent miscarriage and antiphospholipid antibodies. Hum Reprod. 1995;10:3301–4.
14. de Braekeleer M, Dao TN. Cytogenetic studies in couples experiencing repeated pregnancy losses. Hum Reprod. 1990;5:519–28.
15. Clifford K, Rai R, Watson H, Regan L. An informative protocol for the investigation of recurrent miscarriage: preliminary experience of 500 consecutive cases. Hum Reprod. 1994;9:1328–32.
16. Stephenson MD, Sierra S. Reproductive outcomes in recurrent pregnancy loss associated with a parental carrier of a structural chromosome rearrangement. Hum Reprod. 2006;21:1076–82.
17. Franssen MT, Korevaar JC, van der Veen F, Leschot NJ, Bossuyt PM, Goddijn M. Reproductive outcome after chromosome analysis in couples with two or more miscarriages: index [corrected]-control study. BMJ. 2006;332:759–63. Erratum in: BMJ 2006; 332:1012.
18. Carp H, Toder V, Aviram A, Daniely M, Mashiach S, Barkai G. Karyotype of the abortus in recurrent miscarriage. Fertil Steril. 2001;75:678–82.
19. Stephenson MD, Awartani KA, Robinson WP. Cytogenetic analysis of miscarriages from couples with recurrent miscarriage: a case–control study. Hum Reprod. 2002;17:446–51.
20. Grimbizis GF, Camus M, Tarlatzis BC, Bontis JN, Devroey P. Clinical implications of uterine malformations and hysteroscopic treatment results. Hum Reprod Update. 2001;7:161–74.
21. Salim R, Regan L, Woelfer B, Backos M, Jurkovic D. A comparative study of the morphology of congenital uterine anomalies in women with and without a history of recurrent first trimester miscarriage. Hum Reprod. 2003;18:162–6.
22. Acién P. Incidence of Müllerian defects in fertile and infertile women. Hum Reprod. 1997;12:1372–6.
23. Woelfer B, Salim R, Banerjee S, Elson J, Regan L, Jurkovic D. Reproductive outcomes in women with congenital uterine anomalies detected by three-dimensional ultrasound screening. Obstet Gynecol. 2001;98:1099–103.
24. Hanson U, Persson B, Thunell S. Relationship between haemoglobin A1C in early type 1 (insulin-dependent) diabetic pregnancy and the occurrence of spontaneous abortion and fetal malformation in Sweden. Diabetologia. 1990;33:100–4.
25. Mills JL, Simpson JL, Driscoll SG, Jovanovic-Peterson L, Van Allen M, Aarons JH, et al. Incidence of spontaneous abortion among normal women and insulin-dependent diabetic women whose pregnancies were identified within 21 days of conception. N Engl J Med. 1988;319:1617–23.
26. Abalovich M, Gutierrez S, Alcaraz G, Maccallini G, Garcia A, Levalle O. Overt and subclinical hypothyroidism complicating pregnancy. Thyroid. 2002;12:63–8.
27. Bussen S, Sütterlin M, Steck T. Endocrine abnormalities during the follicular phase in women with recurrent spontaneous abortion. Hum Reprod. 1999;14:18–20.

28. Li TC, Spuijbroek MD, Tuckerman E, Anstie B, Loxley M, Laird S. Endocrinological and endometrial factors in recurrent miscarriage. BJOG. 2000;107:1471–9.
29. Esplin MS, Branch DW, Silver R, Stagnaro-Green A. Thyroid autoantibodies are not associated with recurrent pregnancy loss. Am J Obstet Gynecol. 1998;179:1583–6.
30. Rushworth FH, Backos M, Rai R, Chilcott IT, Baxter N, Regan L. Prospective pregnancy outcome in untreated recurrent miscarriers with thyroid autoantibodies. Hum Reprod. 2000;15:1637–9.
31. Rai R, Backos M, Rushworth F, Regan L. Polycystic ovaries and recurrent miscarriage—a reappraisal. Hum Reprod. 2000;15:612–5.
32. Craig LB, Ke RW, Kutteh WH. Increased prevalence of insulin resistance in women with a history of recurrent pregnancy loss. Fertil Steril. 2002;78:487–90.
33. Cocksedge KA, Saravelos SH, Wang Q, Tuckerman E, Laird SM, Li TC. Does free androgen index predict subsequent pregnancy outcome in women with recurrent miscarriage? Hum Reprod. 2008;23:797–802.
34. Wold AS, Arici A. Natural killer cells and reproductive failure. Curr Opin Obstet Gynecol. 2005;17:237–41.
35. Rai R, Sacks G, Trew G. Natural killer cells and reproductive failure—theory, practice and prejudice. Hum Reprod. 2005;20:1123–6.
36. Tuckerman E, Laird SM, Prakash A, Li TC. Prognostic value of the measurement of uterine natural killer cells in the endometrium of women with recurrent miscarriage. Hum Reprod. 2007;22:2208–13.
37. Bombell S, McGuire W. Cytokine polymorphisms in women with recurrent pregnancy loss: meta-analysis. Aust N Z J Obstet Gynaecol. 2008;48:147–54.
38. Regan L, Jivraj S. Infection and pregnancy loss. In: MacLean AB, Regan L, Carrington D, editors. Infection and pregnancy. London: RCOG Press; 2001. p. 291–304.
39. Hay PE, Lamont RF, Taylor-Robinson D, Morgan DJ, Ison C, Pearson J. Abnormal bacterial colonisation of the genital tract and subsequent preterm delivery and late miscarriage. BMJ. 1994;308:295–8.
40. Leitich H, Kiss H. Asymptomatic bacterial vaginosis and intermediate flora as risk factors for adverse pregnancy outcome. Best Pract Res Clin Obstet Gynaecol. 2007;21:375–90.
41. Llahi-Camp JM, Rai R, Ison C, Regan L, Taylor-Robinson D. Association of bacterial vaginosis with a history of second trimester miscarriage. Hum Reprod. 1996;11:1575–8.
42. Ralph SG, Rutherford AJ, Wilson JD. Influence of bacterial vaginosis on conception and miscarriage in the first trimester: cohort study. BMJ. 1999;319:220–3.
43. Rey E, Kahn SR, David M, Shrier I. Thrombophilic disorders and fetal loss: a meta-analysis. Lancet. 2003;361(9361):901–8.
44. Kovalevsky G, Gracia CR, Berlin JA, Sammel MD, Barnhart KT. Evaluation of the association between hereditary thrombophilias and recurrent pregnancy loss: a meta-analysis. Arch Intern Med. 2004;164:558–63.
45. Carp H, Dolitzky M, Tur-Kaspa I, Inbal A. Hereditary thrombophilias are not associated with a decreased live birth rate in women with recurrent miscarriage. Fertil Steril. 2002;78:58–62.
46. Rai R, Backos M, Elgaddal S, Shlebak A, Regan L. Factor V Leiden and recurrent miscarriage—prospective outcome of untreated pregnancies. Hum Reprod. 2002;17:442–5.
47. Jivraj S, Makris M, Saravelos S, Li TC. Pregnancy outcome in women with factor V Leiden and recurrent miscarriage. BJOG. 2009;116:995–8.
48. Stephenson MD, Kutteh W. Evaluation and management of recurrent early pregnancy loss. Clin Obstet Gynecol. 2007;50:1312–45.
49. Royal College of Obstetricians and Gynaecologists, Scientific Advisory Committee, Guideline No. 17. The investigation and treatment of couples with recurrent first-trimester and second-trimester miscarriage. Published May 2011. https://www.rcog.org.uk/globalassets/documents/guidelines/gtg_17.pdf.
50. Practice Committee of the American Society for Reproductive Medicine. Evaluation and treatment of recurrent pregnancy loss: a committee opinion. Fertil Steril. 2012;98:1103–11.

51. Stephenson MD. Frequency of factors associated with habitual abortion in 197 couples. Fertil Steril. 1996;66:24–9.
52. Jaslow CR, Camey JL, Kutteh WH. Diagnostic factors identified in 1020 women with two versus three or more recurrent pregnancy losses. Fertil Steril. 2010;93:1234–43.
53. Mall FP, Meyer AW. Studies on abortuses: a survey of pathologic ova in the Carnegie embryological collection. In: Contributions to embryology, vol. 12. Washington, DC: Carnegie Institution; 1921. p. 1–364.
54. Hertig AT. Human trophoblast. Springfield, IL: Charles C.Thomas; 1968. p. 167.
55. Rushton DI. Simplified classification of spontaneous abortions. J Med Genet. 1978;15:1–9.
56. Bagshawe KD, Dent J, Webb J. Hydatidiform mole in England and Wales 1973–83. Lancet. 1986;2:673–7.
57. Berkowitz RS, Im SS, Bernstein MR, Goldstein DP. Gestational trophoblastic disease. Subsequent pregnancy outcome, including repeat molar pregnancy. J Reprod Med. 1998;43:81–6.
58. Lorigan PC, Sharma S, Bright N, Coleman RE, Hancock BW. Characteristics of women with recurrent molar pregnancies. Gynecol Oncol. 2000;78:288–92.
59. Matsui H, Iitsuka Y, Suzuka K, Seki K, Sekiya S. Subsequent pregnancy outcome in patients with spontaneous resolution of HCG after evacuation of hydatidiform mole: comparison between complete and partial mole. Hum Reprod. 2001;16:1274–7.
60. Sebire NJ, Fisher RA, Foskett M, Rees H, Seckl MJ, Newlands ES. Risk of recurrent hydatidiform mole and subsequent pregnancy outcome following complete or partial hydatidiform molar pregnancy. BJOG. 2003;110:22–6.
61. Sebire NJ, Savage PM, Seckl MJ, Fisher RA. Histopathological features of biparental complete hydatidiform moles in women with NLRP7 mutations. Placenta. 2013;34:50–6.
62. Jauniaux E, Nicolaides KH. Early ultrasound diagnosis and follow-up of molar pregnancies. Ultrasound Obstet Gynecol. 1997;9:17–21.
63. Lazarus E, Hulka CA, Siewert B, Levine D. Sonographic appearance of early complete molar pregnancies. J Ultrasound Med. 1999;18:589–93.
64. Lindholm H, Flam F. The diagnosis of molar pregnancy by sonography and gross morphology. Acta Obstet Gynecol Scand. 1999;78:6–9.
65. Benson CB, Genest DR, Bernstein MR, Soto-Wright V, Goldstein DP, Berkowitz RS. Sonographic appearance of first trimester complete hydatidiform moles. Ultrasound Obstet Gynecol. 2000;16:188–91.
66. Jauniaux E, Kadri R, Hustin J. Partial mole and triploidy: screening in patients with first trimester spontaneous abortion. Obstet Gynecol. 1996;88:616–9.
67. Jauniaux E, Hustin J. Histological examination of first trimester spontaneous abortions: the impact of materno-embryonic interface features. Histopathology. 1992;21:409–14.
68. Fukunaga M, Ushigome S, Fukunaga M, Sugishita M. Application of flow cytometry in diagnosis of hydatidiform moles. Mod Pathol. 1993;6:353–9.
69. Koening C, Demopoulos RI, Vamvakas EC, Mittal KR, Feiner HD, Espiritu EC. Flow cytometric DNA ploidy and quantitative histopathology in partial moles. Int J Gynaecol Pathol. 1993;12:235–40.
70. van Oven MW, Schoots CJ, Oosterhuis JW, Keij JF, Dam-Meiring A, Huisjes HJ. The use of DNA flow cytometry in the diagnosis of triploidy in human abortions. Hum Pathol. 1989;20:238–42.
71. Blocklage TJ, Smith HO, Barlow SA. Distinctive flow histogram pattern in molar pregnancies with elevated maternal serum human chorionic gonadotropin levels. Cancer. 1994;73:2782–90.
72. Kaspar HG, Kraemer BB, Kraus FT. DNA ploidy by image cytometry and karyotype in spontaneous abortion. Hum Pathol. 1998;29:1013–6.
73. Chew SH, Perlmann EJ, Williams R, Kurman RJ, Ronnett BM. Morphology and DNA content analysis in the evaluation of first trimester placentas for partial hydatidiform mole (PHM). Hum Pathol. 2000;31:914–24.

74. Genest DR. Partial hydatidiform mole: clinicopathological features, differential diagnosis, ploidy and molecular studies, and gold standards for diagnosis. Int J Gynecol Pathol. 2001;20:315–22.
75. Fisher RA, Hodges MD, Newlands ES. Familial recurrent hydatidiform mole: a review. J Reprod Med. 2004;49:595–601.
76. Murdoch S, Djuric U, Mazhar B, Seoud M, Khan R, Kuick R, Bagga R, Kircheisen R, Ao A, Ratti B, et al. Mutations in NALP7 cause recurrent hydatidiform moles and reproductive wastage in humans. Nat Genet. 2006;38:300–2.
77. Parry DA, Logan CV, Hayward BE, Shires M, Landolsi H, Diggle C, Carr I, Rittore C, Touitou I, Philibert L, et al. Mutations causing familial biparental hydatidiform mole implicate c6orf221 as a possible regulator of genomic imprinting in the human oocyte. Am J Hum Genet. 2011;89:451–8.
78. Jacques SM, Qureshi F. Chronic intervillositis of the placenta. Arch Pathol Lab Med. 1993;117(10):1032–5.
79. Doss BJ, Greene MF, Hill J, Heffner LJ, Bieber FR, Genest DR. Massive chronic intervillositis associated with recurrent abortions. Hum Pathol. 1995;26:1245–51.
80. Boyd TK, Redline RW. Chronic histiocytic intervillositis: a placental lesion associated with recurrent reproductive loss. Hum Pathol. 2000;31:1389–96.
81. Boog G, Le Vaillant C, Alnoukari F, Jossic F, Barrier J, Muller JY. Combining corticosteroid and aspirin for the prevention of recurrent villitis or intervillositis of unknown etiology. J Gynecol Obstet Biol Reprod. 2006;35:396–404.
82. Rota C, Carles D, Schaeffer V, Guyon F, Saura R, Horovitz J. Perinatal prognosis of pregnancies complicated by placental chronic intervillitis. J Gynecol Obstet Biol Reprod. 2006;35:711–9.
83. Creagh MD, Malia RG, Cooper SM, Smith AR, Duncan SL, Greaves M. Screening for lupus anticoagulant and anticardiolipin antibodies in women with fetal loss. J Clin Pathol. 1991;44:45–7.
84. Hanly JG, Gladman DD, Rose TH, Laskin CA, Urowitz MB. Lupus pregnancy. A prospective study of placental changes. Arthritis Rheum. 1988;31:358–66.
85. Salafia CM, Parke AL. Placental pathology in systemic lupus erythematosus and phospholipid antibody syndrome. Rheum Dis Clin N Am. 1997;23:85–97.
86. Levy RA, Avvad E, Oliveira J, Porto LC. Placental pathology in antiphospholipid syndrome. Lupus. 1998;7(Suppl 2):S81–5.
87. Magid MS, Kaplan C, Sammaritano LR, Peterson M, Druzin ML, Lockshin MD. Placental pathology in systemic lupus erythematosus: a prospective study. Am J Obstet Gynecol. 1998;179:226–34.
88. Ackerman J, Gonzalez EF, Gilbert-Barness E. Immunological studies of the placenta in maternal connective tissue disease. Pediatr Dev Pathol. 1999;2:19–24.
89. Ogishima D, Matsumoto T, Nakamura Y, Yoshida K, Kuwabara Y. Placental pathology in systemic lupus erythematosus with antiphospholipid antibodies. Pathol Int. 2000;50:224–9.
90. Sebire NJ, Fox H, Backos M, Rai R, Paterson C, Regan L. Defective endovascular trophoblast invasion in primary antiphospholipid antibody syndrome associated early pregnancy failure. Hum Reprod. 2002;17:1067–71.
91. Arias F, Romero R, Joist H, Kraus FT. Thrombophilia: a mechanism of disease in women with adverse pregnancy outcome and thrombotic lesions in the placenta. J Matern Fetal Med. 1998;7:277–86.
92. Mousa HA, Alfirevic Z. Do placental lesions reflect thrombophilia state in women with adverse pregnancy outcome? Hum Reprod. 2000;15:1830–3.
93. Rand JH, Wu XX, Guller S, Scher J, Andree HA, Lockwood CJ. Antiphospholipid immunoglobulin G antibodies reduce annexin-V levels on syncytiotrophoblast apical membranes and in culture media of placental villi. Am J Obstet Gynecol. 1997;177:918–23.
94. Khong TY, Liddell HS, Robertson WB. Defective haemochorial placentation as a cause of miscarriage: a preliminary study. Br J Obstet Gynaecol. 1987;94(7):649–55.

95. Michel MZ, Khong TY, Clark DA, Beard RW. A morphological and immunological study of human placental bed biopsies I miscarriage. Br J Obstet Gynaecol. 1990;97(11):984–8.
96. Jauniaux E, Burton GJ. Pathophysiology of histological changes in early pregnancy loss. Placenta. 2005;26(2–3):114–23.
97. Nakashima A, Shiozaki A, Myojo S, Ito M, Tatematsu M, Sakai M, Takamori Y, Ogawa K, Nagata K, Saito S. Granulysin produced by uterine natural killer cells induces apoptosis of extravillous trophoblasts in spontaneous abortion. Am J Pathol. 2008;173(3):653–64.
98. Hiby SE, Apps R, Sharkey AM, Farrell LE, Gardner L, Mulder A, Claas FH, Walker JJ, Redman CW, Morgan L, Tower C, Regan L, Moore GE, Carrington M, Moffett A. Maternal activating KIRs protect against human reproductive failure mediated by fetal HLA-C2. J Clin Invest. 2010;120(11):4102–10.
99. Wu S, Zhang H, Tian J, Liu L, Dong Y, Mao T. Expression of kisspeptin/GPR54 and PIBF/PR in the first trimester trophoblast and decidua of women with recurrent spontaneous abortion. Pathol Res Pract. 2014;210(1):47–54.
100. Tian FJ, Qin CM, Li XC, Wu F, Liu XR, Xu WM, Lin Y. Decreased stathmin-1 expression inhibits trophoblast proliferation and invasion and is associated with recurrent miscarriage. Am J Pathol. 2015;185(10):2709–21.
101. Aplin JD, Haigh T, Vicovac L, Church HJ, Jones CJP. Anchorage in the developing placenta: an overlooked determinant of pregnancy outcome? Hum Fertil. 1998;1(1):75–9.
102. Bulla R, de Guarrini F, Pausa M, Fischetti F, Meroni PL, De Seta F, Guaschino S, Tedesco F. Inhibition of trophoblast adhesion to endothelial cells by the sera of women with recurrent spontaneous abortions. Am J Reprod Immunol. 1999;42(2):116–23.
103. Cinar O, Kara F, Can A. Potential role of decidual apoptosis in the pathogenesis of miscarriages. Gynecol Endocrinol. 2012;28(5):382–5.
104. Lea RG, Underwood J, Flanders KC, Hirte H, Banwatt D, Finotto S, Ohno I, Daya S, Harley C, Michel M, et al. A subset of patients with recurrent spontaneous abortion is deficient in transforming growth factor beta-2-producing "suppressor cells" in uterine tissue near the placental attachment site. Am J Reprod Immunol. 1995;34(1):52–64.
105. Zhao A, Lin Q, Zhou H. [Immunohistochemical study on the decidua vessels in recurrent spontaneous abortion]. Zhonghua Fu Chan Ke Za Zhi. 1997;32(11):674–7.
106. Lea RG, Tulppala M, Critchley HO. Deficient syncytiotrophoblast tumour necrosis factor-alpha characterizes failing first trimester pregnancies in a subgroup of recurrent miscarriage patients. Hum Reprod. 1997;12(6):1313–20.
107. Kwak JY, Beer AE, Kim SH, Mantouvalos HP. Immunopathology of the implantation site utilizing monoclonal antibodies to natural killer cells in women with recurrent pregnancy losses. Am J Reprod Immunol. 1999;41(1):91–8.
108. Emmer PM, Steegers EA, Kerstens HM, Bulten J, Nelen WL, Boer K, Joosten I. Altered phenotype of HLA-G expressing trophoblast and decidual natural killer cells in pathological pregnancies. Hum Reprod. 2002;17(4):1072–80.
109. Quack KC, Vassiliadou N, Pudney J, Anderson DJ, Hill JA. Leukocyte activation in the decidua of chromosomally normal and abnormal fetuses from women with recurrent abortion. Hum Reprod. 2001;16(5):949–55.
110. Askelund K, Liddell HS, Zanderigo AM, Fernando NS, Khong TY, Stone PR, Chamley LW. CD83(+)dendritic cells in the decidua of women with recurrent miscarriage and normal pregnancy. Placenta. 2004;25(2–3):140–5.
111. Mei S, Tan J, Chen H, Chen Y, Zhang J. Changes of CD4+CD25high regulatory T cells and FOXP3 expression in unexplained recurrent spontaneous abortion patients. Fertil Steril. 2010;94(6):2244–7.
112. Ozcimen EE, Kiyici H, Uckuyu A, Yanik FF. Are CD57+ natural killer cells really important in early pregnancy failure? Arch Gynecol Obstet. 2009;279(4):493–7.
113. Wang WJ, Hao CF, Yi-Lin, Yin GJ, Bao SH, Qiu LH, Lin QD. Increased prevalence of T helper 17 (Th17) cells in peripheral blood and decidua in unexplained recurrent spontaneous abortion patients. J Reprod Immunol. 2010;84(2):164–70.

114. Bao SH, Wang XP, De Lin Q, Wang WJ, Yin GJ, Qiu LH. Decidual CD4+CD25+CD127dim/- regulatory T cells in patients with unexplained recurrent spontaneous miscarriage. Eur J Obstet Gynecol Reprod Biol. 2011;155(1):94–8.
115. Li J, Li FF, Zuo W, Zhou Y, Hao HY, Dang J, Jiang M, He MZ, Deng DR. Up-regulated expression of Tim-3/Gal-9 at maternal-fetal interface in pregnant woman with recurrent spontaneous abortion. J Huazhong Univ Sci Technolog Med Sci. 2014;34(4):586–90.
116. Yuan J, Li J, Huang SY, Sun X. Characterization of the subsets of human NKT-like cells and the expression of Th1/Th2 cytokines in patients with unexplained recurrent spontaneous abortion. J Reprod Immunol. 2015;110:81–8.
117. Zhang XX, Kang XM, Zhao AM. Regulation of $CD4^{+}FOXP3^{+}$ T cells by CCL20/CCR6 axis in early unexplained recurrent miscarriage patients. Genet Mol Res. 2015;14(3):9145–54.
118. Wang S, Zhu X, Xu Y, Zhang D, Li Y, Tao Y, Piao H, Li D, Du M. Programmed cell death-1 (PD-1) and T-cell immunoglobulin mucin-3 (Tim-3) regulate CD4+ T cells to induce Type 2 helper T cell (Th2) bias at the maternal-fetal interface. Hum Reprod. 2016;31(4):700–11.
119. Meuleman T, Cohen D, Swings GM, Veraar K, Claas FH, Bloemenkamp KW. Increased complement C4d deposition at the maternal-fetal interface in unexplained recurrent miscarriage. J Reprod Immunol. 2016;113:54–60.
120. Dong F, Zhang Y, Xia F, Yang Y, Xiong S, Jin L, Zhang J. Genome-wide miRNA profiling of villus and decidua of recurrent spontaneous abortion patients. Reproduction. 2014;148(1):33–41.
121. Li D, Li J. Association of miR-34a-3p/5p, miR-141-3p/5p, and miR-24 in decidual natural killer cells with unexplained recurrent spontaneous abortion. Med Sci Monit. 2016;22:922–9.
122. Wang JM, Gu Y, Zhang Y, Yang Q, Zhang X, Yin L, Wang J. Deep-sequencing identification of differentially expressed miRNAs in decidua and villus of recurrent miscarriage patients. Arch Gynecol Obstet. 2016;293(5):1125–35.

Inflammatory Markers and Proteomic Analysis

19

Pakhee Aggarwal

19.1 Introduction

Recurrent pregnancy loss (RPL) is a common pregnancy complication and is defined as three or more consecutive pregnancy losses before the 20th week of gestation. The incidence of RPL is estimated to be <5% with about 1% women of reproductive age group facing three or more consecutive miscarriages [1]. Even so, up to 50% of women with RPL are still reported as unexplained, often because of limited clinical investigations [2]. It is in this subgroup of women that molecular analysis of inflammatory markers and proteomics can have diagnostic and therapeutic implications. Proteomics involves the study of protein markers in serum, blood, pregnancy tissue, or follicular fluid which are differentially expressed between normal pregnancy and RPL. These markers are evaluated using techniques of large-scale protein separation and identification like 2D gel electrophoresis and MALDI-TOF or real-time PCR. Research is ongoing in this area, and each new discovery brings with it a promise of improved diagnosis and treatment of women suffering from RPL.

Pregnancy is a state of immune tolerance to the developing fetus, and the complex interactions between the two are an important area where new directions continue to excite interest in the medical fraternity. Separating the immune from the inflammatory may be difficult due to the natural overlap between the two. Nevertheless, this chapter will try to focus on the inflammatory markers pertaining to RPL. We know that inflammation is vital to both implantation and miscarriage [1].

While inflammatory markers have been studied for a while now, biomarkers and proteomics have come up within the last decade. There is no one marker which stands above the rest, although several have been studied and are the subject of ongoing research.

P. Aggarwal
Obstetrics and Gynaecology, Fortis Healthcare (Fortis Memorial Research Institute, Gurugram and Fortis Flt Lt, Rajan Dhall Hospital, New Delhi, India
e-mail: drpakhee@gmail.com

S. Mehta, B. Gupta (eds.), *Recurrent Pregnancy Loss*,
https://doi.org/10.1007/978-981-10-7338-0_19

The research on molecular causes of RPL can be divided into three types of "omics" [3]:

1. Genomics—immune response, thrombosis, steroid biosynthesis, and apoptosis- and angiogenesis-related genes are responsible.
2. Transcriptomics—immune response and angiogenesis- and apoptosis-related genes are involved.
3. Proteomics—immune response and thrombosis-related proteins are involved.

After excluding the traditional causes of RPL, if immunopathological evaluation of placenta is done, studies show that there is increased inflammatory cell infiltration at the implantation site and fibrin deposition in decidua and perivillous placental membranes. Also, nearly a third of the decidual vessels show evidence of thrombosis, suggesting that inflammation and coagulation go hand in hand [4].

As the fetal-placental unit develops, an immune barrier is set up between the semi-allogenic fetus carrying the paternal antigens and the maternal immune system. This barrier is formed of the peripheral blood lymphocytes (easy to evaluate) and the endometrial lymphocytes (evaluated by endometrial biopsy). While the peripheral blood lymphocytes reflect the systemic immune responses, endometrial lymphocytes indicate the local environment [5].

19.1.1 Peripheral Blood Lymphocytes

At a cellular level, the T lymphocytes are segregated into helper T cells (CD3+ and CD4+) and suppressor T cells (CD3+ and CD8+). The T helper cells can be further characterized by their patterns of cytokine production into T helper 1 (Th1) and 2 (Th2) cells. Th1 secrete TNF-α, IFN-γ, and IL-2 cytokines, while Th2 cells secrete IL-10, IL-5, IL-6, and IL-4. Successful pregnancy is said to be a Th2 cytokine-dominated phenomenon, while Th1 cytokines can lead to pregnancy loss. Th1 cytokines (1) induce cytotoxic activity in uterine NK cells and cytotoxic T cells (CTLs) and (2) cause B cells to release various autoantibodies, including APA, ANA, and ATA. These may cause growth inhibition of the trophoblast and pathogenic thrombosis. In contrast to Th1 cytokines, Th2 cytokines inhibit the activation of uterine NK cells and CTLs. IL-12 induces the secretion of Th1 cytokines and suppresses the secretion of Th2 cytokines [3].

Miscarriage is associated with an increased level of IFN-γ and decreased level of IL-10, and the converse true for the control group as per a study [6]. Several studies show that the percentages of T helper cell (CD3+/CD4+) levels in women with RPL are not different from those of normal fertile women [7], but when the ratios of Th1/Th2 were compared, women with RPL had significantly elevated Th1:Th2 ratios compared to that of normal fertile controls. This is calculated by dividing the proportion of Th1 cytokine-producing cells by the proportion of Th2 cytokine-producing cells with the following combinations: IFNγ/IL-4, IFNγ/IL-10, TNFα/IL-4, and TNFα/IL-10 [8].The same study also demonstrated that although the T suppressor cell (CD3+/CD8+) levels were not different in women with recurrent pregnancy losses compared to controls, the ratio of TNFα to IL-10 was significantly elevated as compared to those of normal controls [7]. Thus, women with RPL have increased Th1 cytokine responses at the systemic level. In addition, regulatory T cells (CD56+) are reduced in women with RPL compared to normal pregnancy or nonpregnant controls indicating that these may play a role in the maintenance of normal pregnancy [9].

At a further molecular level, in peripheral blood of healthy pregnant women, the percentage of T cells with γδ TCR+ was significantly higher ($p < 0.001$) than in that of recurrent aborters or of nonpregnant individuals. These γδ TCR-bearing lymphocytes may have a role in progesterone-dependent immunomodulation [10]. There are two separate subpopulations of these cells, one of which is found in the peripheral blood of healthy pregnant women, while the other is seen in recurrent aborters.

19.1.2 Endometrial Lymphocytes

Lymphocytes are found in the endometrium during all phases of the menstrual cycle. Their levels decline in early pregnancy. Some studies show that patients who had miscarriages had significantly more $CD4^+$, $CD8^+$, $CD14^+$, $CD16^+$, and $CD56^+$ leukocytes in their endometrium on endometrial biopsy than women with live births or women with proven fertility [11]. Sometimes, an alteration in the ratio of CD4/CD8, with decrease in CD8+, has been seen in women with RPL [12]. These indicate that endometrial immune conditions are altered in women with RPL, with the T lymphocytes showing a distinctive profile.

At a cytokine level, helper Th2 and cytotoxic Th2 cells are reduced in the decidua basalis of women with RPL, lending further credence to the fact that successful pregnancy requires a Th2 envoirnment [13].

19.1.3 Natural Killer Cells

The natural killer (NK) cells (CD16+/CD56+), although called so, cannot kill trophoblastic cells, except when activated by Th1 cytokines or in vitro. However activated NK cells can produce cytokines that can induce abortion [5]. Women with RPL have increased peripheral blood NK cells compared to women with normal pregnancy outcomes [14]. When the levels of peripheral blood NK cells were quantified, women with RPL had a significant elevation which was associated with spontaneous abortion of a pregnancy with normal karyotype [15]. Thus, conventional NK cells and failure to suppress NK cell activation play an important role in immunologically preventable spontaneous abortions.

Activated NK cells may also be responsible for implantation failure as they are present in the endometrium at the peri-gestational period. The endometrial NK cells have a different phenotypic expression (CD16-/CD56bright) than peripheral blood

NK cells (CD16+/CD56dim). CD56dim cells show high cytotoxicity and express high level of CD16. On the other hand, CD56bright cells show low cytotoxicity, express low level of CD16, and produce some immunoregulatory cytokines, mainly IFN-γ10 [16]. The main role of endometrial NK cells is the cytotoxicity and production of cytokines that are controlled by HLA class I antigens. When the HLA-G molecule of trophoblast cells interacts with killer activatory receptor (KAR) of uterine natural killer (NK) cells, cytokines released from uterine NK cells attack trophoblast cells. Interaction of HLA-G with killer inhibitory receptor (KIR) has opposite effects [3]. In addition, the decidual NK (dNK) cells initiate decidualization, regulate trophoblast migration and invasion, and also mediate endometrial angiogenesis, thereby playing a role in endometrial angiogenesis and regeneration [17]. Flow cytometric analysis of decidual lymphocytes from normal pregnancy demonstrated that the relative proportion of decidual NK cells was increased to approximately the same extent in normal pregnancy and RPL. But, in women with RPL, the decidual NK activity was much higher [18]. These cells produce many different cytokines such as G-CSF, GM-CSF, M-CSF, TNFα, IFNγ, LIF, and IL-8, and the imbalance between these can predispose to RPL. The percentages of IL-4 and IFNγ-producing NK T cells were significantly higher in the decidua compared with the peripheral blood, indicating that NK cells might control the Th1/Th2 balance by producing IL-4 and IFNγ at the feto-maternal interface [19].

Proinflammatory cytokines also play a central role in the differential effects on the coagulation and fibrinolysis pathways. Conversely, the activation of coagulation may affect inflammatory responses by direct and indirect mechanisms [20]. Increase in proinflammatory cytokines is associated with a decrease in the ability to generate activated protein C (APC). Pregnant women with increased thrombin reserve and resistance to APC have increased levels of TNFα, and this may be important in the risk for adverse pregnancy outcomes [21]. Women with RPL have significantly increased peripheral blood Th1 cells as compared to normal fertile women [8]. The combination of proinflammatory cytokines and an upregulated thrombophilic tendency seems to play a major role in RPL.

Apoptosis is a critical process during placental development and differentiation to maintain tissue homeostasis. It has been shown that the Fas ligand (FasL)—Fas interaction between decidual cells expressing FasL and Fas-bearing leukocytes—leads to apoptosis of activated leukocytes. This leads to downregulation of the production of cytokines, including TGFb and IL-10. This promotes trophoblast invasion. Conversely, when decidual cells lacking FasL are present, extensive leukocyte infiltration and inhibition of trophoblast invasion have been observed. The regulatory mechanisms for expression of FasL in decidual cells need further study [22].

During pregnancy, extensive angiogenesis occurs in the chorionic villi and placenta to provide oxygen and nutrition for the fetus. Aberrant angiogenesis may lead to pregnancy loss or abnormal growth of the fetus. Studies show that the expression levels of angiogenesis-related genes, including matrix metalloproteinase-2 (MMP-2), plasminogen activator inhibitor (PAI), integrin, transforming growth factor-b (TGF-b), vascular endothelial growth factor (VEGF), and basic fibroblast growth factor (bFGF), were lower in chorionic villi derived from RPL patients as compared to normal controls [23], indicating its possible involvement in RPL.

19.2 Human Leukocyte Antigen

Some studies show that aberrant human leukocyte antigen (HLA)-G expression is associated with RPL [24]. HLA-G is a nonclassical MHC class Ib antigen expressed almost exclusively in extravillous trophoblasts at the feto-maternal interface throughout pregnancy and may play a crucial role in immune tolerance of the fetus [25]. The classical MHC class I is not expressed in this tissue. This differential expression of HLA-G and HLA class I molecules suggests a genetic regulation at the microlevel. Indeed, a consistent overexpression of miRNA-133a was found in women who had RPL with normal karyotype; this miRNA-133a targets HLA-G and mediates reduction of HLA-G expression at protein level. Since HLA-G confers feto-maternal immune tolerance, a reduction may be implicated in RPL. Several other polymorphisms have been investigated and need further research in order to be therapeutically useful [26].

An excess of HLA sharing in primary and secondary recurrent aborters has been reported. The primary aborters shared human HLA-A and DQ antigens, and primary and secondary aborters shared three or more of the human leukocyte A, B, DR, and DQ antigens [27]. For HLA class II loci, significantly more couples with RPL shared 2 HLA DQA1 alleles as compared with fertile control couples, who had a significant deficit of HLA DQA1 compatible live born babies [28].

HLA antigens have been associated with the extent of an immune response to specific antigens. Couples with increased HLA sharing and recurrent pregnancy losses often demonstrate lack of anti-paternal cytotoxic antibodies (APCA), anti-idiotypic antibodies (Ab2), and mixed lymphocyte reaction blocking antibodies (MLR-Bf). This finding suggests that a histocompatible pregnancy may evoke maternal autoimmunity and perhaps upregulate Th1 immune responses [5].

19.3 Inflammatory Markers

The evaluation of nongenetic biomarkers in peripheral blood or the uterus may sometimes be unrevealing as they may not necessarily reflect conditions in the compartment of the body where the pregnancy is located; for example, measurement of these biomarkers in the uterus can only be undertaken by endometrial biopsy or uterine flushing, which cannot be done with the pregnancy in situ. During the non-pregnant state, these biomarkers vary with the menstrual cycle and are also different from the first trimester of pregnancy. Cytokine mRNA expression is low in the proliferative and early secretory phases but rises in the mid-secretory phase to peak in the late secretory phase. The expression in early pregnancy is similar to the mid-secretory phase. Testing in a different phase may limit the informative value, to the extent that abnormal biomarkers found in tissue from missed abortions may be the result of the inflammatory process rather than the cause. There may be interlaboratory variations in assessing for these biomarkers, not to mention the inter-assay variations due to the process of evaluation, which is based on enzymatic lysis of the parent endometrial/decidual tissue to isolate the antigens on the lymphocytes or trophoblast cells, which can well modify the antigen expression. These also explain why the test results are not easy to replicate in another setting, despite having encouraging results in one study [29].

As regards genetic biomarkers, most are pertaining to genes which promote excessive inflammatory responses. A recent study showed that during the implantation window, an increase in proinflammatory cytokines (IL-1β, TNFα, and IFNγ) in contrast to anti-inflammatory cytokines (IL-4 and IL-10) resulted in an upregulation of TGFβ which in turn induced the expression of COX-2 gene. The product of this gene, namely, PGE2, was upregulated, which in combination with decrease in VEGF (mediated by a decrease in angiogenic cytokines) made the endometrium inhospitable for implantation. COX-2 gene also upregulates MMP-9 causing excessive matrix degradation and improper remodeling of the endometrium. On endometrial biopsy, the markers of receptivity like leukemia inhibitory factor (LIF), integrins, and cell adhesion molecules are reduced, and the pinopdes are poorly developed. All these can interfere with implantation and lead to RPL. This is a double-edged sword, for although early exposure of proinflammatory cytokines is necessary for stimulating invasion of the blastocyst and formation of new blood vessels during implantation, an exaggerated proinflammatory response and reduced anti-inflammatory cytokines can bring about complications in implantation that can even result in pregnancy loss [30].

Two genetic molecular markers TNF-α (−308) and IFN-γ (+874) are the candidate genes for RPL. Women carrying select polymorphisms of these genes may be genetically predisposed to developing RPL. However, their expression is also influenced by other genes in the region and the environmental factors. This is why the extent of the manifestation varies with different ethnic groups, lifestyle factors, and other population-specific environmental factors [31].

Even before the era of molecular medicine, an older study showed that inflammation was linked to RPL. Women with RPL and normal karyotype had one or more of the following features on histology—chronic intervillositis, increased perivillous fibrin deposition with intermediate trophoblast, decidual plasma cells, deciduitis without plasma cells, and chronic villitis. These features were more common in habitual aborters (31%) as compared to one time aborters (13%) [32].

In a more recent study, women with BMI ≥ 25 kg/m^2 and RPL had a significantly increased endometrial expression of haptoglobin compared to their lean counterparts ($p = 0.01$). These patients also displayed a significant increase in endometrial expression of transthyretin ($p = 0.04$) and beta globulin ($p = 0.04$). Haptoglobin is an important component of the body's response to inflammatory conditions (one such condition being obesity) and is also produced by the endometrium. Transthyretin and beta globin are intravascular products, and their increased expression in the obese miscarriage cohort may indicate some form of vascular or endothelial dysfunction (again as a part of chronic inflammation) in these women. Although the sample size in this study was small, the putative role of inflammation in RPL can be gleaned from the results [33].

When it comes to detecting inflammatory biomarkers in the blood, one recent molecule that has been evaluated is the soluble form of cellular receptor for advanced glycation end products (sRAGE). The cellular form of this receptor (RAGE) is a cell surface receptor which is bound by ligands, including AGEs, eliciting oxidative stress and subsequent inflammatory and thrombogenic reactions in a many cells. Its role in several disorders such as glucose intolerance, cardiovascular disease, cancer cell growth and metastasis, Alzheimer's disease, and osteoporosis is under study. The activation of RAGE results in inflammatory and thrombogenic reactions in the vessels, stimulating the production of soluble forms of intercellular adhesion molecule-1 (sICAM-1), vascular cell adhesion molecule-1 (sVCAM-1), plasminogen activator inhibitor-1 (PAI-1), vascular endothelial growth factor (VEGF), TNFα, IFNγ, monocyte chemoattractant protein-1 (MCP-1), interleukin-8 (IL-8), and insulin resistance, which together play a role in RPL. These effects can be measured using ELISA or commercially available test kits. A prospective study found that the values for sRAGE and metabolic biomarkers were statistically significantly higher in women with RPL compared with the controls. A further multivariate analysis revealed that the levels of insulin, plasminogen activator inhibitor-1, the resistance index of the uterine radial artery, and the ratio of tumor necrosis factor-α/interleukin-10 producing T helper cells were statistically significantly associated with the serum sRAGE level. Thus, sRAGE may contribute to RPL by reducing uterine blood flow and subsequently causing ischemia in the fetus via inflammatory and thrombotic reactions [34].

A recent retrospective study evaluated inflammatory markers (adiponectin, CRP, leptin, and IL-6) and autoimmune markers (total immunoglobulins, ANA, thyroid antibodies, antiphospholipid antibodies) in a group of 55 women with RPL/recurrent implantation failure (RIF) and also correlated it to the presence of chronic endometritis on biopsy. The study revealed a prevalence of systemic inflammation in 32.7%, autoimmunity in 61.8%, and chronic endometritis in 45.5% women with RPL/RIF. However, there was no correlation of systemic inflammatory or autoimmune markers with the presence of endometritis on biopsy [35].

In the peripheral blood, natural cytotoxicity receptors (NCR) are markers which regulate NK cell cytotoxicity and cytokine production. A study which evaluated NCRs and intracellular cytokine expression of peripheral blood NK cells using flow cytometry, in women with RPL/RIF, found a negative correlation between NCRs and intracellular cytokines expression. This observation suggests that excessive pro-inflammatory cytokine expression in NK cells in RPL/RIF may be mediated through the NCRs or interruption of signal transduction processes [36].

In women with RPL, defects in endometrial receptivity also play a role. These could be related to the integrin family-mediated regulation of estrogen and progesterone mediators during the implantation window [37].

19.4 Proteomics

Proteomics refers to the identification and quantification of all the proteins derived from a tissue or the whole genome. Proteomics has been considered as a new technique for investigation of the possible proteins associated with placentation and pregnancy-related disorders like RPL or preeclampsia [38].

For proteomic analysis, the sequence followed to extract and analyze the proteome is as follows: two-dimensional gel electrophoresis to identify protein spots of interest, which are then subject to mass spectrometry (MS). Proteins are then identified by peptide mass fingerprinting and confirmed by matrix-assisted laser desorption ionization (MALDI) – time-of-flight MS (MALDI-TOF MS). Validation of proteomic data is done by quantitative real-time reverse transcriptase-polymerase chain reaction (RT-PCR). The relative expression of mRNA is then quantified and deemed positive when the value is few folds higher than control. This is followed by Western blotting to determine protein levels using their respective monoclonal or polyclonal antibodies. These are expressed as units. Flow cytometry is used to analyze activity (e.g., cytokine activity) in cells of interest.

Research into proteomics showed five aberrantly expressed proteins (complement component C3c chain E, fibrinogen gamma, antithrombin, angiotensinogen, and hemopexin precursor) in follicular fluid from RPL patients with MALDI-TOF-MS and nano-LC MS/MS. Western blot analysis confirmed that the protein expression level of fibrinogen gamma and antithrombin was less in follicular fluid from RPL patients than those from normal controls. Further, semiquantitative RT-PCR and real-time PCR analyses revealed that mRNA level of these coagulation factors was also decreased significantly in chorionic villi of RPL patients compared with normal samples, indicating that these coagulation factors (fibrinogen gamma and antithrombin) play an important role in maintaining normal pregnancy [39].

Another RPL-associated factor studied in the human blood using proteomics is ITI-H4 (inter-α trypsin inhibitor-heavy chain 4). When blood from women with RPL was studied and compared to pooled blood sample of normal women, this protein was highly expressed in Western blot analysis. The preliminary data indicates that this could be a potential proteomic marker with diagnostic and therapeutic implications [40].

Even in patients with antiphospholipid syndrome (APS), few proteins were significantly altered among monocytes from APS patients with thrombosis (annexin I, annexin II, protein disulfide isomerase, Nedd8, RhoA proteins, and Hsp60) which were functionally related to the induction of a procoagulant state as well as to autoimmune-related responses. Proteins reported to be connected to RPL fibrinogen and hemoglobin were also determined to be significantly deregulated in APS patients without thrombosis, thus giving importance to the role of proteomic biomarkers for diagnosis, assessing prognosis, and guiding therapy in APS [41].

Over 5000 proteins are expressed in the placental villi. Focal adhesion is a critical signaling pathway at the interface between cells and the extracellular matrix. Focal adhesion proteins are essential for successful implantation and placentation during early pregnancy. Proteomic analysis revealed that five proteins are altered in women with early pregnancy loss. While Desmin, HistoneH4, and MMP-9 are upregulated, the LaminC/LaminA protein ratio was downregulated in the pregnancy loss group compared to the control group. These proteins may serve as biomarkers for early and recurrent pregnancy loss [42].

In another study involving the placenta of women with unexplained RPL (URPL), at least 19 protein spots were differentially expressed between URPL and normal placentas ($p < 0.05$), of which 12 of them were successfully identified. While only two proteins were downregulated (calumenin and enolase 1), the remaining ten spots (actin gamma 1 propeptide, cathepsin D prepropeptide, heat shock protein gp96, tubulin beta, tubulin alpha 1, glutathione S-transferase, vitamin D-binding protein, prohibitin, actin beta, apolipoprotein A-I) showed increased expression in URPL cases in comparison with normal placentas. Each of these proteins mediates specific functions at a molecular level—cytoskeletal proteins (actin gamma 1 propeptide, actin beta, tubulin alpha and beta), transport/cargo proteins (vitamin D-binding protein, apolipoprotein A-I), endoplasmic reticulum proteins (HSP gp96 precursor, calumenin), a glycolysis protein (enolase 1), migration proteins (cathepsin D prepropeptide, prohibitin), and an antioxidant protein (glutathione S-transferase). The two proteins which were downregulated also have key roles. Calumenin is highly expressed by placental cells and helps in inhibition of coagulation and thrombosis through inhibition of the activity of vitamin k and also helps in prevention of atherosclerosis. Therefore, its downregulation may lead to activation of coagulation and thrombosis, which can induce recurrent abortion. Enolase 1 is a glycolytic enzyme that is overexpressed in normal pregnancy and mediates an adaptive response to placental hypoxia. Its downregulation leads to poor tolerance of hypoxia and hence RPL. Thus, alteration in the expression of proteins involved in proliferation and migration of endothelial cells as well as control of coagulation by these cells might play an important role in the pathogenesis of URPL [43].

In the first trimester of pregnancy, the oxygen tension within the placenta is increased to supply oxygen to the fetus. This increases the production of reactive oxygen substances (ROS) thus creating a situation of oxidative stress within the placenta. The peroxiredoxins (Prxs) family of antioxidant proteins work as natural antioxidants and protect the placenta from adverse effects of oxidative stress. Of this, Peroxiredoxin 3 (Prx3) and Peroxiredoxin 4 (Prx4) are expressed by cytotrophoblast cells and play an important role in the implantation and a normal placentation through their antioxidant activities. A study evaluated the presence of antibodies to these proteins in the sera of women with RPL, using proteomic analysis. These antibodies may enhance the oxidative stress by inhibiting antioxidant enzymatic activity and need to be researched in further detail [44].

The complement system consists of a series of serum proteins that help to regulate the immune response and the inflammatory process by generating fragments that promote chemotaxis, phagocytosis, cell activation, and cell lysis. The placenta expresses high levels of complement regulators throughout gestation. In a study, C3 and C4 levels were higher in women who had a third miscarriage than in women who had a history of two miscarriages and went on to have a successful pregnancy [45].

Thus, the domain of proteomics and inflammatory markers and their role in RPL is an exciting one and shows a lot of promise in further evaluating nearly half the women with RPL in whom the traditional testing does not reveal any positive results. This is an area of ongoing research as novel molecules continue to be discovered and their role elucidated.

Key Points

- Although pregnancy is a state of immune tolerance, in women with RPL, the balance between proinflammatory and anti-inflammatory cytokines is disturbed and leads to an inflammatory reaction.
- This inflammation may be local (at the endometrial level) or systemic (at the peripheral blood level).
- Various cellular and tissue-based markers are under study to better evaluate the inflammation that occurs at these levels.
- Using proteomics, the proteins responsible for RPL can be characterized and isolated and subject to further study.
- Most genetic biomarkers pertain to genes which promote excessive inflammatory responses and activation of the coagulation cascade leading to thrombosis.
- The findings of one study may not be replicated in another study as there are interlaboratory and inter-assay variations, not to mention the variations that occur in different phases of the menstrual cycle or different trimesters of pregnancy.

References

1. Khanna P. Inflammation and immunity in recurrent pregnancy loss: a snapshot. Reprod Immunol. 2016;1(1:5):1–2.
2. Atia TA, Elzaher MA. Natural killer cells, macrophages and inflammatory chemokines in recurrent pregnancy loss: immunohistochemical study. Life Sci J. 2014;11(2):134–42.
3. Baek KH, Lee EJ, Kim YS. Recurrent pregnancy loss: the key potential mechanisms. Trends Mol Med. 2007;13(7):310–7.
4. Kwak JY, Beer AE, Kim SH, et al. Immunopathology of the implantation site utilizing monoclonal antibodies to natural killer cells in women with recurrent pregnancy losses. Am J Reprod Immunol. 1999;41(1):91–8.
5. Kwak-Kim J, Kim JW, Gilman-Sachs A. Immunology and pregnancy losses: HLA, autoantibodies and cellular immunity. Madame Curie Bioscience Database [internet]. Austin, TX: Landes Bioscience; 2000–2013.
6. Jenkins C, Roberts J, Wilson R, et al. Evidence of a T(H)1 type response associated with recurrent miscarriage. Fertil Steril. 2000;73(6):1206–8.
7. Kwak JY, Beaman KD, Gilman-Sachs A, et al. Up-regulated expression of CD56+, CD56+/CD16+, and CD19+ cells in peripheral blood lymphocytes in pregnant women with recurrent pregnancy losses. Am J Reprod Immunol. 1995;34(2):93–9.
8. Kwak-Kim JY, Chung-Bang HS, Ng SC, et al. Increased T helper 1 cytokine responses by circulating T cells are present in women with recurrent pregnancy losses and in infertile women with multiple implantation failures after IVF. Hum Reprod. 2003;18(4):767–73.

9. Yahata T, Kurabayashi T, Honda A, et al. Decrease in the proportion of granulated CD56+ T-cells in patients with a history of recurrent abortion. J Reprod Immunol. 1998;38(1):63–73.
10. Polgar B, Barakonyi A, Xynos I, et al. The role of gamma/delta T cell receptor positive cells in pregnancy. Am J Reprod Immunol. 1999;41(4):239–44.
11. Lachapelle MH, Miron P, Hemmings R, et al. Endometrial T, B, and NK cells in patients with recurrent spontaneous abortion. Altered profile and pregnancy outcome. J Immunol. 1996;156(10):4027–34.
12. Lila N, Rouas-Freiss N, Dausset J, et al. Soluble HLA-G protein secreted by allo-specific CD4+ T cells suppresses the allo-proliferative response: a CD4+ T cell regulatory mechanism. Proc Natl Acad Sci U S A. 2001;98(21):12150–5.
13. Michimata T, Sakai M, Miyazaki S, et al. Decrease of T-helper 2 and T-cytotoxic 2 cells at implantation sites occurs in unexplained recurrent spontaneous abortion with normal chromosomal content. Hum Reprod. 2003;18(7):1523–8.
14. Ntrivalas EI, Kwak-Kim JY, Gilman-Sachs A, et al. Status of peripheral blood natural killer cells in women with recurrent spontaneous abortions and infertility of unknown aetiology. Hum Reprod. 2001;16(5):855–61.
15. Coulam CB, Goodman C, Roussey RG, et al. Systemic CD56+ cells can predict pregnancy outcome. Am J Reprod Immunol. 1995;33(1):40–6.
16. Dosiou D, Giudice LC. Natural killer cells in pregnancy and recurrent pregnancy loss: endocrine and immunologic perspectives. Endocr Rev. 2005;26(1):44–62.
17. Eastabrook G, Hu Y, von Dadelszen P. The role of decidual natural killer cells in normal placentation and in the pathogenesis of preeclampsia. J Obstet Gynecol Can. 2008;30(6):467–76.
18. Chao KH, Yang YS, Ho HN, et al. Decidual natural killer cytotoxicity decreased in normal pregnancy but not in anembryonic pregnancy and recurrent spontaneous abortion. Am J Reprod Immunol. 1995;34(5):274–80.
19. Tsuda H, Sakai M, Michimata T, et al. Characterization of NKT cells in human peripheral blood and decidual lymphocytes. Am J Reprod Immunol. 2001;45(5):295–302.
20. Nawroth P, Stern D. Modulation of endothelial cell hemostatic properties by tumor necrosis factor. J Exp Med. 1986;163(3):740–5.
21. Ku DH, Arkel YS, Paidas MP, et al. Circulating levels of inflammatory cytokines (IL-1 beta and TNF-alpha), resistance to activated protein C, thrombin and fibrin generation in uncomplicated pregnancies. Thromb Haemost. 2003;90(6):1074–9.
22. Qiu Q, Yang M, Tsang BK, et al. Fas ligand expression by maternal decidual cells is negatively correlated with the abundance of leukocytes present at the maternal-fetal interface. J Reprod Immunol. 2005;65(2):121–32.
23. Choi HK, Choi BC, Lee SH, et al. Expression of angiogenesis- and apoptosis related genes in chorionic villi derived from recurrent pregnancy loss patients. Mol Reprod Dev. 2003;66(1):24–31.
24. Hviid TV. HLA-G in human reproduction: aspects of genetics, function and pregnancy complications. Hum Reprod Update. 2006;12(3):209–32.
25. Goldman-Wohl DS, Ariel I, Greenfield C, et al. HLA-G expression in extravillous trophoblasts is an intrinsic property of cell differentiation: a lesson learned from ectopic pregnancies. Mol Hum Reprod. 2000;6(6):535–40.
26. Santamaria X, Taylor H. MicroRNA and gynaecological reproductive diseases. Fertil Steril. 2014;101(6):1545–51.
27. Ho HN, Gil TJ, Nsieh RP, et al. Sharing of human leukocyte antigens in primary and secondary recurrent spontaneous abortions. Am J Obstet Gynecol. 1990;163(1 Pt 1):178–88.
28. Ober C, Steck T, van der Ven K, et al. MHC class II compatibility in aborted fetuses and term infants of couples with recurrent spontaneous abortion. J Reprod Immunol. 1993;25(3):195–207.
29. Christiansen OB, Steffensen R, Nielsen HS, et al. Multifactorial etiology of recurrent miscarriage and its scientific and clinical implications. Gynecol Obstet Investig. 2008;66(4):257–67.
30. Banerjee P, Jana SK, Pasricha P, et al. Proinflammatory cytokines induced altered expression of cyclooxygenase-2 gene results in unreceptive endometrium in women with idiopathic recurrent spontaneous miscarriage. Fertil Steril. 2013;99(1):179–87.

31. Walia GK, Mukhopadhyay R, Saraswathy KN, et al. Immuno-molecular etiology of recurrent pregnancy loss and the anthropological perspective. Int J Hum Genet. 2008;8(1–2):227–35.
32. Redline RW, Zaradgoza M, Hassold T. Prevalence of developmental and inflammatory lesions in nonmolar first-trimester spontaneous abortions. Hum Pathol. 1999;30(1):93–100.
33. Metwally M, Preece R, Thomas J, et al. A proteomic analysis of the endometrium in obese and overweight women with recurrent miscarriage: preliminary evidence for an endometrial defect. Reprod Biol Endocrinol. 2014;12:75.
34. Ota K, Yamagishi S, Kim M, et al. Elevation of soluble form of receptor for advanced glycation end products (sRAGE) in recurrent pregnancy losses (RPL): possible participation of RAGE in RPL. Fertil Steril. 2014;102(3):782–9.
35. Kushnir VA, Solouki S, Sariq-Meth T, et al. Systemic inflammation and autoimmunity in women with chronic endometritis. Am J Reprod Immunol. 2016;75(6):672–7.
36. Fukui A, Ntrivalas E, Fukuhara R, et al. Correlation between natural cytotoxicity receptors and intracellular cytokine expression of peripheral blood NK cells in women with recurrent pregnancy losses and implantation failures. Am J Reprod Immunol. 2009;62(6):371–80.
37. Lessey BA. Endometrial integrins and the establishment of uterine receptivity. Hum Reprod. 1998;13(Suppl 3):247–58.
38. Gharesi Fard B, Zolghadri J, Kamali-Sarvestani E. Proteome differences in the first- and third trimester human placentas. Reprod Sci. 2015;22(4):462–8.
39. Kim YS, Kim MS, Lee SH, et al. Proteomic analysis of recurrent spontaneous abortion: identification of an inadequately expressed set of proteins in human follicular fluid. Proteomics. 2006;6(11):3445–54.
40. Kim MS, Gu BH, Song S, et al. ITI-H4, as a biomarker in the serum of recurrent pregnancy loss (RPL) patients. Mol BioSyst. 2011;7(5):1430–40.
41. Lopez-Pedrera C, Cuadrado MJ, Herandez V, et al. Proteomic analysis in monocytes of antiphospholipid syndrome patients: deregulation of proteins related to the development of thrombosis. Arthritis Rheum. 2008;58(9):2835–44.
42. Xin L, Xu B, Ma L, et al. Proteomics study reveals that the dysregulation of focal adhesion and ribosome contribute to early pregnancy loss. Proteomics Clin Appl. 2016;10(5):554–63.
43. Gharesi Fard B, Zolghadri J, Kamali-Sarvestani E. Alteration in the expression of proteins in unexplained recurrent pregnancy loss compared with those in the normal placenta. J Reprod Dev. 2014;60(4):261–7.
44. Gharesi Fard B, Jafarzadeh L, Ghaderi-shabankareh F, et al. Presence of autoantibody against two placental proteins, peroxiredoxin 3 and peroxiredoxin 4, in sera of recurrent pregnancy loss patients. Am J Reprod Immunol. 2013;69(3):248–55.
45. Sugiura-Ogasawara M, Nozawa K, Nakanishi T, et al. Complement as a predictor of further miscarriage in couples with recurrent miscarriages. HumReprod. 2006;21(10):2711–4.

20 Emotional Support and Psychological Care of Recurrent Pregnancy Loss Couple

Shruti Srivastava and Aparna Goyal

20.1 Introduction

Recurrent pregnancy loss (RPL) has been defined inconsistently since its conception. RPL, recurrent abortion (RA), habitual abortion (HA), and recurrent miscarriage (RM) are all various synonyms that had been used to define RPL in literature. Most commonly used definition described RPL as two or three or more consecutive pregnancy losses less than 20 weeks from last menstrual period. RPL was found to be associated with psychiatric comorbidity, decreased self-esteem, and self-concept [1]. About one third of women with RPL in various studies were found to be depressed and one in five had anxiety levels similar to that seen in general psychiatric population [2]. RPL has been found to affect men too though their grieving period is less than that seen in women [3]. About 40–60% of men have reported an awareness of vulnerability and powerlessness [4]. RPL with infertility and stress to conceive and procreate also found to affect the functioning of couple's relationship. RPL and psychiatric complications are intertwined with each other as studies have been found that they can be a cause of RPL as well as causal for psychiatric disorders in the patients; hence, it becomes necessary to address the psychological factors.

20.2 Epidemiology

Approximately 15% of clinically recognized pregnancies were found to be related with spontaneous pregnancy loss [5]. Considering this RPL was calculated to be 1 in 300 pregnancies [2]. Studies have reported incidence of RPL as high as up to

S. Srivastava (✉) • A. Goyal
Department of Psychiatry, University College of Medical Sciences and Guru Teg Bahadur Hospital, Dilshad Garden, Delhi, India
e-mail: srivastava_shruti@hotmail.com; piku0908@gmail.com

S. Mehta, B. Gupta (eds.), *Recurrent Pregnancy Loss*,
https://doi.org/10.1007/978-981-10-7338-0_20

Table 20.1 Evidence with recurrent pregnancy loss and psychiatric morbidity

Study	Methodology	Scales	Results
Teichman et al. 1993 [9]	77 women planning an abortion, 32 women in their 40th week of pregnancy, and 45 nonpregnant women Case control	Life cycle stage, trait anxiety, contextual factors (ethnicity and religiosity), and private context (Olson, Portner, and Lavee's family adaptability cohesion scale)	Elevated emotional distress and discomfort in couple relationships pre-abortion and reduced levels post-abortion
Broen et al. 2006 [10]	40 women with miscarriage and 80 with induced abortion. Prospective, longitudinal follow-up study	Hospital anxiety and depression scale and the life events scale	Anxiety and depression correlated can be used as predictors for negative response after pregnancy termination
Faramarzi et al. 2008 [11]	89 mild to moderate depressed infertile women Case control. CBT vs pharmacotherapy vs controls	Beck depression inventory and Cattell anxiety inventory	CBT superior to fluoxetine for reducing depression and anxiety
Marcinko et al. 2011 [12]	Pregnant women with previous spontaneous abortion vs pregnant women without previous spontaneous abortion and controls (healthy nonpregnant women)	Beck depression inventory and the Beck anxiety inventory	Pregnant women with history of spontaneous abortion have significant higher anxiety score than pregnant women without history of spontaneous abortion and control group
Nakano et al. 2013 [13]	14 women with RM and depression/anxiety. CBT	Beck depression inventory second edition and state-trait anxiety inventory-state anxiety scores	Individual CBT was found useful in participants

5% specially in women with increased age >35 years [6]. Psychiatric illnesses have been found to have both cause and effect relationship with RPL. Psychiatric comorbidity associated with RPL was studied and was found that about 33% were depressed out of which 10% were in moderate, while 7% in severe depression category [7]. About 1/3 of patient with RPL were found to have levels of anxiety similar to that seen in patient consulting at psychiatry OPD. Other psychiatric conditions seen in patient with RPL were post-traumatic stress disorder, erectile dysfunction, and impaired sexual function. In a population-based study by Toffol et al. (2002), it was concluded that the higher the number of miscarriage, the worse is the mood state, and frequency of psychiatric disorder is increased [8]. The various psychiatric morbidities have been summarized in Table 20.1.

20.3 Risk Factors

Multiple risk factors and etiologies have been identified. Commonly seen risk factors in RPL with psychiatric disorders are:

1. Cigarette smoking: It has an adverse effect on trophoblast function which is linked with increased risk of miscarriage.
2. Cocaine use has been shown to have an independent risk on pregnancy loss.
3. Alcohol: Moderate intake of even 3–5 units/week has been shown to have adverse effect on pregnancy as well as fetal outcome.
4. Caffeine consumption: It is considered to be dose dependent. Increase intake of >3000 mg has been found to be associated with miscarriage.
5. Drugs: Antidepressant drugs during preconceptual phase and psychotropics and benzodiazepines used during pregnancy can also have an effect on the outcome of pregnancy.
6. Psychiatric disorders like depression: Studies have reported controversial findings with some reporting increased risk while some studies showing no risk at all.
7. Schizophrenia and psychosis: These have also been shown to be associated with risk factor for stillbirth.
8. Post-traumatic stress disorder (PTSD): Higher risk based on known behavioral and neuroendocrine sequelae of traumatic stress including ectopic pregnancy, spontaneous abortion, hyperemesis, preterm contractions, and excessive fetal growth.

20.4 Etiology

At present, only a small number of etiologies have been accepted for RPL. These include chromosomal abnormalities, untreated hypothyroidism, uncontrolled diabetes mellitus, certain uterine anatomic abnormalities, and antiphospholipid antibody syndrome. Other probable or possible etiology includes endocrine disorders, heritable or acquired thrombophilias, infections, immunological abnormalities, and environmental factors. Unexplained causes for miscarriage were also hypothesized to be due to Th1/Th2 cytokine imbalance at the fetomaternal interface. Psychoneuroimmuno endocrine network was also found to be contributory to miscarriage. Stress and depression have found to have an effect on the hypothalamic pituitary adrenal axis (HPA) and sympathetic nervous system.

Raised levels of CD8+ T cells, TNF alpha, and tryptase positive mast cells have been reported in the endometrium of women with sporadic miscarriage and a high stress score.

Stress activates HPA axis and triggers a cascade of adrenocorticotropic hormones, corticotrophin-releasing hormone, and maternal glucocorticoids. This will release placental prostaglandins, increase the effect of oxytocin on uterus, and upregulate proinflammatory cytokines which can cause early labor and preterm birth (Fig. 20.1). In addition several substances like transforming growth factor beta and granulocyte-macrophage colony-stimulating factor, low neuroticism, low depression scale score, and high self-esteem contribute to natural killer K activity among women with RPL.

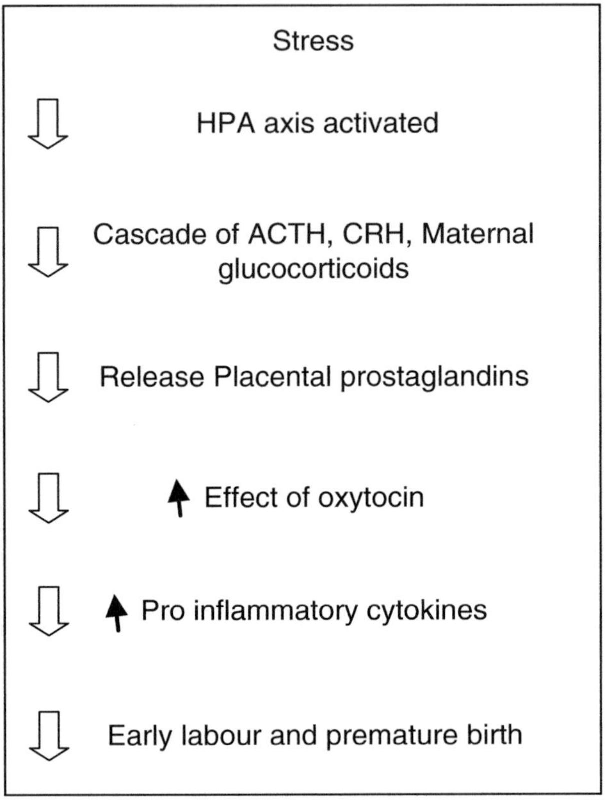

Fig. 20.1 Stress and HPA axis

Psychiatric researchers have recognized the role of mental illness that can cause physiological changes in patients, but the relationship between mental health and pregnancy is likely to be more complex. For example, depressed patients would seek less medical help and less prenatal care, have less physical activity, and are less compliant with medical treatment during pregnancy as compared to pregnant females without depression. They may also carry other potential risk factors such as greater toxic or occupational exposures, higher paternal age, or increased obesity.

20.5 Clinical Features

RPL, which is distressing to affected families and also to the couple seeking parenthood, makes the job of treating physician difficult. Miscarriage can induce pronounced emotional responses such as anxiety, depression, denial, anger, marital disruption, and a sense of loss and inadequacy.

In a Nova Scotia study, two types of women were found to be especially abortion prone: the immature, dependent psychosexually retarded type with a stern father and an inadequate mother and the other is independent frustrated women with ambivalent feelings about their feminine role. Women with dependency traits but a dominating mother and stressed paternal inadequacy were also at risk of repetitive abortions [14].

20.6 Screening Tools

The woman can be evaluated with different screening questionnaire for assessment including General Health Questionnaire (GHQ 12) [15], Patient Health Questionnaire (PHQ 9) [16], Perinatal Grief Scale [17], Impact of Event Scale [18], and Edinburgh Postnatal Depression Scale (EPDS) [19]. Questionnaire like GHQ 12 and EPDS can be used but are criticized for being sensitive to recent stress and confounding distress, grief, and depression.

General Health Questionnaire 12 is a sensitive tool to assess patient's mental well-being, and with scores of more than 2, it is advisable to refer/consult the patient to a psychiatrist for further exploration of patient's mental status. Perinatal Grief Scale (PGS) includes three subscales—active grief, difficulty coping, and despair. Although it has a high reliability and convergent validity, it has been criticized for having too much overlap with symptoms of a depressive episode. PHQ 9 is a nine-item questionnaire, rating the severity of depressive symptoms over the past 2 weeks. Besides its ease of administration and brevity, PHQ is also found effective in monitoring depression over time.

EPDS has been validated for its use in pregnant and postpartum women. It contains ten questions which cover more regarding mood and anhedonia as compared to somatic symptoms. EPDS have been found more effective than PHQ 9. Impact of Event Scale has been widely used as measure of stress after a traumatic event. The IES is a 15-item questionnaire evaluating experiences of avoidance and intrusion which attempts to reflect the intensity of the post-traumatic phenomena.

Other scales that may be used include Hospital Anxiety and Depression Scale (HADS), Beck Depression Inventory-II, and GRID-Hamilton Depression Rating Scale (GRID-HAMD) [20–22]. The various tools have been summarized in Fig. 20.2.

- ✓ *General Health Questionnaire 12 (GHQ 12)*
- ✓ *Patient Health Questionnaire 9 (PHQ 9)*
- ✓ *Perinatal grief scale*
- ✓ *Edinburgh post natal depression scale (EPDS)*
- ✓ *Impact of event scale*
- ✓ *Hospital Anxiety and Depression Scale (HADS)*
- ✓ *Beck Depression Inventory-II (BDI –II)*
- ✓ *GRID-Hamilton Depression Rating Scale (GRID-HAMD)*

Fig. 20.2 Screening tools for psychiatric disorders in RPL

Screening is challenging in women with RPL specially when interviewing in period of acute loss as it is difficult to distinguish grief from depression, and normal grief reactions can vary widely in how long they persist. It is important to be aware of risk factors for persisting distress following perinatal loss and monitor women with risk factors more closely, and assessment should be done routinely by providers.

20.7 Management

20.7.1 Non-pharmacological

It forms the mainstay of treatment. Relaxation exercises, Jacobson's progressive muscle relaxation, yoga, mindfulness therapy, and supportive therapy can be done for management of the symptoms. Pregnancy and medications use have always been controversial, be it due to lack of sufficient randomized controlled trials or the reluctance by patient to use medications during pregnancy. Hence alternative options should always be kept in mind for management of patient with pregnancy and RPL. Studies have also reported that counseling and increased regular checkups in the beginning of pregnancy itself can improve fertility rate. Psychological assessment and intervention/counseling are associated with successful delivery in RPL couple [23] (Fig. 20.3).

Psychiatric history taking along with complete medical history will enable to identify other comorbid disorders such as obesity, smoking, substance abuse, etc. **Diagnostic formulation (DF)** is a useful technique that describes in brief the relevant positive and negative points from the history and mental state examination and relevant investigations that enable us to arrive at psychiatric diagnosis based on the clinical criteria. A multiaxial approach that encompasses psychiatric diagnosis, personality traits or disorder, psychosocial stressors, global assessment of functioning, life events, and complete medical diagnosis should be carried out first.

Non pharmacological

- Cognitive Behavior Therapy
- Jacobson Progressive Muscle Relaxation
- Mindfulness therapy
- Supportive therapy
- Yoga
- Relaxation exercises
- Motivational interviewing
- Psycho-educative group sessions
- E-Self help groups
- Grief resolution
- Eye movement desensitization and reprocessing

Fig. 20.3 Non-pharmacologic therapy

An example is given in Box 20.1. The differential diagnosis of the case was kept as dissociative disorder (F44) and vomiting associated with other psychological causes (F 50.5) (Box 20.1).

Sturmey (2009) [24] had described several approaches of how to proceed for a clinical **case formulation** for psychotherapy. An eclectic approach that includes precipitating factors, current situations and ongoing stressors, interpersonal relationships with family and friends, pre-morbid personality, coping styles, personality makeup, behaviors (adaptive and maladaptive), and faulty cognitions needs to be assessed. Detailed assessments also include whether the client is ready to undergo sessions on individual, couple, or in a group basis. A sample case formulation is given in Box 20.2.

Motivational interviewing should be carried out by asking questions about how the client contemplates the overall situation, whether willing for any type of interventions, lifestyle changes, or compliance and adherence to treatment modalities. In a study carried out on obese women for weight loss prior to receiving fertility treatment, 64 women who received motivational support by phone call or email showed better results in mean weight loss and reduction in body mass index [25] (Box 20.3).

Both the preference of the client and case formulation should help to decide what type of sessions is useful**. Self-help groups or support groups** should be made as they provide moral support and help the individuals exchange useful information from their peer groups about the clinical condition leading to decreased worry and stress perception [26]. Mental health workers in collaboration with the

Box 20.1: Diagnostic Formulation of a Case Vignette

A 35-year-old married educated middle-aged female from middle socioeconomic status diagnosed with systemic lupus erythematosus with antiphospholipid antibody on regular treatment with anticoagulants currently with one living child, spontaneous abortions presenting with complaints of recurrent nonprojectile vomiting, and anorexia for 2 months. Vomiting was seen postprandial preceded by nausea, mostly after solid intake, constituting gastric contents, associated with weight loss, not relieved with antiemetic medications. On examination patient was conscious, oriented, and cooperative, and has anxious affect, pessimistic thoughts, and preoccupations with fear of vomiting after meals. The history, examination, and investigations could not identify any organic cause of vomiting; investigations on ultrasound of the abdomen, barium swallow, and upper GI endoscopy were normal; anticardiolipin antibody was negative; anti-beta-2-glycoprotein was normal; double-stranded DNA 394, routine blood investigations, complete hemogram, liver function test, renal function test, and erythrocyte sedimentation rate were normal; and lupus anticoagulant was positive. Patient was managed with anxiolytics, cognitive restructuring, activity scheduling, dietary advice, and yoga.

Box 20.2: Case Formulation

A middle aged graduate female, currently unemployed due to family refusal, is citing reasons of child care and household work. She exhibited, anticipatory anxiety and negative cognitions like "I will never be pregnant"and "I have no control." As a result she is engaged in menial household tasks, often subdued by a domineering mother in law, demanding constant attention. The joint family system has changed her role from an independent working woman to a disadvantaged social status of a homemaker who constantly struggles throughout the day in an environment of criticism, hostility, and at times overinvolvement from mother-in-law and sisters-in-law. As a consequence she has impaired decision-making, and she indulges in maladaptive behaviors of bouts of vomiting subsequent to her meals. She is preoccupied with persistent thought restricted to vomiting which often distract her from other tasks. She engages in activities such as preparing special meals for herself like soups, liquids, and semiliquid diets. Her premorbid personality is well adjusted. She is sociable and ambitious. Currently she appears anxious with irritable mood with negative views about self, present situation, and future. No contributory genetic factors were present.

Box 20.3: Non-pharmacological/Individualized Intervention Module of Case Vignette

Agenda	Module
1	Case formulation and rating scales are to be assessed in each setting. Subjective feelings, for example, distress, Likert scoring 0–10. Negative thoughts, and dysfunctional schemas identified
2	Motivational interviewing, treatment compliance, and patient preference in choosing the type of intervention
2	Activity scheduling, yoga, daily recordings comprising (negative) thoughts, feelings, behaviors, and actions. Module is tailored as per the client
3	Cognitive restructuring—Negative thought (cognition) was identified in the patient as "I will never become pregnant". Information was provided by therapist that how many cases of RPL have successfully conceived and completed term pregnancy by giving ample examples over three sessions. She simultaneously received treatment for RPL and compliance was emphasized. She gained confidence over sessions and became hopeful. Explanations provided by the therapist challenging the patient's negative thought helped in restoring her self esteem over the sessions and made her optimistic.
4	Behavioral tasks—Maladaptive behaviors are curtailed, for example, using remedies like pinching salt or putting finger in throat for self-induced vomiting. Clients are assigned homework
5	Gradually, the client masters the skills, carries out daily schedule in time-bound manner, becomes focused, restores self-confidence and happy mood, and replaces to positive cognition "I can manage my life"
6	Family/spouse intervention—Negative emotions are to be curtailed like criticism. Nurture positive (optimistic) thoughts, improve communication skills, and enhance social support
7	Impart skills that will help in relapse prevention at the termination

gynecologists need to actively monitor these self-help groups. **Psychoeducative group sessions** should include medical information that is evidence based, different therapeutic approaches, costs and time and efforts, success/failure rates of different options, adoption, and in vitro fertilization. Informed decision-making will help the individual cope better with the ongoing stressors of lengthy treatment process. Antenatal counseling and psychological support found to achieve higher pregnancy success rates of 86% compared to 33% of those who did not receive specific antenatal care [27].

E-self-help groups can be made after taking informed consent and keeping into account the laws of the land, privacy, confidentiality, copyright issues, and anonymity of the individuals. Several such **websites** are available wherein the individuals can raise their queries and answers can be provided. Group therapist should have empathetic attitude, be gentle, and create emotional warmth so that the support can be provided to individuals who are suffering. The information about several such websites that already exists can also be provided to the clients where they can carefully go through the cyber laws, privacy, disclaimer for such website, and confidentiality. The clients are likely to benefit from self-help support groups by gaining information/resources across the globe. Often, clients are unable to gather such information from busy clinicians due to their hesitancy, shortage of allocated time, or an individual simply forgot to ask.

Individuals with poor coping skills suffer from **grief** reaction. The psychiatrist should help the individual complete the process of complete **resolution** of grief by allowing the patient to ventilate the pent-up emotions. Initially, after a recent pregnancy loss, there is a denial and shock. Acceptance with reality of the loss comes in the next stage. They often feel the emptiness, loneliness, irritability, and depressed mood along with physical symptoms such as headaches and backaches. Gradually, as the healing occurs with passage of time, the individual restores the usual level of functioning [28].

Often, guilt and shame should be dealt with by the therapist. Enhance coping skills with family and friends should be carried out [29]. At every step, instillation of hope and empathy should be priority.

Assessment of grief in RPL can be carried out using Perinatal Grief Scale that has high internal consistency (reliability) and good convergent validity for the association of mental health, social support, and marital satisfaction [30].

Mindfulness-based therapy can also be used as a therapeutic option in RPL couple for managing anxiety and depressive disorder. It has been successfully tried for perinatal grief after stillbirth in a study carried out in rural India [31].

Cognitive behavioral therapy and counseling have been found to be effective in dealing couples with infertility as supportive treatment interventions [32]. Adaptive behaviors need to be discussed, and cognitive restructuring is often required in patients with depression. The therapist identifies the negative automatic thoughts and notes them down. These negative thoughts are challenged, and the client is provided with an alternate explanation. Activity scheduling of all the clients needs to be carried out. This helps in meaningfully structuring the daily routines of the clients with sufficient time for leisure and recreation. The therapist engages the clients in homework assignments that are reviewed in the subsequent visits. During the course of CBT sessions, the clients master the skills that help them overcome the negative thoughts, feelings, and behaviors linked with these negative thoughts. Finally, the client identifies the future risks and learns the skills so that they can prevent themselves from a relapse.

Patient with depression and anxiety has been shown to have benefited from cognitive behavioral therapy and brief interpersonal therapy and can be considered in the initial treatment management. CBT, in collaboration with other therapeutic modalities, can decrease depression and/or anxiety of patients with recurrent miscarriage [13]. However, for patient with moderate to severe symptoms, physician should not only consider risk of medications but also think about the risk to fetal exposure to untreated or inadequately treated anxiety or depression. Hence it seems reasonable and ethical for obstetrical and primary care providers to try to assist pregnant women with treatment for active issues.

At risk women or those who have psychiatric manifestations require close clinical monitoring and evidence-based psychotherapeutic options that are available. The clinical decision-making of whether to prescribe pharmacotherapy should necessarily involve the severity of illness and complications [33]. The dictum should be that, as far as possible, the drugs should be avoided in preconception period and in the first trimester. Clinical cases of increased severity such as complicated grief or depression with suicidal ideas or plans, pharmacotherapy should be prescribed. The complex drug-drug interaction of the hormonal preparations and other drugs used in RPL can be avoided if caution is exercised in prescribing antidepressants or anxiolytic drugs.

In a qualitative interview, infertility-related communication strategy (secrecy, formal communication, open-minded) was identified in a cohort of couples seeking treatment. Formal communication strategy that involves not discussing about the emotional aspects of infertility was associated with high fertility problem stress. Active avoidance coping and faulty partner communication were associated with high fertility problem stress [34]. Improving interpersonal communication between the partners helps in mitigating stress and in turn helps in improving the clinical outcome of RPL. This enhances emotional support of the couple. They need to be encouraged to talk about problem-solving and reciprocating positive emotions rather than indulge in criticism, over-involvement, and hostility with each other. Stress is a known etiology that triggers RPL and a useful measure that, if managed effectively, will improve the course and outcome of the clinical condition of RPL. Regular exercise, walks, inculcating hobbies, time management, cognitive restructuring, **and yoga** are all known to mediate stress**. Improving the communication among the partners** will help develop interpersonal relationship thereby contributing to better marital adjustment [35]. In a study carried out on psychiatric inpatients, yoga and exercise intervention was found beneficial and demonstrated improvement in clinical symptoms [36]. Eye movement desensitization and reprocessing (**EMDR**) is a useful psychotherapeutic technique that helps lower the distress in post-traumatic stress disorder by reprocessing the traumatic events [37].

Conclusions

Non-pharmacological management constitutes the mainstay of treatment in RPL couple with psychiatric disorders or stress. Screening tools assist in the early detection of psychiatric morbidity in RPL couple. Healthcare professionals need to be sensitized to pick up both at risk and the patients suffering from several psychiatric disorders. A systematic workup of a clinical case helps to reach a psychiatric diagnosis and highlights other relevant parameters that need to be the focus of clinical attention. A consultation-liaison psychiatry unit services will ensure better management of psychosocial stressors/psychiatric disorders, thereby enhancing the success rate of pregnancy in RPL couple. Self-help groups, counseling, cognitive therapy, yoga and exercise intervention, improving communication skills, stress management, and successful resolution of grief are some of the interventions. Caution needs to be exercised in prescribing pharmacotherapy, but a physician should always weigh the risk-benefit ratio of pharmacotherapy versus non-treating the psychiatric illness on fetal outcome. However, in the context of RPL, several non-pharmacological measures like relaxation exercises, yoga and exercise interventions, couple therapy, EMDR, and behavior therapy need to be extrapolated with a randomized controlled trial.

Key Points

- RPL has a cause and effect relationship with psychological factors/psychiatric disorders.
- Early detection of psychiatric disorders should be routinely carried out.
- Several screening tools are available that help in early detection of psychological morbidity.
- At risk cases, moderate to severe psychiatric disorders, comorbid substance abuse, suicidal risk or attempt, and significant family history of psychiatric disorder or past history should be referred.
- Consultation-liaison psychiatric services help in better management of psychosocial stressors/mental disorders.
- Motivational interviewing, counseling, cognitive therapy, yoga and exercise intervention, self-help groups, grief resolution, mindfulness-based interventions, eye movement desensitization and reprocessing, and stress management are some of the intervention measures.
- Studies provide evidence that the chances of reaching a successful term pregnancy in RPL are improved if psychological problems are better dealt with.

References

1. Serrano F, Lima ML. Recurrent miscarriage: psychological and relational consequences for couples. Psychol Psychother. 2006;79:585–94.
2. Rai R, Regan L. Recurrent miscarriage. Lancet. 2006;368:601–11.

3. Klier CM, Geller PA, Ritsher JB. Affective disorders in the aftermath of miscarriage: a comprehensive review. Arch Womens Ment Health. 2002;5:129–49.
4. Speraw SR. The experience of miscarriage: how couples define quality in health care delivery. J Perinatol. 1994;14:208–15.
5. Ford HB, Schust DJ. Recurrent pregnancy loss: etiology, diagnosis, and therapy. Rev Obstet Gynaecol. 2009;2(2):76–83.
6. Branch DW, Gibson M, Silver RM. Clinical practice. Recurrent miscarriage. N Engl J Med. 2010;363:1740–7.
7. Craig M, Tata P, Regan LJ. Psychiatric morbidity among patients with recurrent miscarriage. Psychosom Obstet Gynaecol. 2002;23(3):157–64.
8. Toffol E, Koponen P, Partonen T. Miscarriage and mental health: results of two population-based studies. Psychiatry Res. 2013;205(1–2):151–8.
9. Teichman Y, Shenhar S, Segal S. Emotional distress in Israeli women before and after abortion. Am J Orthopsychiatry. 1993;63(2):277–88.
10. Broen AN, Moum T, Bödtker AS, Ekeberg O. Predictors of anxiety and depression following pregnancy termination: a longitudinal five-year follow-up study. Acta Obstet Gynecol Scand. 2006;85(3):317–23.
11. Faramarzi M, Alipor A, Esmaelzadeh S, Kheirkhah F, Poladi K, Pash H. Treatment of depression and anxiety in infertile women: cognitive behavioral therapy versus fluoxetine. J Affect Disord. 2008;108(1–2):159–64.
12. Marcinko VM, Marcinko D, Dordević V, Oresković S. Anxiety and depression in pregnant women with previous history of spontaneous abortion. Coll Antropol. 2011;35(Suppl 1):225–8.
13. Nakano Y, Akechi T, Furukawa TA, Sugiura-Ogasawara M. Cognitive behavior therapy for psychological distress in patients with recurrent miscarriage. Psychol Res Behav Manag. 2013;6:37–43.
14. Sharma S, Sonawalla S, Parikh F, Parikh R. Psychiatric disorders associated with pregnancy. J Obstet Gynecol India. 2005;55(3):218–27.
15. Goldberg D. General health questionnaire (GHQ-12). Windsor, UK: NFER-Nelson; 1992.
16. Kroenke K, Spitzer R, Williams W. The PHQ-9: validity of a brief depression severity measure. JGIM. 2001;16:606–16.
17. Toedter LJ, Lasker JN, Alhadeff JM. The perinatal grief scale: development and initial validation. Am J Orthopsychiatry. 1988;58(3):435.
18. Horowitz M, Wilner N, Alvarez W. Impact of event scale: a measure of subjective stress. Psychosom Med. 1979;41(3):209–18.
19. Cox JL, Holden JM, Sagovsky R. Detection of postnatal depression: development of the 10-item Edinburgh Postnatal Depression Scale. Br J Psychiatry. 1987;150:782–6.
20. Zigmond AS, Snaith RP. The hospital anxiety and depression scale. Acta Psychiatr Scand. 1983;67:361–70.
21. Beck AT, Steer RA, Brown GK. Manual for the Beck depression inventory-II. San Antonio, TX: Psychological Corporation; 1996.
22. Williams JB, Kobak KA, Bech P, Engelhardt N, Evans K, Lipsitz J, et al. The GRID-HAMD: standardization of the Hamilton Depression Rating Scale. Int Clin Psychopharmacol. 2008;23(3):120–9.
23. Sills ES, Perloe M, Stamm LJ, Kaplan CR, Tucker MJ. Medical and psychological management of recurrent abortion, history of postneonatal death, ectopic pregnancy and infertility: successful implementation of IVF for multifactorial reproductive dysfunction. A case report. Clin Exp Obstet Gynecol. 2004;31(2):143–6.
24. Sturmey P. Clinical case formulation: varieties of approaches. Chichester, West Sussex: Wiley; 2009.
25. Karlsen K, Humaidan P, Sørensen LH, Alsbjerg B, Ravn P. Motivational interviewing: a part of the weight loss program for overweight and obese women prior to fertility treatment. Gynecol Endocrinol. 2013;29(9):839–42.
26. Mosalanejad L, Khodabakshi Koolee A. Looking at infertility treatment through the lens of the meaning of life: the effect of group logotherapy on psychological distress in infertile women. Int J Fertil Steril. 2013;6(4):224–31.

27. Stray-Pedersen B, Stray-Pedersen S. Etiologic factors and subsequent reproductive performance in 195 couples with a prior history of habitual abortion. Am J Obstet Gynecol. 1984;148(2):140–6.
28. Perry SE. Perinatal loss and grief. Chapter 38. In: Carter R, Gower LK, editors. Maternity and women's health care. 10th ed. St. Louis, MO: Elsevier Mosby Inc; 2012. p. 931–50.
29. Griebel CP, Halvorsen J, Golemon TB, Day AA. Management of spontaneous abortion. Am Fam Physician. 2005;72(7):1243–50.
30. Toedter LJ, Lasker JN, Janssen HJ. International comparison of studies using the perinatal grief scale: a decade of research on pregnancy loss. Death Stud. 2001;25(3):205–28.
31. Roberts LR, Montgomery SB. Mindfulness-based intervention for perinatal grief after stillbirth in rural India. Issue Ment Health Nurs. 2015;36(3):222–30.
32. Luk BH, Loke AY. A review of supportive interventions targeting individuals or couples undergoing infertility treatment: directions for the development of interventions. J Sex Marital Ther. 2016;42(6):515–33.
33. Bhat A, Byatt N. Infertility and perinatal loss: when the bough breaks. Curr Psychiatry Rep. 2016;18(3):31.
34. Schmidt L. Infertility and assisted reproduction in Denmark. Epidemiology and psychosocial consequences. Dan Med Bull. 2006;53(4):390–417.
35. Srivastava S. Stress and its management. In: Jiloha RC, Bhatia MS, editors. Psychiatry for general practitioners. New Delhi: New Age International Publishers; 2010. p. 95–100.
36. Srivastava S, Bhatia MS, Gautam P, Saha R, Chauhan J. Yoga and exercise intervention study in psychiatry inpatients from a tertiary care teaching hospital. Delhi Psychiatry J. 2015;18(1):138–41.
37. Srivastava S. Eye movement desensitization and reprocessing (EMDR) - A review in Indian context using clinical case. Delhi Psychiatry J.2013;16(1):190–195.

Pregnancy After Recurrent Pregnancy Loss

21

Divya Pandey

21.1 Introduction

Management strategy of a pregnancy care following a miscarriage or with history of recurrent pregnancy loss (RPL) depends on the underlying cause of miscarriage.

The risk of recurrence of pregnancy loss goes on increasing with successive pregnancy losses and with advancing maternal and paternal age.

These pregnancies need precise antenatal surveillance and delivery at a center with specialized obstetrics and neonatal intensive care facilities. This is because women with RPL are also at risk of pregnancy complications like preeclampsia, fetal growth retardation, preterm labor, perinatal loss, and need for operative delivery.

21.2 Definition of RPL

Spontaneous pregnancy loss occurs in 12–15% antenatal women with one-third losses occurring between implantation and 6 weeks [1]. It has been estimated that 5% females experience two consecutive pregnancy losses, while only 1% experience three or more [2]. The *American Society of Reproductive Medicine (ASRM)* has taken this figure into account while formulating the definition of RPL. ASRM guidelines have replaced the ACOG Guidelines. *ASRM* defines the *recurrent pregnancy loss (RPL)* as a distinct disorder with two or more failed clinical pregnancies [3]. But the fallacy of this definition is the non-defining of the upper limit of gestational age.

D. Pandey
Obstetrics and Gynecology, Vardhman Mahavir Medical College and Safdarjung Hospital, Delhi, India
e-mail: dr_devya1@yahoo.co.in

S. Mehta, B. Gupta (eds.), *Recurrent Pregnancy Loss*,
https://doi.org/10.1007/978-981-10-7338-0_21

On the other hand, The *Royal College of Obstetricians and Gynecologists (RCOG) guidelines*, which have been updated in 2011, have defined RPL or recurrent miscarriage (RM) as loss of three or more consecutive pregnancies. Miscarriage refers to spontaneous pregnancy loss before viability, i.e., before 24 weeks of gestation [4].

21.3 Available Guidelines for Management of RPL

There are various extensive protocols in literature for management of RPL. Almost all protocols treat RPL as a homogenous condition and suggest a battery of investigations or treatment based on evidence and experience. *These guidelines give conflicting statements without stressing that patient-specific approach is the best.*

The aim of this chapter is to provide evidence-based yet clinically relevant approach for antenatal care of a pregnancy after RPL.

21.4 Presentation

Woman carrying pregnancy after RPL can reach the clinicians with two different timings of presentation:

1. At time of third or more order miscarriage.
2. Pregnancy with history of RPL.

21.5 At Time of the Third or More Order Miscarriage

1. **Approach**
   The couple must be approached together with sympathy and sensitivity. Tender loving care must be administered to all.
2. **Documentation**
   It is very important to document the pattern and gestational age of the pregnancy loss.
   (a) Make a record whether a live fetus was present.
   (b) Clinical and ultrasound features are also important to be noted.
   (c) During surgical evacuation, it's important to make note of any suspected uterine anomaly, e.g., submucous fibroid or presence of septum.
3. **Testing products of conception (POCs)**
   Send products of conception for histology or autopsy and karyotyping. Cytogenetic abnormalities account for 2–4% of causes of RPL.
4. **Follow-up**
   Follow-up assessment and counselling has to be offered to all.

21.6 Pre-Pregnancy Assessment and Counselling After the Third Miscarriage

(a) **History**

- **Obstetric history**—A thorough obstetric history is a must to confirm the diagnosis of "recurrent pregnancy loss." It's important to note the pattern of losses, period of gestation at which previous losses occurred, and confirmation of the pregnancy by biochemical, ultrasonographic, and/or histologic means.

  In case of recurrent midtrimester pregnancy losses, most common factor cited is cervical incompetence. Factors in the history suggestive of cervical incompetence are a painless midtrimester delivery, history of previous major cervical surgery like conization or large loop excision, documented cervical trauma in previous pregnancy, and a history of prelabor preterm rupture of membranes.
- **Medical history**
  - History of features suggestive of autoimmune diseases, e.g., joint pains, skin rash, allergy, etc.
  - Features of antiphospholipid syndrome (APS), e.g., migraine, epilepsy, joint pain, vascular thrombosis, and Raynaud's phenomena
  - Features associated with thrombophilia, e.g., family history of vascular thrombosis like stroke and deep venous thrombosis (DVT)
  - Exposure to environmental toxins or drugs
  - Surgery on uterus, cervix, or ovary
- **Family history**
  - Family h/o RPL, PCOS, diabetes, genetic disorders, thrombophilia, early-onset cardiovascular disease like stroke.

(b) **Physical examination**

- Look for signs of gynecologic or endocrine disorders.
- Can do opportunistic screening of the patient like blood pressure, cervical cytology, and breast palpation.

(c) **Investigations and treatment**

1. **Royal College of Obstetricians and Gynecologists (RCOG) guidelines, 2012** [4]

   These guidelines recommend fetal karyotyping, 3D ultrasound, hydrosonography/hysteroscopy for uterine abnormalities, antiphospholipid testing, and diagnosis based on Sapporo criteria and treatment with heparin and aspirin.

   Parental karyotyping is no longer recommended except in the presence of unbalanced chromosomal abnormality in the products of conception. Moreover assessment of thyroid function, antithyroid antibodies, alloimmune testing, immunotherapy, and assessment of TORCH and other infective agents are also not recommended. There is no role of assessment of bacterial vaginosis (BV) and progesterone and HCG supplementation. These guidelines suggest that although there may be association of factor V Leiden deficiency or other hereditary thrombophilia with the second trimester pregnancy loss but not with the first trimester loss. These guidelines also denounce the use of empirical treatment in unexplained RPL cases.

RCOG has not taken into account specific types of pregnancy losses and does not distinguish between different types of patients.

2. **American Society of Reproductive Medicine (ASRM) guidelines** [5]
These guidelines clearly warrant the investigation after two recurrent pregnancy losses. Unlike RCOG, ASRM clearly suggests that management can be tailored depending on the needs of individual patient, available resources, and limitations of particular institution or type of practice.

   In contrast to RCOG guidelines, ASRM recommends parental karyotyping, and prenatal diagnosis should be offered if one of the patients is having chromosomal abnormality. It also recommends karyotyping of the abortus. Uterine cavity assessment should be done, and septum should be resected if present, for second trimester loss. Screening of antiphospholipid antibodies is recommended with treatment with aspirin and unfractionated heparin rather than low molecular weight heparin. These guidelines recommend against screening for antithyroid antibodies and infective agents like chlamydia, mycoplasma or BV, alloimmune testing, parental leucocyte immunization, or intravenous immunoglobulin (IVIg). The role of HCG supplementation is not mentioned.
3. **European Society of Human Reproduction and Embryology (ESHRE) guidelines, 2006** [6]
Like RCOG, ESHRE (2006) has also restricted the definition of recurrent miscarriage (pregnancy loss) to three or more consecutive miscarriages.

   It takes account of different types of patients. These guidelines discuss the investigations of cause and treatment interventions separately and don't figure level of evidence for its recommendation unlike RCOG. It recommends testing of blood sugar levels, thyroid testing, antiphospholipid antibodies (LAC and ACL), parental karyotyping, and uterine cavity assessment by pelvic ultrasound or hysterosalpingography. Laparoscopy and hysteroscopy are categorized under "advanced investigations," but the "group of patients" whom to subject to these advanced investigations has not been mentioned. A new category of investigations under "framework of clinical trial" include fetal karyotyping, natural killer (NK) cell testing, luteal phase endometrial biopsy, and homocysteine levels. Treatment interventions are mentioned separately. Tender loving care (TLC) and abstinence from alcoholism and smoking and reduction of coffee intake have been described as established treatments. As per ESHRE, the following modalities require well-designed RCTs before making recommendations: aspirin and low molecular weight heparin for antiphospholipid syndrome, anticoagulants for inherited thrombophilia, progesterone supplementation, intravenous immunoglobulin, folic acid in hyperhomocystenemia, and immunization with third-party leucocytes.

However, the ESHRE Early Pregnancy Guideline Development Group has released a draft of updated guidelines for review in July 2017 [7].

As per this draft, diagnosis of recurrent pregnancy loss is to be considered after loss of two or more pregnancies. The recommendations given here are based on level of evidence in contrast to the 2006 guidelines. The salient changes suggested through this draft have been mentioned in Table 21.1. Table 21.1 compares the recommendations by various societies regarding investigation and management of RPL. The recommendations will soon be released after the review.

Complete dependability on these guidelines will leave the clinicians in quandary, regarding which investigations to be done and what treatment to be offered. Thus there is need to follow a tailored approach depending on the patient clinical profile.

(d) **Key counselling points**

1. The couple should be seen together with a sympathetic and sensitive approach.
2. They should be counselled that after three consecutive losses, intensive investigation will identify a cause in only less than 50% cases.
3. The majority of cases are due to repeated fetal chromosomal abnormalities occurring consecutively by chance.
4. They should be emphasized that the chances of future successful pregnancy can exceed 60% in cases of unexplained RPL depending on maternal age and parity [8, 9]. The success rates are lower in women with antiphospholipid syndrome and those with activated protein C resistance.
5. Advance maternal and paternal age and previous reproductive history are important risk factor for further pregnancy loss [4].
6. Recurrent pregnancy loss is associated with significant psychological morbidity.
7. Role of psychological stress is unclear.

Table 21.1 Comparing the investigation and treatment according ESHRE, RCOG, and ASRM guidelines

Investigation/treatment option	*ESHRE (2006)* [4]	*ESHRE (2017)* [7]	*RCOG (2012)* [5]	*ASRM (2012)* [6]
Karyotyping				
Parental	R	NR[a]	NR	R
Fetal	Trials needed	NR	R	R
Assessment of uterine cavity	R	R	R	IE
Resection of uterine septum	–	IE	IE	Should be considered
Antiphospholipid assessment (ACA and LAC)	R	R	R	R
Treatment of APS with heparin and aspirin	IE	R	R	R
Infective agents				
TORCH	NR	–	NR	NR
Bacterial vaginosis	–	–	IE	NR
Thyroid function tests	R	R	–	R
Glucose challenge tests	R	–[b]	–	–
Prolactin estimation	–	R[c]	–	R
Investigation of luteal phase defect	IE		–	NR
Progesterone supplementation	IE	IE	IE	IE
HCG supplementation	–	IE	IE	–
Hereditary thrombophilias Screening	Recommended as advanced investigation	NR	Recommended for midtrimester losses	NR
Anticoagulants for hereditary thrombophilia	IE	NR	IE	–
Alloimmune testing	IE	NR	NR	NR
Immunotherapy	IE; RCTs needed for IVIg and third-party leucocytes; no proven effect of paternal leucocyte injection	NR	NR	NR
Tender loving care	R	R	IE	R
Diet modification	R	R	–	–
Abstaining from smoking and alcohol	NR	R	–	–
Vitamin supplementation	IE	NR	–	–

Table 21.1 (continued)

Investigation/treatment option	*ESHRE (2006)* [4]	*ESHRE (2017)* [7]	*RCOG (2012)* [5]	*ASRM (2012)* [6]
Folic acid for hyperhomocysteinemia	NR	–	NR	NR
Steroids	–	NR	NR	NR

RCOG Royal College of Obstetricians and Gynecologists; *ESHRE* European Society of Human Reproduction and Embryology; *APS* antiphospholipid syndrome; *RCT* randomized controlled trial; *IVIg* intravenous immunoglobulin; *TORCH Toxoplasma, Rubella, Cytomegalovirus, Herpes*, and others; *ACA* anticardiolipin antibody; *LAC* lupus anticoagulant; *R* recommended; *NR* not recommended; *IE* insufficient evidence

[a]Not routinely recommended; needs to be individualized

[b]Fasting insulin and fasting glucose test in women with PCOS with RPL-NR

[c]Prolactin test in women with RPL in absence of clinical symptoms of hyperprolactinemia-NR

21.7 Pre-pregnancy Treatment Options

(a) **Lifestyle, environmental, and occupational factors**
Cigarette smoking, cocaine use, alcohol consumption (three to five drinks per week), and increase in coffee consumption have been associated with risk of miscarriage [10]. Obesity is another factor which has been linked with sporadic pregnancy loss. Stress on avoidance of these unhealthy lifestyle habits and controlling obesity is important part of preconception counselling of these couples.

(b) **Tender loving care approach**
The couples with RPL should be dealt with a “tender loving care” and sympathetic approach [11].

(c) **No role of empirical treatment**
RCOG guidelines recommends that there is no role of empirical treatment [4].

(d) **Genetic counselling**
In case structural genetic cause is identified, genetic counselling becomes very important. The chance of a successful pregnancy outcome depends on the involvement and type of rearrangement of chromosomes. When one of the parents is identified to have a structural genetic abnormality, options of chorionic villus sampling (CVS) and amniocentesis should be offered to the couple. Preimplantation genetic diagnosis, transfer of unaffected embryo, and use of donor gametes are the treatment options available for specific chromosomal translocations. However, there is insufficient evidence suggesting “in vitro fertilization with preimplantation genetic diagnosis” improves the rates of successful pregnancy outcomes in couples with RPL or with structural genetic abnormality [12]. Currently, routine preimplantation embryo aneuploidy screening is not justified [13].

(e) **Uterine abnormalities**

Subserosal and intramural fibroids that do not distort the cavity have no deleterious effect on the pregnancy outcome; however, fibroids with submucosal or intracavitary component have been associated with decreased implantation rates and miscarriage rates.

There is inconclusive evidence that surgical management of RPL patients with Asherman syndrome/intrauterine synechiae, fibroids, or polyps reduces the risk of pregnancy loss. In absence of randomized controlled trials, general consensus is that surgical correction of significant uterine defects should be done [5].

(f) **Folic acid supplementation**

Folate supplementation (4 mg/day) should be given to allay the chance of congenital abnormalities especially neural tube defects.

21.8 Management During Pregnancy After RPL

21.8.1 Etiology-Specific Management

21.8.1.1 Cervical Incompetence

Cervical cerclage is to be applied in these women. Recommended indications of cerclage are [14, 15]:

1. History of three or more previous preterm and/or second trimester loss but not indicated with two or fewer previous preterm or second trimester losses.
2. History of second trimester pregnancy loss associated with painless cervical dilation without labor or abruption.
3. History of spontaneous preterm birth before 34 weeks or if cervical length is less than 25 mm before 24 weeks in current pregnancy.
4. Having painless dilation in current pregnancy.
5. History of cerclage in previous pregnancy due to painless dilation.

However, cerclage is not recommended in ultrasound diagnosed short cervix (<25 mm) in women without history of spontaneous preterm birth.

21.8.1.2 Antiphospholipid Syndrome

Although antiphospholipid antibodies are positive in 5–20% women with RPL, the actual reported range is between 8 and 42% [16, 17]. Women with APS should be offered aspirin and low-dose heparin treatment [13, 18]. Low-dose aspirin (75 g/day) and heparin should be started as soon as the urine pregnancy test is positive. Low molecular weight heparin scores over unfractionated heparin owing to the advantage of once daily injection due to its longer half-life and increased bioavailability. Moreover it is associated with fewer bleeding episodes, a more predictable therapeutic response, a lower risk of heparin-induced thrombocytopenia, a longer half-life, and less bone mineral density loss [19, 20]. Although there is significant improvement in the live birth rates in the women who are treated with aspirin and heparin till 34 weeks, they are still at risk of preeclampsia, fetal growth restriction, abruption, and preterm delivery [21].

21.8.1.3 Thrombophilia

Low-risk thrombophilia (factor V Leiden heterozygous, prothrombin G20210A heterozygous, protein C or protein S deficiency) can be managed during antepartum period with surveillance without anticoagulation therapy or prophylactic low molecular weight heparin (LMWH) or unfractionated heparin (UFH). Those with additional risk factors (obesity, prolonged immobilization, or first-degree relative with history of thrombotic episode) or with history of episode of venous thromboembolism in self require postpartum anticoagulation therapy [22].

Those with high-risk thrombophilia (antithrombin deficiency, double heterozygous for prothrombin gene mutation G20210A, and factor V Leiden mutation homozygous or prothrombin G20210A mutation homozygous) need prophylactic antepartum anticoagulation therapy along with postpartum anticoagulation therapy with LMWH/UFH for 6 weeks [22].

Thrombophilia with two or more episodes of venous thromboembolism should receive therapeutic dose of LMWH or UFH along with postpartum therapeutic dose heparin therapy for 6 weeks (who were not on long-term anticoagulation therapy) and for lifelong (who were on long-term anticoagulation therapy) [22].

21.9 General Management for Pregnancy with RPL

21.9.1 First Trimester

These couples are anxious and thus need constant reassurance and support in addition to the "tender loving care approach." "Unproven treatment" should not be advocated.

There is no evidence of benefit of any immunologic therapy [5]. A recent meta-analysis has shown that there is no beneficial effect of paternal white blood cell immunization therapy [23]. Several trials and meta-analysis have shown that there is no benefit of treatment with intravenous immunoglobulin [24–26]. Patients with diabetes mellitus should achieve good metabolic control.

Ultrasound in early pregnancy is a must to confirm fetal viability and fetal heart activity. This will also provide maternal reassurance. Transvaginal ultrasound can detect the fetal cardiac activity at 6 weeks, yolk sac at 5.5 weeks, and intrauterine gestational sac at 5 weeks. Early anomaly scan (11–14 weeks) should be done as a routine. Besides ruling out congenital malformation, it also assures fetal growth thereby reassuring the parents. Aneuploidy screening (biochemical and ultrasonographic) should be done in all cases. TIFFA scan (targeted imaging for fetal anomalies) should be done routinely between 16–20 weeks. Apart from ruling out congenital abnormalities of fetus, one can also assess the cervical length. This is especially important for the women who have history recurrent second trimester losses associated with painless cervical dilation without labor or abruption or spontaneous preterm birth before 34 weeks.

21.9.2 Second Trimester

Uterine artery Doppler ultrasound at 22–24 weeks can predict preeclampsia and fetal growth restriction, especially in APS pregnancies, especially those with circulating LA and high titres of IgG anticardiolipin antibodies [21]. A glucose tolerance test at 28 weeks is especially important to be done in patients with PCOS due to increased risk of GDM.

21.9.3 Third Trimester

Antepartum fetal surveillance can be initiated no earlier than 32 0/7 weeks of gestation. However, in presence of other comorbid high-risk condition (e.g., chronic hypertension with suspected fetal growth restriction), surveillance can be started at gestation when delivery would be considered for perinatal benefit [27].

When clinical condition which has prompted clinician to start antepartum fetal surveillance persists, the test can be repeated to monitor for continued fetal well-being until delivery. If the maternal medical condition is stable and test results are reassuring, tests of fetal well-being (non-stress test, modified biophysical profile) can be typically repeated at weekly intervals.

Serial growth scans staring from 28 weeks onwards and umbilical artery Doppler study is advisable [21], as the women with history of RPL especially those who with APS and thrombophilia are at increased risk of developing fetal growth retardation. The growth restricted fetuses and umbilical artery Doppler velocimetry use in conjunction with standard fetal surveillance, like NST or BPP or both, are associated with improved outcomes.

Antenatal corticosteroids for fetal lung maturity should be given to all women at risk of iatrogenic or spontaneous preterm birth from 26 to 34^{+6} weeks of gestation [28, 29]. Current evidence supports the use of dexamethasone as the first choice of treatment: four 6 mg doses given 12 hourly. However, if dexamethasone is not available, betamethasone may be used: two 12 mg doses can be given 24 hourly. A rescue course of four doses of 6 mg dexamethasone or two doses of 12 mg should be considered only where first course was given at less than 26 weeks of gestation [28]. Corticosteroids should be given to reduce the risk of respiratory morbidity in all babies delivered by elective Cesarean section prior to 38 + 6 weeks of gestation.

The women, who have cervical stitch in situ, need removal of the same between 37 and 38 weeks of gestation.

21.9.4 Induction of Labor (IOL)

Induction of labor (IOL) needs to be considered when risk-benefit analysis indicates that delivering the baby is a safer option for the baby, the mother, or both rather than continuing the pregnancy and when there are no clear indications for Cesarean section and no contraindications for vaginal delivery, [30]. In general there is no clear cut indication of exact gestation for IOL in these group of patients.

In uncomplicated or low-risk pregnancy, it has been seen that maternal complications of pregnancy increase after 40 weeks of gestation [31]. In low-risk patients, preventive use of IOL prior to possible development of uteroplacental insufficiency or cephalo-pelvic disproportion can improve pregnancy outcomes and can reduce Cesarean section rates [32, 33]. So these patient can be offered induction of labor at 38 weeks. In the setting of uncomplicated isolated and persistent oligohydramnios (deepest vertical pocket; DVP <2 cm), delivery at 36–37 weeks of gestation is recommended [34].

21.9.5 Delivery

In the absence of obstetric contraindications, the delivery of the fetus with abnormal antepartum fetal testing is done by induction of labor as already discussed. And these patients need continuous intrapartum monitoring of the fetal heart rate and uterine contractions [34].

Women who are self-administering the anticoagulants must be instructed to stop the drug, if there are any signs of labor. If she goes in labor while on medication, and the aPTT is in the therapeutic range near time of delivery, protamine sulfate can be given to decrease the risk of excessive blood loss. In cases of planned delivery, prophylactic heparin is to be discontinued 24 h before delivery. Those who are on therapeutic doses of LMWH can be reduced to prophylactic doses a day before delivery. Regional anesthesia like spinal or epidural should not be used until at least 12 h of last prophylactic dose of LMWH or 24 h of the last therapeutic dose of LMWH or 6 h of dose of UFH. The postpartum prophylactic dose is to be given at least 3 h after vaginal delivery or 4 h after removal of epidural catheter. Therapeutic dose can be resumed 12 h later. The epidural cannula should be removed only after 10–12 h of the last dose of heparin, and further doses are to be started after 4 h of removal.

21.9.6 Postpartum

Postpartum anticoagulant therapy should be given in thrombophilia as already discussed. In women with APS with no symptoms other than RPL, there is no evidence to justify routine thrombo-prophylaxis. In women with APS without any additional thrombotic risk factors, postnatal thrombo-prophylaxis is not recommended.

21.9.7 Breastfeeding

Postpartum anticoagulant therapy can be continued with either heparin or warfarin. After initial overlapping with heparin, warfarin can be continued. Breastfeeding is not contraindicated with warfarin, as this drug does not induce an anticoagulant effect in the breastfed infant.

Table 21.2 This table shows the Medical Eligibility Criteria (MEC) for different contraceptive methods in women with history/ongoing thromboembolism event

Contraceptive methods	h/o DVT/pulmonary embolism/other risk factors	Acute DVT	h/o stroke
COCs and CICs	MEC 4	MEC 4	MEC 4
POPs	MEC 2	MEC 3	MEC 2
DMPA/NETEN	MEC 2	MEC 3	MEC 3
Implants	MEC 2	MEC 3	MEC 2
Copper IUCD	MEC 1	MEC 1	MEC 1
LNG IUCD	MEC 2	MEC 3	MEC 2

MEC category 1 = **Yes**: Use the method in any circumstance
MEC category 2 = **Yes**: Generally use the method
MEC category 3 = **No**: Use of the method not usually recommended unless other more appropriate methods are not available or acceptable
MEC category 4 = **No**: Method NOT to be used

21.9.8 Contraception

Contraceptive advice needs caution especially in women who have history of thromboembolism (e.g., deep venous thrombosis (DVT), acute DVT, or stroke). Medical eligibility criteria [35] as laid down in Table 21.2 should be followed.

Conclusion

The management of pregnancy after recurrent pregnancy loss needs tender loving care along with a systematic approach. Of the many risk factors, parental karyotype abnormalities, APS, activated protein C resistance, and cervical incompetence are the only established etiologies of RPL. Of all treatment options for women with RPL, only low-dose aspirin with heparin therapy in APS has proven role. In spite of thorough evaluation, in more than 50% of the women with RPL, etiology remains unexplained. In these unexplained cases, prognosis remains good, and tender loving care approach appears to play an important role. Empirical treatment should be avoided. Introduction of new treatments should be done after judging their benefits through properly designed controlled trials. So, the aim of the management is to identify the etiology and treat it. Different guidelines available differ in the approach leaving the treating clinicians in dilemma. There might be a single or multiples etiologies for RPL in single woman. So the approach needs to be individualized and tailored according to the patient for the optimum outcome.

References

1. Jeve YB, Davies W. Evidence based management of recurrent miscarriages. J Human Reprod Sci. 2014;7(3):159–69. https://doi.org/10.4103/0974–1208.142475.
2. Stirrrat GM. Recurrent miscarriage. Lancet. 1990;336:673–5.
3. Vanden Boogard E, Kaanclorp SP, Franssen T, Mol BW, Leschot NJ, et al. Consecutive or non-consecutive recurrent miscarriage: is there any difference in carrier status? Hum Reprod. 2010;25:1411–4.

4. The Investigation and treatment of couples with recurrent first trimester and second trimester miscarriage. Greentop guideline no. 17. April 2011.
5. Practice Committee of the American Society for Reproductive Medicine. Evaluation and treatment of recurrent pregnancy loss: a committee opinion. Fertil Steril. 2012;98:1103–11.
6. Jauniaux E, Farquharson RG, Christiansen OB, Exalto N. Evidence based guidelines for the investigation and medical treatment of recurrent miscarriage. Hum Reprod. 2006;21(9):2216–22.
7. Recurrent Pregnancy loss. ESHRE Early Pregnancy Development Group July 2017. https://www.eshre.eu/Guidelines/Guidelines/Guidelines in development/ESHRE guideline on Recurrent Pregnancy loss open for review. Last accessed on 1 Aug 2017.
8. Lund M, Kamper-Jorgenson M, Nielson HS, Lidegaard Ø, Andersen AM, Christiansen OB. Prognosis for live birth in women with recurrent miscarriage: what is the best measure of success? Obstet Gynecol. 2012;119:37–43.
9. Anderson AN, Wohlfart J, Chistens P, Olsen J, Melbye M. Maternal age and fetal loss: population based register linkage study. BMJ. 2000;320:1708–12.
10. Ness RB, Grisso JA, Hirshinger N, Markovic N, Shaw LM, et al. Cocaine and tobacco use and the risk of spontaneous abortion. N Engl J Med. 1999;340:333–9.
11. Brigham SA, Conlon C, Farquharson RG. A longitudinal study of pregnancy outcome following idiopathic recurrent miscarriage. Hum Reprod. 1999;14:2868–71.
12. Franssen MTM, Musters AM, van der Veen F, Repping S, Leschot NJ, et al. Reproductive outcome after PGD in couples with recurrent miscarriage in specific chromosomal abnormality: a systematic review. Hum Reprod Update. 2011;17:467–75.
13. Vissenberg R, Goddijn M. Is there a role of assisted reproductive technology in recurrent miscarriage? Sem Reprod Med. 2011;29:548–56.
14. Cervical Cerclage. Greentop Guidelines no. 60. May 2011.
15. American College of Obstetricians and Gynecologists. ACOG Practice Bulletin No. 142: cerclage for the management of cervical insufficiency. Obstet Gynecol. 2014:123(2 Pt 1):372–379. https://doi.org/10.1097101.AOG.0000443276.68274.CC.
16. Antiphospholipid syndrome. ACOG Practice Bulletin, No 118. January 2011.
17. Yetman DL, Kutteh WH. Antiphospholipid antibody panels and recurrent pregnancy loss: prevalence of anticardiolipin antibodies compared with other antiphospholipid antibodies. Fertil Steril. 1996;66:540–6.
18. Empson M, Lassere M, Craig J, Scott J. Prevention of recurrent miscarriage for women with antiphospholipid antibody or lupus anticoagulant. Cochrane Database Syst Rev. 2005;3.
19. Sanson BJ, Lensing AW, Prins MH, Ginsberg JS, Barkagan ZS, Lavenne-Pardonge E, et al. Safety of low-molecular weight heparin in pregnancy: a systematic review. Thromb Haemost. 1999;81:668–72.
20. Pettila V, Leinonen P, Markkola A, Hiilesmaa V, Kaaja R. Postpartum bone mineral density in women treated for thromboprophylaxis with unfractionated heparin or LMW heparin. Thromb Haemost. 2002;87:182–6.
21. James DK, Steer PJ, Weiner CP, Gonik B, Crowther C, Robson S. Chapter 6. Recurrent miscarriage. In: High risk pregnancy, management options. 4th ed. London: Elsevier; 2011. p. 75–96.
22. Thromboembolism in pregnancy. ACOG Practice Bulletin number 123. September 2011.
23. Porter TF, LaCoursiere Y, Scott JR. Immunotherapy for recurrent miscarriage. Cochrane Database Syst Rev. 2006;(2):CD000112.
24. Stephensen MD, Dreher K, Houlihan E, Wu V. Prevention of unexplained recurrent abortion using intravenous immunoglobulin: a prospective randomized, double blind, placebo-controlled trial. Am J Reprod Immunol. 1998;39:82–8.
25. Ata B, Tan SL, Shehata F, Holzer H, Buckett W. A systematic review of intravenous immunoglobulin for treatment of unexplained recurrent miscarriage. Fertil Steril. 2011;95:1080–5.
26. Hutton B, Sharma R, Fergusson D, Tinmouth A, Hebert P, Jamieson J, Walker M. Use of intravenous immunoglobulin for treatment of recurrent miscarriage: a systematic review. Br J Obstet Gynecol. 2007;114:134–42.
27. ACOG Practice Bulletin Number 145: antepartum fetal surveillance, July 2014. Obstet Gynecol. 2014;124:182–92.

28. Antenatal corticosteroids to reduce neonatal morbidity and mortality. Green Top Guidelines No 7. October 2010.
29. Hofmeyr GJ. Antenatal corticosteroids foe women at risk of preterm birth: RHL commentary (Last Revised: 2 February 2009). The WHO Reproductive Health Library; Geneva: World Health Organization.
30. Goonewardene M, Rameez MFM, Kaluarachchi A, Perera H. WHO recommendations for induction of labour: RHL commentary (Last Revised: 1 November 2011). The WHO Reproductive Health Library; Geneva: World Health Organization.
31. Caughey AB, Bishop JT. Maternal complications of pregnancy increase beyond 40 weeks of gestation in low risk women. J Perinatol. 2006;26:540–5.
32. Nicholson MD, Kellar LC, Bennet I, et al. The active management of risk in multiparous pregnancy at term: association between a higher prevention labour induction rate and improved birth outcomes. Am J Obstetr Gynaecol. 2009;200:250.e1–250.e13.
33. Nicholson MD, Kellar LC, Cronholm PF, Macones GA. Active management of risk in pregnancy at term in an urban population: an association between a higher induction of labor rate and a lower caesarean delivery rate. Am J Obstetr Gynaecol. 2004;191:1516–28.
34. ACOG Practice Bulletin. Antepartum surveillance. Number 145. July 2014.
35. Medical Eligibility Criteria (MEC) for different contraceptive methods (Medical Eligibility Criteria for contraceptive use). 5th ed. 2015.

Future Research Strategies and Directions in Recurrent Pregnancy Loss

22

Sruthi Bhaskaran and Amita Suneja

Recurrent pregnancy loss (RPL) is defined as two or more consecutive pregnancy losses in the first or early second trimester [1]. The overall incidence of RPL is approximately 3%, whereas that of recurrent miscarriage (RM; 3 or more miscarriages) is approximately 1% of the population [2]. Most of research in this area has focused on maternal factors such as meiotic error, oocyte quality, obesity, uterine architecture, metabolic factors, infection, and immunology. Even after a thorough evaluation, and due to the complex etiology involved in miscarriages, the potential cause remains unexplained in one third to one half of the cases, and one must acknowledge that despite the remarkable innovations over years, there are still open questions.

RM is generally multifactorial and current research is focused on finding the multiple etiologies which may be related to the process of implantation, trophoblast invasion, and placentation and also to elucidate embryopathic factors and in possible therapies for unexplained RM.

22.1 Biomarkers

Gene polymorphisms (almost 90 genes) as an etiology for RM has been investigated in various studies. The most frequently addressed genes are those associated with the developing immunotolerance (HLA-A,B, HLA-C, HLA-E, HLA-G, HLA-DPB1, HLA-DQA1, HLA-DQB1, KIR) [3–15], inflammation (IL1B, IL6, IL10, IFNγ, TNFα, etc.) [16, 17], and those controlling the maternal metabolism and blood coagulation (ANXA5, APOB, F2, F5, MTHFR, PAI-1, TGFB1, VEGF, factor V Leiden, prothrombin gene) [18–30].

S. Bhaskaran • A. Suneja (✉)
Obstetrics and Gynecology, University College of Medical Sciences and GTB Hospital, Delhi, India
e-mail: Amita_suneja@yahoo.co.in; sruthi_bhaskaran@yahoo.co.in

S. Mehta, B. Gupta (eds.), *Recurrent Pregnancy Loss*,
https://doi.org/10.1007/978-981-10-7338-0_22

But metaanalysis of studies investigating association of these factors in relation to RM risk has resulted in controversial results. This could be due to:

- Different definitions of RM and control group.
- The partner is not included in many studies.
- Small sample size.
- Ethnic variation in the study populations.
- Lifestyle and environmental factors play a confounding role on the pregnancy course.
- Secondary pathways leading to discrepancies between genotype and respective protein levels [31].

Over the years focus has gradually switched from maternal factors to the genes involved in the function of placenta, carrying maternally and paternally originated gene copies.

22.1.1 Advances and Future Directions in Genetics

In order to predict the genetic risk factors and biomarkers for RM, advances are needed in clinic as well as in the research strategies [31]:

- A detailed history with emphasis on obstetric history should be taken for the couples included as study or control group.
- The male partners should be evaluated by andrologists.
- Including mother–placenta and fetus as 2 units (duos) or including father also, i.e., trios (mother–father–placenta/fetus) would further help in validation of the studies.
- Studies should use collected material (DNA, RNA, and protein studies) from the same recruited family.
- Large multicentric trials involving a network of targeted clinics would facilitate carrying out validation of novel identified biomarkers.
- Copy number variations (CNVs) involving one or several loci generally have a stronger effect on the phenotype compared to SNPs. An ongoing study in Estonian and Danish population using genome-wide genotyping data to map common CNVs showed that couples with RM had significantly more frequent prevalence of a 52.4kb locus duplication on chromosome 5 [32]. So, further studies on role of CNVs in etiology of RM need to be undertaken.

  Role of biomarkers in RM also needs to be elucidated [33].

22.1.2 Genetics and Epigenetics Integration

Placental development depends on epigenetic control of gene expression [34]. There still has been no targeted microRNA expression profiling for RMrelated tissues.

The placenta specific miRNAs can cross the placental barrier, and their levels in maternal plasma can serve as an indicator for pregnancy complications. In women with RM, a 3′ UTR polymorphism controlling the expression of HLAG and exhibiting allele-specific affinity to microRNAs miR148a, miR148b, and miR152 has been studied [35, 36]. Research related to miRNA expression may help in discriminating disease samples with high accuracy.

22.1.3 Implications for Clinical Practice

In the future, combining information about important clinical history, genetic biomarkers, their individual strengths of association with RM, and their degree will clinicians to decide whether the etiology is immunological, thrombophilic, endocrine, or fetal [37]. Accordingly, optimal treatment which will benefit the patient maximally can be provided.

Research centers and RM clinics have to work in tandem so that research in biomolecular markers, gene, and genomic studies translates into newer treatment options for patients (e.g., gene and protein expression, epigenetic regulation).

22.2 Newer Molecular Markers

22.2.1 Leptins

Leptin hormone which modulates satiety and energy was originally thought to be produced only by adipocytes [38]. However, now it is known to be produced in many other tissues and is responsible for specific events in the reproductive maturity and fertility, e.g., implantation, maternal physiological changes, regulation of conceptus development, and fetal growth [39, 40].

Leptin levels increase during pregnancy. Lage et al. showed that leptin levels in women who had a miscarriage were lower than women with a normal pregnancy in first trimester and nonpregnant women. As these women were actually in the first trimester of pregnancy when the miscarriage occurred, so higher levels of leptin were expected [41]. According to Larid et al., leptin plays an important role in continuation of pregnancy and prevents miscarriage, and this hormone could be used as a predictor of pregnancy continuation [42].

22.2.2 Insulin Resistance and Hyperinsulinemia

Insulin resistance (IR) and hyperinsulinemia have been implicated as potential causes of the high rate of pregnancy loss and have been linked to the metabolic and endocrine abnormalities associated with the pathophysiology of RPL [43, 44]. Tian found frequent pregnancy loss in patients with insulin resistance [45]. Celik also found higher mean values for fasting glucose, fasting insulin, and insulin resistance in pregnant women with recurrent pregnancy loss when compared to the control group which included normal pregnant women [46]. The fasting glucose/fasting insulin ratio in the study by Celik et al. was lower in the pregnant women with RPL than women in the control group. Studies indicate insulin resistance may be a risk factor for spontaneous miscarriage in pregnant women with RPL [47, 48]. The use of oral hypoglycemic drugs to counteract the elevated insulin level before and even during pregnancy decreases the miscarriage rate in women with history of RPL [49–51]. Estimation of the serum levels of insulin hormones could be used in cases of RPL as a predictor of pregnancy continuation. Further studies are needed to confirm these results.

22.2.3 Cytokine Response in Blood and Tissue

Implantation is managed by a complex interaction between the endometrium and blastocyst in which several cytokines and adhesion molecules play a vital role in midsecretory phase of the menstrual cycle. This period is also known as the implantation window [52]. During the implantation window, specific expressions of adhesion molecules and cytokines can be observed [53]. It has been suggested that the TH2-type cytokine response is vital for a successful pregnancy, whereas an augmented TH1-type cytokine response may result in pregnancy loss [54]. This is also known as the TH1/TH2 paradigm. The paradigm postulates that the fetus is not rejected by the maternal immune system because pregnancy is a predominance of anti-inflammatory mediators (TH2-type immunity), which overrules TH1-type immunity and subsequently protects the fetus in the maternal uterus.

Comba C et al. evaluated these markers in women with RM and found that blood and tissue 1 levels of IL-18, LIF, and MIF and tissue levels of IL-12, IFN-g, and ICAM-1 correlated well with the prognosis [55]. If an effective treatment could be developed that normalizes immunologic parameters in patients with RPL, such parameters could be monitored during and/or after treatment. Therefore, patients could plan to become pregnant when the parameters are normalized. Clinical use of markers to evaluate endometrial receptivity has been hypothesized to improve the management of recurrent abortion and the implantation rate in women with previous failed in vitro fertilization cycles [56]. Noninvasive blood measurement would be preferable to more invasive endometrial tissue sampling because the blood and tissue levels of IL-12, IL-18, LIF, and MIF are strongly correlated.

22.3 Male Contribution

Evaluation of male factor in RM couple has been largely ignored, and only the basic investigation of semen analysis and karyotyping is routinely done in them. Assessment of sperm functionality which plays an important role is mostly ignored [57]. Varying original reports on factors such as Y-chromosome microdeletions, sperm oxidative stress, sperm DNA fragmentation, sperm concentration, morphology, and function have been reported [58]. A normal constitutional male karyotype does not exclude the presence of chromosome abnormalities in spermatozoa. Such abnormalities could arise de novo in the germ cell line, and several data indicate that moderate but significant increases in a given type of disomy are related to an increase in aneuploidy in the offspring [59]. Therefore, cytogenetic studies on spermatozoa are of great interest to assess their chromosomal constitution. The FISH assay is an accurate technique to detect the most common aneuploidies in decondensed sperm nuclei [59]. The choice of treatment strategies also depends on the specific chromosome abnormalities found in the male partner.

More recently, a systematic review and meta-analysis reported that DNA fragmentation was indeed significantly associated with miscarriage and concluded that using methods to select sperm without DNA damage may reduce miscarriage in assisted conception treatment [60]. The implications of these findings for the unexplained RPL population are still open to debate.

22.4 The Endometrium

Another focus in the recent years has been the endometrium and its ability to distinguish between good-quality and poor-quality embryos [61]. Any abnormality during decidualization might lead to implantation failure and early embryo failure. The "window of natural embryo selection," which was described by Teklenburg et al. refers to the role of stromal cells of decidua to assess the quality of the developing embryo and to dispose the embryos of poor quality by closing the window [61]. A preliminary study showed that women with RPL expressed increased levels of proimplantation cytokines, which rendered approximately 40% of them superfertile [62]. The investigators hypothesized that this superfertility disables the natural selection of healthy embryos and allows implantation of poor-quality embryos, which subsequently inevitably leads to pregnancy loss. A subsequent study attempted to investigate this further by looking at endometrial stromal cell migratory activity in response to high-quality and low-quality human embryos [63]. In women with RPL, the migratory activity did not differ between high-quality and low-quality embryos, whereas in the fertile control group, the migratory activity was inhibited in low-quality embryos in comparison with high-quality embryos.

It is hoped that future studies focusing on the mechanisms by which low-quality embryos inhibit human stromal cell migratory activity will provide further insight into the embryo-endometrial interactions that control implantation and ultimately determine the pregnancy outcome.

Mucin1 prevents adhesion and helps in maintaining barrier at the luminal epithelium. Women with RM have been found to express lower levels of this molecule [64–66]. Another research showed that women with RM had higher levels of prok1, a cytokine that promotes endometrium receptivity, and lower levels of prolactin which is a marker of decidualizing endometrial cells [62].

By targeting the endometrial decidual response prior to pregnancy or immediately after implantation, early pregnancy loss can be prevented.

22.5 Therapy

22.5.1 Immunotherapy

Forty percent of all RPL cases are due to immunological causes. For pregnancy to be successful, an immune-tolerant state is required which can be achieved through suppression of the mother's immune system [67]. The maternal immune system is primarily composed of myelomonocytic cells, T cells, and decidual natural killer (dNK) cells. The dNK cells are the most important in this process [68]. The cellular immunity is influenced by type-1 cytokines(IFN-γ, TNF-α, TNF-β, and IL-2), and humoral immunity is controlled by type-2 cytokines (IL-4, IL-5, IL-6, IL-10, and IL-13). The balance between these two is essential for fetal and placental growth.

TNF-α which is a type-1 cytokine can be inhibited by antibodies against the TNF-α molecule (adalimumab) or against soluble TNF-α receptors (etanercept) [69, 70]. In a study by Winger et al., pregnant women with history of RM were treated with TNF-α blockers administered with or without anticoagulants or anticoagulants + IVIG treatments (control groups). The study group which received treatment with TNF-α blockers had a higher live birth rate of approximately 71%, compared to 19% and 54% in the control group [71]. TNF-α blockers improved the implantation rate in women undergoing IVF also. G-CSF which decreases IFN-γ secretion of dNK cells and reduces the synthesis of various cytokines (especially TNF-α) also has a positive effect on pregnancy outcome [72]. A randomized controlled trial in which women with RM were treated with G-CSF or a placebo showed that live birth rate increased from 48.5% (placebo group) to 82.8% (G-CSF group) [73]. In another study, treatment with G-CSF increased the live birth rate from 13 to 32% [74]. The results of these few clinical studies reveal that it is essential to maintain a balance between type 1 and type 2 cytokines in early pregnancy.

22.5.2 Vitamin D Supplementation

Deficiency of vitamin D is one of the immunological causes for RPL. Deficiency of vitamin D can cause APA syndrome and other autoimmune disorders as they cause a disturbance in the ratio of Th1 and Th2 and also effect the B and NK cell immunity. Study by Ota K showed increased prevalence of APA with increased odds of positive APA (OR 2.22), anti-nuclear antigen antibody (OR 2.81), anti-ssDNA (OR 3.76), and TPO antibody (OR 2.68) in women with low levels of vitamin D [75]. Various other studies have also confirmed that deficiency of vitamin D is seen in women with APA. [76, 77] Also, vitamin D decreases type 1 cytokine production and increases type 2 and growth factors from NK cells. The therapeutic role of vitamin D needs to be assessed further for management of women with RPL.

Key Points

- Future directions in investigating biomolecular risk factors for RM rely on integrating alternative approaches (DNA variants, gene and protein expression, epigenetic regulation) in studies of individual genes as well as whole genome analysis.
- Leptin may play a role in preventing miscarriage and could be used as a predictor of pregnancy continuation.
- Clinical use of markers to evaluate endometrial receptivity and serum measurments of IL-1, 8, TNF alpha has been hypothesized to improve the management of recurrent abortion.
- Therapeutic interventions include monoclonal antibodies against the TNF-α molecule (adalimumab) or against soluble TNF-α receptors (etanercept). G-CSF was also found to have a positive effect on RPL patients.
- G-CSF reduces the cytotoxicity and IFN-γ secretion of dNK cells and reduces the synthesis of various cytokines.

References

1. Practice Committee of American Society for Reproductive Medicine. Definitions of infertility and recurrent pregnancy loss: a committee opinion. Fertil Steril. 2013;99:63.
2. Regan L, Rai R. Epidemiology and the medical causes of miscarriage. Baillieres Best Pract Res Clin Obstet Gynaecol. 2000;14(5):839–54.
3. Beydoun H, Saftlas AF. Association of human leucocyte antigen sharing with recurrent spontaneous abortions. Tissue Antigens. 2005;65:123–35. https://doi.org/10.1111/j.13990039.2005.00367.
4. Kolte AM, Nielsen HS, Moltke I, Degn B, Pedersen B, Sunde L, Nielsen FC, Christiansen OB. A genome widescan in affected sibling pairs with idiopathic recurrent miscarriage suggests genetic linkage. Mol Hum Reprod. 2011;17:379–85.
5. Faridi RM, Agrawal S. Killer immunoglobulinlike receptors (KIRs) and HLAC allo recognition patterns implicative of dominant activation of natural killer cells contribute to recurrent miscarriages. Hum Reprod. 2011;26:491–7.
6. Hiby SE, Apps R, Sharkey AM, Farrell LE, Gardner L, Mulder A, Claas FH, Walker JJ, Redman CW, Morgan L, Tower C, Regan L, Moore GE, Carrington M, Moffett A. Maternal activating KIRs protect against human reproductive failure mediated by fetal HLAC2. J Clin Invest. 2010;120:4102–10.
7. Kanai T, Fujii T, Keicho N, Tokunaga K, Yamashita T, Hyodo H, Miki A, Unno N, Kozuma S, Taketani Y. Polymorphism of human leukocyte antigenE gene in the Japanese population with or without recurrent abortion. Am J Reprod Immunol. 2001;45:168–73.
8. Mosaad YM, Abdel-Dayem Y, El-Deek BS, El-Sherbini SM. Association between HLAE *0101 homozygosity and recurrent miscarriage in Egyptian women. Scand J Immunol. 2011;74:205–9.
9. Aruna M, Sudheer PS, Andal S, Tarakeswari S, Reddy AG, Thangaraj K, Singh L, Reddy BM. HLAGpolymorphism patterns show lack of detectable association with recurrent spontaneous abortion. Tissue Antigens. 2010;76:216–22.
10. Cecati M, Giannubilo SR, Emanuelli M, Tranquilli AL, Saccucci F. HLAG and pregnancy adverse outcomes. Med Hypotheses. 2011;76:782–4.
11. Takakuwa K, Hataya I, Arakawa M, Kikuchi A, Higashino M, Yasuda M, Kurabayashi T, Tanaka K. Possible susceptibility of the HLADPB1*0402 and HLADPB1*04 alleles to

unexplained recurrent abortion: analysis by means of polymerase chain reactionrestricted fragment length polymorphism method. Am J Reprod Immunol. 1999;42:233–9.
12. Aruna M, Nagaraja T, Andal Bhaskar S, Tarakeswari S, Reddy AG, Thangaraj K, Singh L, Reddy BM. Novel alleles of HLADQ and DR loci show association with recurrent miscarriages among South Indian women. Hum Reprod. 2011;26:765–74.
13. Kruse C, Steffensen R, Varming K, Christiansen OB. A study of HLADR and DQ alleles in 588 patients and 562 controls confirms that HLADRB1*03 is associated with recurrent miscarriage. Hum Reprod. 2004;19:1215–21.
14. Faridi RM, Das V, Tripthi G, Talwar S, Parveen F, Agrawal S. Influence of activating and inhibitory killer immunoglobulinlike receptors on predisposition to recurrent miscarriages. Hum Reprod. 2009;24:1758–64.
15. Hiby SE, Regan L, Lo W, Farrell L, Carrington M, Moffett A. Association of maternal killer-cell immunoglobulinlike receptors and parental HLAC genotypes with recurrent miscarriage. Hum Reprod. 2008;23:972–6.
16. Bombell S, McGuire W. Cytokine polymorphisms in women with recurrent pregnancy loss: metaanalysis. Aust N Z J Obstet Gynaecol. 2008;48:147–54.
17. Daher S, Shulzhenko N, Morgun A, Mattar R, Rampim GF, Camano L, DeLima MG. Associations between cytokine gene polymorphisms and recurrent pregnancy loss. J Reprod Immunol. 2003;58:69–77.
18. Bogdanova N, Horst J, Chlystun M, Croucher PJ, Nebel A, Bohring A, Todorova A, Schreiber S, Gerke V, Krawczak M, Markoff A. A common haplotype of the annexin A5 (ANXA5) gene promoter is associated with recurrent pregnancy loss. Hum Mol Genet. 2007;16:573–8.
19. Miyamura H, Nishizawa H, Ota S, Suzuki M, Inagaki A, Egusa H, Nishiyama S, Kato T, Pryor-Koishi K, Nakanishi I, Fujita T, Imayoshi Y, Markoff A, Yanagihara I, Udagawa Y, Kurahashi H. Polymorphisms in the annexin A5 gene promoter in Japanese women with recurrent pregnancy loss. Mol Hum Reprod. 2011;17:447–52.
20. Hohlagschwandtner M, Unfried G, Heinze G, Huber JC, Nagele F, Tempfer C. Combined thrombophilic polymorphisms in women with idiopathic recurrent miscarriage. Fertil Steril. 2003;79:1141–8.
21. Yenicesu GI, Cetin M, Ozdemir O, Cetin A, Ozen F, Yenicesu C, Yildiz C, Kocak N. A prospective casecontrol study analyzes 12 thrombophilic gene mutations in Turkish couples with recurrent pregnancy loss. Am J Reprod Immunol. 2009;63:126–36.
22. Kovalevsky G, Gracia CR, Berlin JA, Sammel MD, Barnhart KT. Evaluation of the association between hereditary thrombophilias and recurrent pregnancy loss: a metaanalysis. Arch Intern Med. 2004;164:558–63. https://doi.org/10.1001/archinte.164.5.558.
23. Silver RM, Zhao Y, Spong CY, Sibai B, Wendel G Jr, Wenstrom K, Samuels P, Caritis SN, Sorokin Y, Miodovnik M, O'Sullivan MJ, Conway D, Wapner RJ. Prothrombin gene G20210A mutation and obstetric complications. Obstet Gynecol. 2010;115:14–20.
24. Ren A, Wang J. Methylene tetrahydrofolate reductase C677T polymorphism and the risk of unexplained recurrent pregnancy loss: a metaanalysis. Fertil Steril. 2006;86:1716–22.
25. Toth B, Vocke F, Rogenhofer N, Friese K, Thaler CJ, Lohse P. Paternal thrombophilic gene mutations are not associated with recurrent miscarriage. Am J Reprod Immunol. 2008;60:325–32.
26. Goodman C, Hur J, Goodman CS, Jeyendran RS, Coulam C. Are polymorphisms in the ACE and PAI1 genes associated with recurrent spontaneous miscarriages? Am J Reprod Immunol. 2009;62:365–70.
27. Sotiriadis A, Makrigiannakis A, Stefos T, Paraskevaidis E, Kalantaridou SN. Fibrinolytic defects and recurrent miscarriage: a systematic review and metaanalysis. Obstet Gynecol. 2007;109:1146–15.
28. Prigoshin N, Tambutti M, Larriba J, Gogorza S, Testa R. Cytokine gene polymorphisms in recurrent pregnancy loss of unknown cause. Am J Reprod Immunol. 2004;52:36–41.
29. von Linsingen R, Bompeixe EP, Bicalho Mda G. A casecontrol study in IL6 and TGFB1 gene polymorphisms and recurrent spontaneous abortion in southern Brazilian patients. Am J Reprod Immunol. 2005;53:94–9.
30. Traina E, Daher S, Moron AF, Sun SY, Franchim CS, Mattar R. Polymorphisms in VEGF, progesterone receptor and IL1 receptor genes in women with recurrent spontaneous abortion. J Reprod Immunol. 2011;88:53–7.

31. Rull K, Nagimaja L, Laan M. Genetics of recurrent miscarriage: challenges, current knowledge, future directions. Front Genet. 2012;3:34.
32. Nagirnaja L, Kasak L, Palta P, Rull K, Christiansen OB, Esko T, Remm M, Metspalu A, Laan M. Role of DNA copy number variations in genetic predisposition to recurrent pregnancy loss. J Reprod Immunol. 2011;90:145.
33. Baek KH, Lee EJ, Kim YS. Recurrent pregnancy loss: the key potential mechanisms. Trends Mol Med. 2007;13:310–7.
34. Nelissen EC, van Montfoort AP, Dumoulin JC, Evers JL. Epigenetics and the placenta. Hum Reprod Update. 2011;17:397–417.
35. Tan Z, Randall G, Fan J, Camoretti-Mercado B, Brockman-Schneider R, Pan L, Solway J, Gern JE, Lemanske RF, Nicolae D, Ober C. Allelespecific targeting of microRNAs to HLAG and risk of asthma. Am J Hum Genet. 2007;81:829–34.
36. Scholer N, Langer C, Kuchenbauer F. Circulating microRNAs as biomarkers—true blood? Genome Med. 2011;3:72.
37. Christiansen OB, et al. Multifactorial etiology of recurrent miscarriage and its scientific and clinical implications. Gynecol Obstet Investig. 2008;66(4):257–67.
38. Kershaw EE, Flier JS. Adipose tissue as an endocrine organ. J Clin Endocrinol Metab. 2004;89:2548–56.
39. Bajoria R, Sooranna SR, Ward BS, Chatterjee R. Prospective function of placental leptin at maternal-fetal interface. Placenta. 2002;23:103–15.
40. Moschos S, Chan JL, Mantzoros CS. Leptin and reproduction: a review. Fertil Steril. 2002;77:433–4.
41. Lage M, et al. Serum leptin levels in women throughout pregnancy and the postpartum period and in women suffering spontaneous abortion. Clin Endocrinol. 1999;50(2):211–6.
42. Laird S, et al. Leptin and leptin-binding activity in women with recurrent miscarriage: correlation with pregnancy outcome. Hum Reprod. 2001;16(9):2008–13.
43. Banu J, Fatima P, Sultana P, Chowdhury MA, Begum N, Anwary SA, et al. Association of infertile patients having polycystic ovarian syndrome with recurrent miscarriage. Mymensingh Med J. 2014;23(4):770–3.
44. Li ZL, Xiang HF, Cheng LH, Cao YX, Wei ZL, Liu C, Hu JJ, et al. Association between recurrent miscarriages and insulin resistance: a meta-analysis. Reprod Med Center. 2012;47(12):915–9.
45. Tian L, Shen H, Lu Q, Norman RJ, Wang J. Insulin resistance increases the risk of spontaneous abortion after assisted reproduction technology treatment. J Clin Endocrinol Metab. 2007;92(4):1430–3.
46. Celik N, Evsen MS, Sak ME, Soydinc E, Gul T. Evaluation of the relationship between insulin resistance and recurrent pregnancy loss. Ginekol Pol. 2011;82(4):272–5.
47. Craig L, Ke R, Kutteh W. Increased prevalence of insulin resistance in women with history of recurrent pregnancy loss. Fertil Steril. 2002;78:487–90.
48. Diejomaoh M, Jirous J, Al-Azemi M, Gupta M, Al-Jaber M, Farhat R, et al. Insulin resistance in women with recurrent spontaneous miscarriage of unknown etiology. Med Princ Pract. 2007;16(2):114–8.
49. Jakubowicz DJ, Iuorno MJ, Jakubowicz S, Roberts KA, Nestler JE. Effects of metformin on early pregnancy loss in the polycystic ovary syndrome. J Clin Endocrinol Metab. 2002;87(2):524–9.
50. Khattab S, Mohsen IA, Foutouh IA, Ramadan A, Moaz M, Al-Inany H. Metformin reduces abortion in pregnant women with polycystic ovary syndrome. Gynecol Endocrinol. 2006;22:680–4.
51. Nawaz FH, Khalid R, Naru T, Rizvi J. Does continuous use of metformin throughout pregnancy improve pregnancy outcomes in women with polycystic ovarian syndrome? J Obstet Gynaecol Res. 2008;34(5):832–7.
52. Psychoyos A. Hormonal control of ovoimplantation. Vitam Horm. 1973;31:201–56. 5.
53. Hoozemans DA, Schats R, Lambalk CB, Homburg R, Hompes PG. Human embryoimplan tation:currentknowledgeandclinicalimplicationsinassisted reproductive technology. Reprod Biomed Online. 2004;9:692–715.
54. Bates MD, Quenby S, Takakuwa K, Johnson PM, Vince GS. Aberrant cytokine production by peripheral blood mononuclear cells in recurrent pregnancy loss? Hum Reprod. 2002;17:2439–44.

55. Comba C, Bastu E, Dural O, et al. Role of inflammatory mediators in patients with recurrent pregnancy loss. Fertil Steril. 2015;104(6):1467–1474.e1.
56. Patel BG, Lessey BA. Clinical assessment and management of the endometrium in recurrent early pregnancy loss. Semin Reprod Med. 2011;29:491–506.
57. Kavitha P, Malini SS. Positive association of sperm dysfunction in the pathogenesis of recurrent pregnancy loss. J Clin Diagn Res. 2014;8:7–10.
58. Vissenberg R, Goddijn M. Is there a role for assisted reproductive technology in recurrent miscarriage? Semin Reprod Med. 2011;29(6):548–56.
59. Egozcue J, Blanco J, Vidal F. Chromosome studies in human sperm nuclei using fluorescence in-situ hybridization (FISH). Hum Reprod Update. 1997;3:441–52.
60. Robinson L, Gallos ID, Conner SJ, et al. The effect of sperm DNA fragmentation on miscarriage rates: a systematic review and meta-analysis. Hum Rep. 2012;27(10):2908–17.
61. Teklenburg G, Salker M, Molokhia M, et al. Natural selection of human embryos: decidualizing endometrial stromal cells serve as sensors of embryo quality upon implantation. PLoS One. 2010;5(4):e10258.
62. Salker M, Teklenburg G, Molokhia M, et al. Natural selection of human embryos: impaired decidualization of endometrium disables embryo-maternal interactions and causes recurrent pregnancy loss. PLoS One. 2010;5(4):e10287.
63. Weimar CH, Kavelaars A, Brosens JJ, et al. Endometrial stromal cells of women with recurrent miscarriage fail to discriminate between high- and low-quality human embryos. PLoS One. 2012;7(7):e41424.
64. Serle E, et al. Endometrial differentiation in the peri-implantation phase of women with recurrent miscarriage: a morphological and immunohistochemical study. Fertil Steril. 1994;62(5):989–96.
65. Aplin J, Hey N, Li T. MUC1 as a cell surface and secretory component of endometrial epithelium: reduced levels in recurrent miscarriage. Am J Reprod Immunol. 1996;35(3):261–6.
66. Hey N, et al. MUC1 in secretory phase endometrium: expression in precisely dated biopsies and flushings from normal and recurrent miscarriage patients. Hum Reprod. 1995;10(10):2655–62.
67. Warning JC, McCracken SA, Morris JM. A balancing act: mechanisms by which the fetus avoids rejection by the maternal immune system. Reproduction. 2011;141(6):715–24.
68. Vacca P, et al. Origin, phenotype and function of human natural killer cells in pregnancy. Trends Immunol. 2011;32(11):517–23.
69. Weinblatt ME, et al. Adalimumab, a fully human anti–tumor necrosis factor α monoclonal antibody, for the treatment of rheumatoid arthritis in patients taking concomitant methotrexate: the ARMADA trial. Arthritis Rheum. 2003;48(1):35–45.
70. Moreland LW, et al. Etanercept therapy in rheumatoid arthritis: a randomized, controlled trial. Ann Intern Med. 1999;130(6):478–86.
71. Winger EE, Reed JL. Treatment with tumor necrosis factor inhibitors and intravenous immunoglobulin improves live birth rates in women with recurrent spontaneous abortion. Am J Reprod Immunol. 2008;60(1):8–16.
72. Würfel W. Treatment with granulocyte colony- stimulating factor in patients with repetitive implantation failures and/or recurrent spontaneous abortions. J Reprod Immunol. 2015;108:123–35.
73. Scarpellini F, Sbracia M. Use of granulocyte colony-stimulating factor for the treatment of unexplained recurrent miscarriage: a randomised controlled trial. Hum Reprod. 2009;24(11):2703–8.
74. Santjohanser C, et al. Granulocyte-colony stimulating factor as treatment option in patients with recurrent miscarriage. Arch Immunol Ther Exp. 2013;61(2):159–64.
75. Ota K, Dambaeva S, Han AR, et al. Vitamin D deficiency may be a risk factor for recurrent pregnancy losses by increasing cellular immunity and autoimmunity. Hum Reprod. 2014;29(2):208–19.
76. Orbach H, Zandman-Goddard G, Amital H, Barak V, Szekanecz Z, Szucs G, Danko K, Nagy E, Csepany T, Carvalho JF, et al. Novel biomarkers in autoimmune diseases: prolactin, ferritin, vitamin D, and TPA levels in autoimmune diseases. Ann N Y Acad Sci. 2007;1109:385–400.
77. Agmon-Levin N, Blank M, Zandman-Goddard G, Orbach H, Meroni PL, Tincani A, Doria A, Cervera R, Miesbach W, Stojanovich L, et al. Vitamin D: an instrumental factor in the anti-phospholipid syndrome by inhibition of tissue factor expression. Ann Rheum Dis. 2011;70:145–50.

Counselling of an RPL Couple

23

Seema Singhal and Juhi Bharti

23.1 Introduction

Spontaneous pregnancy loss or miscarriage is defined as naturally failed pregnancy before 20 weeks gestation. Approximately 15% of all clinical pregnancies result in miscarriage [1]. The definition of recurrent pregnancy loss (RPL) or habitual abortion is not consistent. Historically, it is defined as three consecutive pregnancy losses before 20 weeks gestation. As per the Practice Committee guidelines of the American Society for Reproductive Medicine (ASRM), RPL is defined as two or more failed clinical pregnancies [2], whereas, Royal College of Obstetrics and Gynaecologists (RCOG) has defined RPL as three or more consecutive pregnancy losses affecting 1% of couples trying to conceive [3]. The loss may be primary (in women who has never carried to viability) or secondary (after a previous live birth).

Sometimes, the psychological impact is as high as that of a perinatal loss [4, 5]. Therefore, proper counselling has a very important effect on future pregnancies and is important to change their perspective towards life and subsequent pregnancies. All RPL couples are anxious to get themselves evaluated to know any pre-existing cause. Specific counselling and treatment can improve the chances of a successful pregnancy in case of an identifiable cause. But even in the absence of any cause, reassurance and counselling sessions are very valuable.

S. Singhal (✉) • J. Bharti
Department of Obstetrics and Gynecology, All India Institute of Medical Sciences, New Delhi, India
e-mail: drseemasinghal@gmail.com

S. Mehta, B. Gupta (eds.), *Recurrent Pregnancy Loss*,
https://doi.org/10.1007/978-981-10-7338-0_23

23.2 Psychological Impact

Even a single miscarriage has a significant impact on psychological health of a couple. The couples with recurrent miscarriages experience negative psychological reactions including sadness, depression, guilt and mental stress [6–8]. Trauma in recurrent miscarriage is a type of "strain" trauma because the after effects persist for a longer period of time with the anticipation of further loss [9]. The degree of impact may differ with some experiencing minimal emotional upset; in others it may last for months, and few develop chronic psychiatric morbidity [8, 10, 11]. In a questionnaire-based study by M. Kagami et al. in 2012, they found quite higher levels of depression, stress and anxiety among women as compared to men. Out of 76 women, 39.5% were found to have mild depression, 3.9% suffered from severe depression as compared to just 14.9% of men [12].

Women with supportive partners and social networks and those with compassionate health-care providers do better emotionally than women without such support [13, 14]. Men can also have severe emotional reactions after the miscarriage but present in a different way as compared to women. Besides all this, it is equally important to acknowledge and empathize with an older child who was awaiting the birth of his or her sibling. Children are also affected by their parent's psychological status [15].

23.3 Aetiology of RPL

The various causes of RPL include genetic factors, uterine anomalies, endocrine factors, infections, male factors, immunologic and environmental. However, despite all advances, up to 50% of cases are idiopathic.

23.3.1 Idiopathic or Unexplained RPL

The aetiology remains unknown in about 50% of couples with RPL despite complete investigations. These are the patients where counselling, education and reassurance are important to achieve successful pregnancy. Special emphasis has to be made that their chances of successful pregnancy reach 50–60% depending on age and other factors [16, 17]. These couples especially the female partner require tender loving care that includes psychological and emotional support along with frequent ultrasounds and medical examinations. It has been seen that this improves live birth rates in couples with recurrent miscarriage with no identifiable pathology. The importance of psychological support in optimizing pregnancy result has not been evaluated in the form of a randomized controlled trial. However, several non-randomized studies have suggested that a dedicated early pregnancy clinic improves the pregnancy outcome, although the mechanism is not clearly known [18, 19].

23.3.2 Genetic Factors

A chromosome abnormality has been recognized in 50–70% of the products of conception (POC) in case of a miscarriage [20]. The most common chromosomal abnormalities include autosomal trisomies (13–16, 21 or 22), monosomy X and polyploidies [21]. But, the vast majority of the parental karyotypes are normal. An important aspect to understand is that usually trisomies are related to maternal age and risk increases if age >35 years. Therefore, in such cases, a miscarriage due to foetal aneuploidy is usually sporadic with minimal recurrence risk. In couples with recurrent miscarriage, one of the partners harbours a balanced structural chromosomal anomaly in around 2–5% of cases, most commonly a balanced reciprocal or Robertsonian translocation [22]. These couples should be referred to a genetic clinic for counselling and necessary tests.

In addition to foetal chromosomal analysis of the POC, the foetus and placenta also should be evaluated thoroughly according to the recommendations from the College of American Pathologists [23].This approach may detect associated malformations (e.g., neural tube defects like spina bifida or foetal hydrops, etc.) that may be suggestive of an underlying genetic syndrome. Knowledge of the karyotype of the POC is important to make an informed prognosis for a future pregnancy outcome. The couple should be counselled that while a sporadic foetal chromosome abnormality is the most common cause of any single miscarriage, if the karyotype of the miscarried pregnancy is normal, the next pregnancy bears a better prognosis [24].

Genetic counselling of these couples not only pertains to identify the causes and hence to prognosticate but also to discuss various management options available to them. When a structural chromosome abnormality is diagnosed in one of the partners, the treatment options include preimplantation genetic diagnosis (PGD) or use of donor gametes. PGD requires the couples to undergo in vitro fertilization (IVF) and genetic testing of the embryos for any abnormality. The affected embryos would then be discarded and the healthy ones would be transferred. There are no definitive studies comparing the role of PGD in RPL to the other option of natural conception and observation. The lack of randomized controlled trials in this area makes it difficult to take a decision for both the clinicians and the patients. A systematic review conducted by Franssen et al. concluded that live birth rate per couple in case of a natural conception ranged between 33 and 60% (median 55.5%), whereas after PGD this figure ranges between 0 and 100% (median 31%) [25]. They state that at present, data is not sufficient enough to encourage PGD in couples with RPL. Moreover it is invasive and costly and might require prenatal invasive testing (amniocentesis or chorionic villous sampling) to further rule out any genetic abnormality.

The other option for these couples is use of donor gametes especially useful in case of one partner being a carrier of Robertsonian translocation involving homologous chromosomes. In such cases, it is bound to result in unbalanced gametes, and use of donor gametes is recommended. Thorough counselling of the couples is required to explain them the impact of this condition before offering them option of donor gametes. Many couples get insecure with the feeling that they cannot contribute to a normal pregnancy.

The last but not the least option for these couples is to go for a natural pregnancy and get prenatal testing done to look for any genetic abnormality in the foetus. In the presence of any chromosomal anomaly in the foetus, the couples have the option of terminating the pregnancy. This has to be emphasized and reinforced that couples still have a 50% chance of live birth after natural conception which is higher than PGD/IVF-ICSI cycle.

23.3.3 Anatomic Abnormalities

Uterine anatomic abnormalities like septate, bicornuate and uterus didelphys account for about 15–27% of recurrent second trimester miscarriages [9].

As per RCOG, pelvic ultrasound should be done in all women with recurrent first-trimester losses and with one or more second-trimester miscarriages. In the presence of septa or fibroids, patients should be counselled in a way that they understand the evidence is lacking in this area. But, recent reports of hysteroscopic septal resection appear promising, and they might benefit from this surgery [26].

The role of cervical cerclage in cases of midtrimester miscarriages has been a controversial issue, and couples should be counselled regarding risks and benefits of the procedure. They should be counselled regarding the current indications of cerclage, route of administration, options of laparoscopy and need for adjuvant therapy like tocolytics, bed rest, etc. The risks that need to be explained include failure of cerclage, abortion, preterm labour or infection, suture cut through, haemorrhage and cervical trauma.

23.3.4 Environmental

Many environmental factors have been associated with isolated or recurrent miscarriages. This area deserves special attention as they are avoidable. Basic teratology counselling has to be done regarding the dose of exposure, period of gestation and knowledge of "all-or-nothing" law. Several factors that are said to result in miscarriages include medications (antineoplastics, few anaesthetic agents, etc.), X-rays or other ionizing radiations, heavy metals, etc. But three substances—alcohol, cigarettes and caffeine—are the most implicated ones. Alcohol consumption up to three drinks per week in the first trimester results in increased pregnancy losses [27]. Cigarette and caffeine are also associated with adverse pregnancy outcomes. A prospective cohort study in 2008 found that increased daily caffeine intake (>200 mg/day) increased the risk of miscarriage accounting to adjusted hazard ratio of 2.23 [28]. Though these can cause sporadic pregnancy losses, chronic habits may contribute to recurrent miscarriages. Extensive counselling with the help of support groups is required to recommend lifestyle changes including reduction of work stress and abstaining from alcohol, tobacco and other drug abuse to improve chances of a successful pregnancy. Counselling of the couples who are overstressed should include meditation sessions, family holidays, music therapy, etc.

23.3.5 Endocrine Factors

Endocrine disorders like diabetes mellitus, thyroid disease, hyperprolactinemia and luteal phase defects have been linked to recurrent miscarriages. Therefore, these women should be evaluated for these disorders and treated accordingly. Insulin resistance leads to hyperandrogenemia and increases miscarriage rate by increasing free testosterone levels and hyperhomocysteinemia [29]. High glycosylated haemoglobin A1C levels (HbA1c) increase the rate of miscarriage, and women with uncontrolled diabetes mellitus have to be counselled to optimize blood sugar control during preconceptional period [30]. Women should also be counselled regarding the risk of anomalies, need for insulin therapy, etc. Thyroid dysfunction especially due to the presence of thyroid autoantibodies (i.e. anti-thyroglobulin, thyroid peroxidase) has been implicated in recurrent miscarriage.

23.3.6 Male Factors

Even in the presence of normal semen analysis, male partners in couples with RPL could have genetic abnormalities in sperm DNA like sperm aneuploidies or DNA fragmentation [31]. The diagnostic tests recommended in the evaluation of these men are DNA fragmentation index (DFI) and fluorescence in situ hybridization (FISH). Genetic counsellors play a very important role to help decide the couples regarding the management plan. They have to be educated about the option of preimplantation genetic screening/IVF-ICSI to increase the chance of live birth and the need of donor sperm and even adoption. They have to be counselled regarding need of prenatal testing since these pregnancies are at increased risk for aneuploidy.

23.3.7 Immunologic

Most therapies available for immunological causes of RPL have an experimental role, and the evidence is inconclusive. But success rate is 90% with use of heparin (low molecular weight or unfractionated) plus aspirin in cases of antiphospholipid antibody syndrome. The women should be told that in these cases, live birth rate without any therapy has is very low (10%) [32]. On the other hand, treatment significantly reduces the miscarriage rate by 54%:RR0.46, 95% CI 0.29– 0.71) [33]. They have to be counselled to be compliant with the treatment as it has a significant impact on the outcome. They also need to be counselled regarding other risks of pregnancy like preeclampsia or preterm labour.

23.4 Cultural and Social Implications of RPL

The counsellors and health-care providers should listen to the cultural and social concerns of the couples suffering from recurrent miscarriages. One has to respect their beliefs and strategies to cope up with the loss. There exist cultural and religious differences in response to a miscarriage in different parts of the world. While some women are not allowed to even talk about their experience of a perinatal loss, others believe and perform religious activities to prevent further miscarriage [34–36]. But the couple's personal opinion may differ from the cultural practices, and counselling is to be directed towards personal concerns. Also, beliefs about the reason behind miscarriage is varied including some kind of demonic activity, angering ancestral spirits, committing sins in the past, eating forbidden foods, family conflicts and misconduct [37]. In such condition, educating not only the couples but all the family members becomes important.

23.5 One-Stop RM Clinic

It is a concept of a dedicated clinic to offer the best and fast care to couples with recurrent miscarriage. It is a multidisciplinary approach involving expert gynaecologists, nursing staff, genetic counsellor and psychologists. It not only will help in allaying anxiety, but the couples can also get the investigations faster and plan for future pregnancy accordingly. A study by Habayeb and Konje found that the concept of one-stop clinic led to reduction in the interval of visits to clinic by 36% (206.6–130.4 days, $P < 0.001$), and total number of visits were reduced by 60% (2.5–1, $P < 0.002$) [38]. There was a significant impact on the waiting time after the referral was made.

23.6 Counselling in Special Scenarios

23.6.1 Interpregnancy Interval After a Miscarriage

There is no data in support of delaying conception after a miscarriage. A prospective study conducted by DaVanzo et al. in Bangladesh in 9214 women noted that live birth rate was higher in pregnancies conceived ≤3 months after a miscarriage (adjusted relative risk ratio (RRR) of 0.70, 95% CI 0.57–0.86) [39]. ACOG also recommends abstinence from vaginal intercourse for just 1–2 weeks after an early pregnancy loss to reduce chances of infection.

The couples experiencing RPL have to be counselled to complete their investigations before planning next pregnancy. But once the results of the investigations are available, there is no need to delay the pregnancy. Women should be started on preconceptional medications like folic acid and drugs like aspirin, metformin, etc. wherever indicated.

23.6.2 Counselling Regarding Prevention of Alloimmunization

ACOG recommends 50 μg of anti-D injection in cases of Rh (D) negative and unsensitized pregnancy within 72 h of miscarriage (<12 weeks). Anti-D of 300 μg has to be given in pregnancies >12 weeks.

To conclude, counselling of couples with recurrent miscarriage must include understanding their emotional concerns and providing realistic figures about chances of future successful pregnancies. Genetic counsellors and clinicians should respect their religious and cultural beliefs and have to educate them without hurting their sentiments. In cases of unexplained pregnancy losses, family members have to be sensitized to provide tender loving care to the woman. When a genetic abnormality is detected in the parents, it is the responsibility of genetic counsellors to explain the implications. Referrals to support groups have to be made as appropriate.

Key Points

- Recurrent pregnancy loss can lead to depression, stress and anxiety more among women as compared to men.
- Detailed counselling of the couple should aim to establish aetiology, offer treatment and offer care and sympathy and psychological and emotional support.
- For genetic causes options like preimplantation genetic diagnosis, donor gamete, in vitro fertilization and adoption should be explained.
- One-stop RPL clinics play an important role in providing the required support to the couple.
- Counselling of the family is important to address the cultural and social taboos associated with RPL.

References

1. Chen BA, Creinin MD. Contemporary management of early pregnancy failure. Clin Obstet Gynecol. 2007;50:67–88.
2. Practice Committee of American Society for Reproductive Medicine. Evaluation and treatment of recurrent pregnancy loss: a committee opinion. Fertil Steril. 2012;98(5):1103–11.
3. The investigation and treatment of couples with recurrent first-trimester and second-trimester miscarriage. RCOG Green–top guideline No. 17, April 2011, 1–18.
4. Lee C, Slade P. Miscarriage as a traumatic event: a review of the literature and new implications for intervention. J Psychosom Res. 1996;40(3):235–44.
5. Stirtzinger R, Robinson GE. The psychologic effects of spontaneous abortion. CMAJ. 1989;140:799–801.
6. Brier N. Grief following miscarriage: a comprehensive review of the literature. J Women's Health. 2008;17:451–64.
7. Freda MC, Devine KS, Semelsberger C. The lived experience of miscarriage after infertility. Am J Matern Child Nurs. 2003;28(1):16–23.
8. Madden ME. The variety of emotional reactions to miscarriage. Women Health. 1994;21(2–3):85–104.

9. Katz VL, Kuller JA. Recurrent miscarriage. Am J Perinatol. 1994;11(6):386–97.
10. Corbet-Owen C, Kruger LM. The health system and emotional care: validating the many meanings of spontaneous pregnancy loss. Fam Syst Health. 2001;19(4):411–27.
11. Craig M, Tata P, Regan L. Psychiatric morbidity among patients with recurrent miscarriage. J Psychosom Obstet Gynaecol. 2002;23(3):157–64.
12. Kagami M, Maruyama T, Koizumi T, Miyazaki K, Nishikawa-Uchida S, Oda H, et al. Psychological adjustment and psychosocial stress among Japanese couples with a history of recurrent pregnancy loss. Hum Reprod. 2012;27(3):787–94.
13. Hori S, Nakano Y, Yamada A, Azuma H, Noda Y, Sugiura M, et al. Personality, social support, coping and emotional distress after repeated spontaneous abortions. J Psychosom Obstet Gynaecol. 2002;23(2):133–40.
14. Toedter LJ, Lasker JN, Janssen HJ. International comparison of studies using the perinatal grief scale: a decade of research on pregnancy loss. Death Stud. 2001;25(3):205–28.
15. Weil J. Psychosocial genetic counseling. New York: Oxford University Press Inc.; 2000.
16. Andersen AN, Wohlfahrt J, Christens P, Olsen J, Melbye M. Maternal age and fetal loss: population based register linkage study. BMJ. 2000;320:1708–12.
17. Lund M, Kamper-Jorgensen M, Nielsen HS, Lidegaard O, Andersen AM, Christiansen OB. Prognosis for live birth in women with recurrent miscarriage: what is the best measure of success? Obstet Gynecol. 2012;119:37–43.
18. Clifford K, Rai R, Regan L. Future pregnancy outcome in unexplained recurrent first trimester miscarriage. Hum Reprod. 1997;12:387–9.
19. Brigham SA, Conlon C, Farquharson RG. A longitudinal study of pregnancy outcome following idiopathic recurrent miscarriage. Hum Reprod. 1999;14:2868–71.
20. Hogge WA, Byrnes AL, Lanasa MC, Surti U. The clinical use of karyotyping spontaneous abortions. Am J Obstet Gynecol. 2003;189(2):397–400.
21. Gardner R, Sutherland G. Chromosome abnormalities and genetic counseling. 3rd ed. New York: Oxford University Press Inc.; 2004.
22. Franssen MT, Korevaar JC, van der Veen F, Leschot NJ, Bossuyt PM, Goddijn M. Reproductive outcome after chromosome analysis in couples with two or more miscarriages: index [corrected]-control study. BMJ. 2006;332:759–63. Erratum in: BMJ 2006; 332:1012.
23. College of American Pathologist. The examination of the placenta: patient care and risk management. Arch Pathol Lab Med. 1991;115:660721.
24. Carp H, Toder V, Aviram A, Daniely M, Mashiach S, Barkai G. Karyotype of the abortus in recurrent miscarriage. Fertil Steril. 2001;75:678–82.
25. Franssen MT, Musters AM, Van der Veen F, Repping S, Leschot NJ, Bossuyt PM, et al. Reproductive outcome after PGD in couples with recurrent miscarriage carrying a structural chromosome abnormality: a systematic review. Hum Reprod Update. 2011;17(4):467–75.
26. Homer HA, Li TC, Cooke ID. The septate uterus: a review of management and reproductive outcome. Fertil Steril. 2000;73:1–14.
27. Kesmodel U, Wisborg K, Olsen SF, Henriksen TB, Secher NJ. Moderate alcohol intake in pregnancy and the risk of spontaneous abortion. Alcohol. 2002;37:87–92.
28. Weng X, Odouli R, Li DK. Maternal caffeine consumption during pregnancy and the risk of miscarriage: a prospective cohort study. Am J Obstet Gynecol. 2008;198(3):279.
29. Hong Y, Xie QX, Chen CY, Yang C, Li YZ, Chen DM, et al. Insulin resistance in first-trimester pregnant women with pre-pregnant glucose tolerance and history of recurrent spontaneous abortion. J Biol Regul Homeost Agents. 2013;27:225–31.
30. Jovanovic L, Knopp H, Kim H, Cefalu WT, Zhu XD, et al. Elevated pregnancy losses at high and low extremes of maternal glucose in early pregnancies in diabetics. Diabetes Care. 2005;28:1113–7.
31. Aitken RJ, De Iuliis GN. Origins and consequences of DNA damage in male germ cells. Reprod Biomed Online. 2007;14:727–33.
32. Rai RS, Clifford K, Cohen H, Regan L. High prospective fetal loss rate in untreated pregnancies of women with recurrent miscarriage and antiphospholipid antibodies. Hum Reprod. 1995;10:3301–4.

33. Empson M, Lassere M, Craig J, Scott J. Prevention of recurrent miscarriage for women with antiphospholipid antibody or lupus anticoagulant. Cochrane Database Syst Rev. 2005;(2):CD002859.
34. Hsu M, Tseng Y, Kuo L. Transforming loss: Taiwanese women's adaptation to stillbirth. J Adv Nurs. 2002;40:387–95.
35. McGreal D, Evans BJ, Burrows GD. Gender differences in coping following loss of a child through miscarriage or stillbirth: a pilot study. Stress Med. 1997;13(3):159–65.
36. Van P, Meleis A. Coping with grief after involuntary pregnancy loss: perspectives of African American women. J Obstet Gynecol Neonatal Nurs. 2003;32:28–39.
37. Cecil R, editor. The anthropology of pregnancy loss: comparative studies in miscarriage, stillbirth and neonatal death. Washington, DC: Berg Publishers; 1996.
38. Habayeb OMH, Konje JC. The one-stop recurrent miscarriage clinic: an evaluation of its effectiveness and outcome. Hum Reprod. 2004;19(12):2952–8.
39. DaVanzo J, Hale L, Rahman M. How long after a miscarriage should women wait before becoming pregnant again? Multivariate analysis of cohort data from Matlab, Bangladesh. BMJ Open. 2012;2:e001591.

Part IV

Management Options in RPL: Hype or Hope

Progestogens/hCG Supplementation: A Vital Role?

24

Nisha Singh

24.1 Introduction

Once a woman is labeled as a case of recurrent pregnancy loss, every effort is made to protect her from any adversity in her next pregnancy. Among the various preventive and therapeutic steps, hormonal supplementation in the form of progestogens or hCG is widely used. Most of the women with threatened abortion are given progesterone as a tocolytic [1, 2]. Though in developing countries, there is dearth of latest reliable information on effective care, yet progesterone is commonly prescribed in India for cases of threatened abortion and recurrent miscarriage [3]. Hence, it is important to justify their use with all pros and cons. There is a definite need to discuss and ascertain the role of progestogen and hCG supplementation for continuation of pregnancy and preventing another loss.

This chapter has been written with the help of all possible evidence required to understand the usefulness of hormonal supplementation in recurrent pregnancy loss.

24.2 Normal Physiology of Conception and Pregnancy

To understand the usefulness of hormonal supplementation, we must have a look at the normal physiology of conception and pregnancy. Progesterone and hCG are important hormones that act throughout pregnancy from fertilization to implantation and fetal development.

N. Singh
Department of Obstetrics and Gynecology, King George Medical University, Lucknow, India
e-mail: nisha.kgmc@gmail.com

S. Mehta, B. Gupta (eds.), *Recurrent Pregnancy Loss*,
https://doi.org/10.1007/978-981-10-7338-0_24

24.2.1 Role of Progesterone

During menstrual cycles, progesterone acts every month, on the uterine endometrium, to bring about secretory changes that make it suitable for implantation, in case pregnancy happens. The primary source of progesterone is the corpus luteum, where the theca and granulosa lutein cells act under the influence of luteinizing hormone (LH).

The corpus luteum is formed from the avascular Graafian follicle by the process of luteinization under the effect of LH (Leutinising Hormone). The basement membrane between granulosa cells and theca cells breaks down, and neovascularization in this area leads to formation of a vascular corpus luteum, which in turn secretes progesterone in addition to estrogen and androstenedione [4].

Progesterone stimulates the endometrium under the influence of hCG during the luteal phase of the cycle [5].

Mechanism of action of progesterone:

- Progesterone stimulates production of T-helper 2, cytokines and C3 and C4.
- It increases nitric oxide production, which causes vasodilatation, and improves blood flow and oxygen to the endometrium [6–8].
- It acts as a uterine tocolytic and reduces myometrial contractility at the time of the implantation [9, 10].
- Dihydrogesterone is an immunomodulator which helps in the production of progesterone-induced blocking factors (PIBF). PIBF acts as an immunoprotector for pregnancy by inhibiting cell-mediated cytotoxicity and natural killer cell activity.

The corpus luteum solely maintains pregnancy up to 6–7 weeks until the placenta takes over. Surgical removal of the corpus luteum (luteotomy) before 6–7 weeks of pregnancy is known to be associated with abortion. After 9 weeks of gestation, there is luteal-placental shift in which the placental trophoblasts become the sole producer of progesterone [11]. Serum progesterone levels gradually increase throughout pregnancy, and daily production at term is around 250 mg. Progesterone is released in a pulsatile fashion, and this makes it difficult to assess and prove progesterone deficiency as the cause of recurrent miscarriage in a woman. Unlike estrogen levels, placental progesterone production does not immediately fall with fetal demise, ligation of umbilical cord, or anencephaly.

24.2.2 Role of Human Chorionic Gonadotropin

Human chorionic gonadotropin (hCG) is also known as the "pregnancy hormone" since it is almost exclusively secreted by the placenta. It is a glycoprotein containing α and β subunits. The structural similarity with LH, FSH, and TSH is due to the sharing of α subunit. The distinct characteristics of β subunit make it a special pregnancy hormone.

hCG is detectable in maternal plasma 7–9 days after the preovulatory LH surge. Both cytotrophoblasts and syncytiotrophoblasts produce hCG up to 5 weeks of pregnancy. Later, it is produced only by the syncytiotrophoblasts. Peak levels of hCG are reached at 8–10 weeks of gestation and then start falling up to 16 weeks. A plateau level of 10–20 IU/mL is maintained throughout pregnancy [4]. The initial function of hCG is to maintain the corpus luteum and hence progesterone production. The second role is fetal testicular stimulation for testosterone production in male fetus. Thus, hCG actually maintains pregnancy through progesterone, and hCG supplementation will also lead to increased progesterone production and function. *Despite the knowledge of these basic physiological functions of progesterone and hCG in early pregnancy, we need to discuss whether the deficiency or lack of these hormones will be a definite cause of recurrent pregnancy loss.*

24.3 Progesterone Deficiency as a Cause of Recurrent Abortion

Eight to twelve percent of recurrent abortions are caused by endocrine factors. Thyroid autoimmunity and uncontrolled diabetes are well-known endocrine causes. Progesterone deficiency may produce abortions through luteal phase defect (LPD), but this, as an endocrine cause of recurrent abortions, is a controversial topic [12].

In LPD there is insufficient progesterone to maintain a normal secretory endometrium, and so normal implantation does not take place [13]. Before we can prove that LPD can cause recurrent abortions, it's important to be able to diagnose LPD.

Randomized controlled trials have proven that histological evaluation of the endometrium is not accurate in differentiating fertile women from women with LPD and infertility [13]. Ultrasonographic features like endometrial thickness >7 mm, triple-layered endometrium, and power Doppler have been assessed as parameters to confirm uterine receptivity, but their absence as diagnostic parameter for LPD also have not stood the test of time. Serum levels of progesterone fluctuate frequently, and its levels peak 6–8 days after the ovulation [14], so it cannot be used to define a "fertile" luteal phase.

McCord et al. correlated serum progesterone levels with miscarriage rates and found some positive correlation. The miscarriage rates were 85.5%, 65.8%, 31.3%, 9.8%, and 7.7% with serum progesterone levels of <5 pg/mL, 5–10 pg/mL, 10–15 pg/mL, 15–20 pg/mL, and 20–25 pg/mL, respectively [15].

Another study conducted by Hilgers et al. studied 610 patients who were receiving progesterone supplementation during the course of their pregnancy. The study evaluated 830 pregnancies and 8545 serum progesterone levels [10]. They found that progesterone levels in first and second trimester spontaneous abortions were statistically low. The data suggests that it is the second and third trimester which is significantly affected by progesterone deficiency. With paucity of literature supporting easy diagnosis of LPD, Royal College of Obstetricians & Gynaecologists (RCOG) guidelines [16] for infertility do not recommend the use of basal body temperature charts or endometrial sampling to evaluate the luteal phase in routine infertility investigation. They recommend measurement of serum progesterone in the mid-luteal phase of the cycle. According to the American Society for Reproductive Medicine (ASRM), there is no reliable diagnostic test for luteal phase insufficiency [13].

Thus, as per the current knowledge, diagnosis of LPD is neither easily possible nor routinely recommended. *Since it is not easy to prove the presence of LPD and hence its implication in causing recurrent abortions, more investigators have focused on the role of progesterone supplementation in preventing recurrent abortions.*

24.4 Role of Progestogen Supplementation in Preventing Miscarriage: The Evidence

The positive role of progesterone supplementation in early pregnancy in women with RPL has been shown in the study done at the Pope Paul VI Institute [10]. They also recommended the measurement of serum progesterone levels in early pregnancy to assess the future of the index pregnancy. Another systematic review concluded that standardised laboratory protocols are required to select women who would benefit from progesterone therapy and more randomised trials are needed to confirm the usefulness of progesterone therapy [17]. Thach TS (2008) [18] reviewed 15 trials involving 2118 women who were perceived to be at an increased risk of miscarriage due to previous obstetric history including a trial in which 180 women with recurrent miscarriage were randomized to receive oral dydrogesterone, intramuscular human chorionic gonadotropin, or no treatment (controls). They did not find any statistically significant difference in the risk of miscarriage between the three groups [OR 0.98; 95% confidence interval (CI) 0.78–1.24]. The review also included four small studies which suggested that progestogen therapy could be beneficial in management of women with RPL.

Hussain et al. (2012) [19] conducted a 9-year cohort study of women with unexplained recurrent miscarriages in whom 203 pregnancy cycles were studied. Women who had inadequate endogenous progesterone secretion were treated with vaginal pessaries (containing 200 mg of endogenous progesterone) 12-hourly until 12 weeks of gestation. They found a decrease in the miscarriage rate in the treated women.

The latest Cochrane review (2013) [20] included 14 randomized controlled trials (2158 women) and found no evidence of progestogens preventing miscarriage in early to midpregnancy in cases of sporadic pregnancy loss. However, in women with RPL, they suggested that treatment might be given as it reduced the rates of miscarriage in the treatment group with no significant maternal and fetal adverse effects. The outcome did not depend on the route of administration of progestogen (oral, intramuscular, vaginal) versus placebo or no treatment.

Gallot et al. (2014) [21] reviewed the evaluation protocols and management of early recurrent miscarriage and concluded that progesterone supplementation should be included in the first quarter of pregnancy of women with history of unexplained early recurrent miscarriage. Kumar et al. (2014) showed that daily supplementation of 20 mg dydrogesterone in early pregnancy in women with history of recurrent miscarriage reduces the risk by 2.4 times [22]. Howard JA Carp (2015) [23] conducted meta-analysis of 3 RCTs on the role of progesterone in recurrent abortions and showed a statistically significant OR of 3.18 for a live birth with the use of progesterone therapy.

Tsur A et al. (2015) [24] concluded that progestogens have a potent anti-inflammatory and immune-modulatory action and thus may maintain healthy pregnancy through both endocrine and immunologic actions.

The results of the much-awaited large multicenter **PROMISE trial** (progesterone in miscarriage treatment trial) were published in NEJM in November 2015 [25]. The trial which was done across 36 hospitals in the UK and 9 in Netherlands included 826 women with history of unexplained RPL. Women were grouped as one receiving twice-daily vaginal suppositories containing 400 mg of micronized and those who received a placebo. The treatment was carried up to 12 weeks of gestation. The trial concluded that the women who received micronized progesterone treatment in early pregnancy were no less likely to miscarry than those who received a placebo. Live birth after 24 weeks was taken as the primary, and it was comparable in both the groups, 65.8% (262 of 398 women) in the progesterone group and 63.3% (271 of 428 women) in the placebo group (relative rate, 1.04; 95% confidence interval [CI]).

With lack of supportive evidence in favor of preventive progesterone therapy for recurrent pregnancy loss, it remains the last and empirical choice for clinical practice.

24.5 Evidence on Role of hCG in Preventing Miscarriage: The Evidence

In 1992, Blumenfeld Z and Ruach M compared twice-weekly hCG (2500 IU) administration (249) to no treatment (198) in high-risk cases up to 8 weeks of pregnancy and found that it significantly decreased the pregnancy wastage rate in cases with high risk of luteal inadequacy [26]. Morley LC et al. (2013) showed a statistically significant reduction in miscarriage rate using hCG. Their study included 5 studies (of which two were of weak methodology) and involved 596 women. The results did not show a statistically significant benefit (risk ratio 0.74; 95% confidence interval 0.44–1.23) when the two weak studies were removed. Thus, the results of the Cochrane review on the role of hCG supplementation are equivocal [27].

Since the availability of wide variety and higher safety of progesterone preparations, hCG supplementation has lost its role in the prevention of recurrent pregnancy loss. Most of the hCG-related evidence is available from the past when micronized progesterone was not available. *As per the current evidence, there is no role of hCG support to women in early pregnancy except for in research trials.*

24.6 Role of Progestogens/hCG in ART and IVF Cycles: The Evidence

As per ASRM guidelines (2008), IVF cycles which require downregulation with a long-acting GnRH agonist, supplementation with either injectable OHPC preparation (50 mg/day) or vaginal micronized progesterone (200–600 mg/day) increases the pregnancy rates significantly compared to treatment with placebo or no treatment [11].

Cochrane review concluded that progesterone increased the live birth rate in women with history of RPL (OR 2.95, 95% CI 1.02–8.56) [28]. For clinical pregnancy rates also, the results were in favor of progesterone (OR 1.83, 95% CI 1.29–2.61). They also recommended progesterone for treatment of luteal phase defects. In all the studies, synthetic progesterone showed better results than micronized progesterone. hCG supplementation was not beneficial in this group of women, and it led to significantly higher risk of ovarian hyperstimulation syndrome (OHSS) (OR 3.62, 95% CI 1.85–7.06).

Baker VL et al. (2014) [29] compared vaginal progesterone with aqueous subcutaneous progesterone for luteal support in IVF cycles and found comparable results.

Evidence is limited to determine the optimal dose of progesterone in non-IVF-controlled ovarian stimulation cycles with gonadotropins. A very recent RCT by Biberoglu EH et al. (2016) [30] evaluated two doses of vaginal progesterone for IUI cycles in terms of fecundability rates. They found that duration and dose of gonadotropin used, number of follicles, endometrial thickness, and the total, ongoing, and multiple pregnancy rates were comparable in both groups. Hence, they concluded that 300 mg of intravaginal micronized progesterone should be the maximum dose for luteal phase support (LPS) in IUI cycles.

Stefano Palomba et al. [5] reviewed the literature and found improvement of reproductive outcomes with treatment of LPD with progesterone supplementation, in all gonadotropin COS/COH cycles for IVF and non-IVF cycles. Progesterone levels peak around fifth day after oocyte retrieval and then fall rapidly; the increase following that of hCG rise though slightly more slowly. This creates a window during which progesterone lacks hCG stimulation to reach the threshold of 80–100 nmol/L, necessary to maintain the pregnancy. Progesterone support during this period is vital for continuation of pregnancy.

The optimal dose, route of administration, and timing of progesterone supplementation have still not been defined. No statistical difference has been found in results when progesterone has been administered intramuscular, vaginal rectal, or oral. As per the ASRM committee opinion (2015) [13], though it is difficult to confirm LPD, it is commonly associated with thyroid and prolactin disorders, obesity, PCOS, and during COS for IVF cycles. Thus progesterone support seems logical in these clinical conditions. In the absence of any of these, it is an empiric therapy. Treatment of LPD during natural and unstimulated cycles has not shown to improve pregnancy outcomes. *Assisted reproduction is thus one area where progesterone supplementation in early pregnancy is supported by almost all evidence.*

24.7 Role of Progestogens in Later Pregnancy

Recurrent pregnancy loss beyond 20 weeks occurs mainly due to preterm labor. Progesterone levels usually fall before onset of labor, and numerous studies have been done over the years to assess the role of progesterone supplementation in preventing preterm birth. Most of them used 17-hydroxyprogesterone caproate, and the results are conflicting. Hilgers T.W. et al. noticed a decrease in serum progesterone levels at onset of labor and concluded that progesterone has a tocolytic effect. So they supported the administration of progesterone in later pregnancy in their study [10]. Exogenous progesterone can be used to prevent preterm labor, and a meta-analysis by O'Brien et al. [31] showed a significant reduction in risk of preterm labor in women with a short cervix (<25 mm).

There are numerous well-defined causes of preterm labor that must be looked for and treated accordingly. Progesterone supplementation may be added in diagnosed cases of short cervix.

24.8 Safety of Progestogens/hCG in Pregnancy

Vaginal progesterone is considered safe in the first trimester of pregnancy as sufficient evidence is available from pregnancies conceived on ART. The FDA has approved the marketing of vaginal progesterone for luteal support in the first trimester of pregnancy, and there is no difference in adverse effects compared to placebo. A 2-year follow-up evaluation of fetuses who were exposed to progesterone in utero was completed by O'Brien et al., and no differences between vaginal progesterone and placebo were reported [31].

Regarding the use of 17 –oh Progesterone caproate, FDA only recommends for use in prevention of preterm labor and not RM as a trial by Meis et al. reported a nonsignificant increased rate of stillbirth and miscarriages in women who received 17-OHPC [32].

As per the ASRM committee's opinion (2008) [11], increased risk of hypospadias has been seen in women exposed to exogenous progestogens during early pregnancy; but this is limited to treatment with progestins that bind to the androgen receptor. This association does not appear to be significant as there were only a few such cases and they were also in women who had been exposed to high doses of progestins derived from androgens. Luteal phase supplementation with progesterone is better as it does not lead to OHSS as often as treatment with hCG [11]. The Cochrane analysis of 2013 [27] did not find any documented adverse effects of using hCG in early pregnancy.

Thach TS in the Cochrane review (2009) [18] concluded that progestogen therapy was safe and not associated with any adverse effects on the women. The fetal/neonatal adverse events (fetal abnormalities and neonatal deaths) were slightly more among women receiving progestogens, but the numbers were far too small to qualify as a potential risk.

24.9 Progesterone Supplements in Pregnancy

There are three types of progesterone preparations used in pregnancy. All are derived from plant steroids found in *Dioscorea mexicana*, a plant of yam family found in Mexico. To make it therapeutically usable, the plant product is micronized (micronized progesterone), treated with UV light (dydrogesterone), or compounded with 17-OHPC (hydroxyprogesterone caproate or acetate).

Synthetic progestins have androgenic effects that include fluid retention, reduction of HDL cholesterol levels, headaches, and mood disturbance. They are not preferred in pregnancy.

Progesterone supplementation can be given through various routes. Micronized progesterone can be given as oral or vaginal tablets, vaginal gel, and inserts. 17-OHPC preparations are given as intramuscular or subcutaneous injections. Dydrogesterone is available as oral tablet.

Vaginal gel (4% and 8%) is the only once-daily progesterone preparation, which is FDA-approved for ART cases up to 12 weeks of pregnancy. This micronized progesterone in emulsion system is available with brand names like **Crinone or Prochieve**.

Vaginal suppositories are wax-based preparations of micronized progesterone. They are used two to three times a day, but they are not FDA-approved.

Vaginal inserts are FDA-approved for progesterone supplementation but not for progesterone replacement. They are effective in women under 35 years. One hundred milligram preparation is used two to three times a day. The common side effects are bloating, breast tenderness, constipation, cramping, drowsiness, and fluid retention.

Progesterone tablets or capsules can be used both orally and vaginally. They are not formulated or FDA-approved for vaginal use. They are prescribed two to three times a day, most commonly 400 mg daily in divided doses. Oral route has low absorption rates. Vaginal route has advantages of rapid absorption and higher bioavailability in addition to local effects on endometrium. Side effects include nausea, headache, and sleepiness.

Injections: Oil-based solutions (50 mg/day) are the most established method of progesterone delivery. As the injection needs to penetrate the skin and subcutaneous fat, so a long thick needle is required. Injections may be painful, and skin reactions are common. The pharmacokinetic properties of intramuscular route allow a wider implantation window, but these preparations are not available in all countries.

Two large multicenter RCTs concluded that the 25 mg subcutaneous progesterone administered once daily (similar to amount produced daily) is effective and well tolerated [33].

24.10 hCG Supplements Available

Injectable hCG has been traditionally prepared from urine of pregnant women. These preparations are available in various concentrations ranging from as low as 11% to 92%. Nowadays, Recombinant hCG is prepared from Chinese hamster ovary-cultured cell. This CHO cell recombinant hCG is 100% hCG and contains minimal impurities.

24.11 Summary

The use of progesterone for recurrent miscarriages is still not clearly established. Various trials have shown some level of benefit in pregnancy outcome without any compromise on maternal or fetal health. The decision should be based on clinician's discretion until strong evidence is available to recommend routine use.

Key Points

- Progesterone has important functions in pregnancy including stimulation of uterine growth, maturation of the endometrium into secretory type, and decidualization of the endometrium for implantation and tocolysis.
- Early pregnancy (up to 7 weeks) is dependent on progesterone coming from the corpus luteum. From 9 weeks the placental trophoblasts take over the function completely.
- Progesterone supplementation may be needed only in first 10 weeks of pregnancy.
- Documentation of progesterone deficiency and diagnosis of LPD are difficult and not recommended.
- There are conflicting evidences on the role of progesterone supplementation for prevention of recurrent pregnancy loss.
- One Cochrane review (2013) has supported the use of progesterone supplementation, but the recently published large multicenter PROMISE trial (2015) does not show any benefit of micronized progesterone supplementation in early pregnancy for women with history of recurrent pregnancy loss.
- There is a definite evidence-based role of progesterone supplementation up to 12 weeks in women conceiving with ART.
- hCG, though an important pregnancy hormone, is not recommended as supplement in early pregnancy for prevention of recurrent pregnancy loss due to the risk of OHSS, intramuscular route, and lack of supportive evidence.
- The natural progesterones are safe for use in pregnancy.

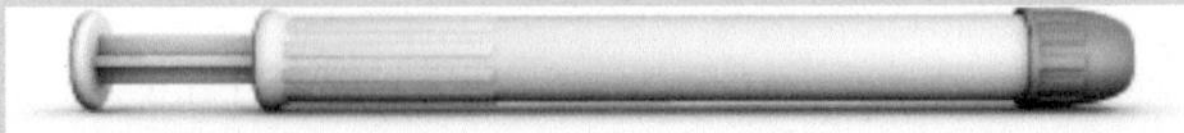

(a) Vaginal gel applicator

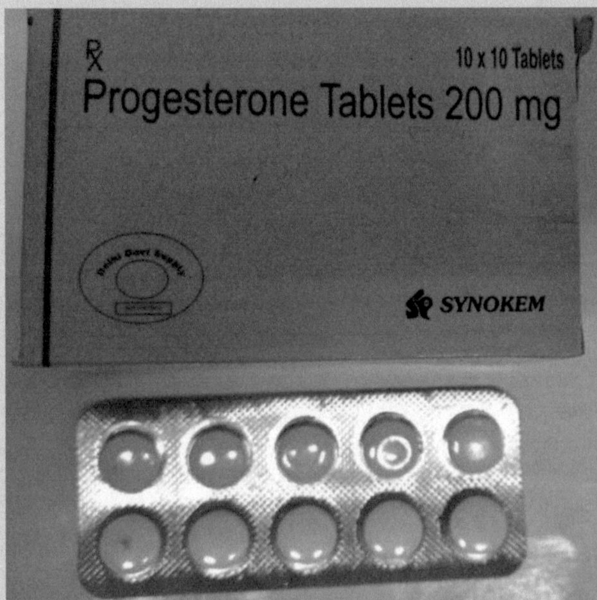

(b) Progesterone vaginal inserts

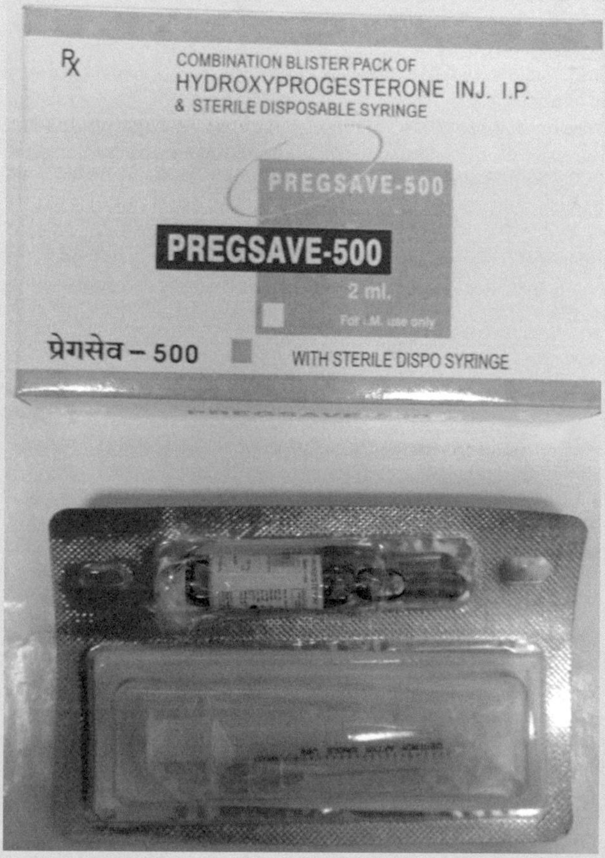

(c) 17-OHPC injectable progesterones

References

1. Beyens MN, Guy C, Ratrema M, Ollagnier M. Prescription of drugs to pregnant women in France: the HIMAGE study. Therapie. 2003;58:505–11.
2. Donati S, Baglio G, Spinelli A, Grandolfo ME. Drug use in pregnancy among Italian women. Eur J Pharmacol. 2000;56:323–8.
3. Villar J, Gulmezoglu AM, Khanna J, Carroli G, Hofmeyr GJ, Schulz K, et al. Evidence-based reproductive health in developing countries. The WHO Reproductive Health Library, No. 2. Geneva: World Health Organization. 1999 (WHO/RHR/HRP/RHL/2/99).

4. Implantation and placental development. In: Cunningham F, Leveno KJ, Bloom SL, Spong CY, Dashe JS, Hoffman BL, Casey BM, Sheffield JS, editors. Williams obstetrics. 24th ed. McGraw Hill Education; 2014. p. 80–115.
5. Palomba S, Santagni S, La Sala GB. Progesterone administration for luteal phase deficiency in human reproduction: an old or new issue? J Ovarian Res. 2015;8:77.
6. Druckmann R, Druckmann MA. Progesterone and the immunology of pregnancy. J Steroid Biochem Mol Biol. 2005;97:389–96.
7. Szekeres-Bartho J, Wilczynski JR, Basta P, Kalinka J. Role of progesterone and progestin therapy in threatened abortion and preterm labour. Front Biosci. 2008;13:1981–90.
8. Simoncini T, Caruso A, Garibaldi S, XD F, Giretti MS, Baldacci C, et al. Activation of nitric oxide synthesis in human endothelial cells using nomegestrol acetate. Obstet Gynecol. 2006;108:969–78.
9. Hill MJ, Whitcomb BW, Lewis TD, Wu M, Terry N, De Cherney AH, et al. Progesterone luteal support after ovulation induction and intrauterine insemination: a systematic review and meta-analysis. Fertil Steril. 2013;100:1373–80.
10. Hilgers TW. The medical & surgical practice of NaProTechnology. Copyright 2016, Pope Paul VI Institute for the Study of Human Reproduction. 2004.
11. The Practice Committee of the American Society for Reproductive Medicine and the Society for Reproductive Endocrinology and Infertility. Progesterone supplementation during the luteal phase and in early pregnancy in the treatment of infertility: an educational bulletin. Fertil Steril. 2008;90:S150–3.
12. Abortion. In: Cunningham F, Leveno KJ, Bloom SL, Spong CY, Dashe JS, Hoffman BL, Casey BM, Sheffield JS, editors. Williams obstetrics, 24th ed. McGraw Hill Education; 2014. p. 350–95.
13. Practice Committee of the American Society for Reproductive Medicine. Current clinical irrelevance of luteal phase deficiency: a committee opinion. Fertil Steril. 2015;103:e27–32.
14. McGovern PG, Myers ER, Silva S, Coutifaris C, Carson SA, Legro RS, et al. Absence of secretory endometrium after false-positive home urine luteinizing hormone testing. Fertil Steril. 2004;82:1273–7.
15. McCord ML, Muram D, Buster JE, et al. Single serum progesterone as a screen for ectopic pregnancy. Exchanging specificity and sensitivity to obtain optimal test performance. Fertil Steril. 1996;66:513–6.
16. National Collaborating Centre for Women's and Children's Health (UK) Fertility. Assessment and treatment for people with fertility problems. London: RCOG Press; 2004.
17. Szekeres-Bartho J, Balasch J. Progestagen therapy for recurrent miscarriage. Hum Reprod Update. 2008;14(1):27–35.
18. Thach TS. Progestogen for preventing miscarriage: RHL commentary (Last Revised: 2 February 2009). The WHO Reproductive Health Library; Geneva: World Health Organization.
19. Hussain M, El-Hakim S, Cahill DJ. Progesterone supplementation in women with otherwise unexplained recurrent miscarriages. J Hum Reprod Sci. 2012;5(3):248–51.
20. Haas DM, Ramsey PS. Progestogen for preventing miscarriage. Cochrane Database Syst Rev. 2013;(10): Art. No.: CD003511.
21. Gallot V, Nedellec S, Capmas P, et al. [Early recurrent miscarriage: evaluation and management. J Gynecol Obstet Biol Reprod (Paris). 2014;43(10):812–41.
22. Kumar A, Begum N, Prasad S, Aggarwal S, Sharma S. Oral dydrogesterone treatment during early pregnancy to prevent recurrent pregnancy loss and its role in modulation of cytokine production: a double blind randomized parallel placebo controlled trial. Fertil Steril. 2014;102(5):1357–1363.e3.
23. Carp HJA. Opinion: progestogens in recurrent miscarriage. In: Carp HJA, editor. Recurrent pregnancy loss causes, controversies and treatment. 2nd ed. London: CRC Press/Taylor and Francis Group; 2015.
24. Tsur A, Hughes GC, Shoenfeld Y, Carp H. Interdisciplinary exchange of ideas: progestogens for autoimmunity, biologics for pregnancy complications. Immunol Res. 2015;61(1–2):31–4.

25. Coomarasamy A, Williams H, Truchanowicz E, Seed PT, Small R, Quenby S, et al. A randomized trial of progesterone in women with recurrent miscarriages. N Engl J Med. 2015;373:2141–8.
26. Blumenfeld Z, Ruach M. Early pregnancy wastage: the role of repetitive human chorionic gonadotropin supplementation during the first 8 weeks of gestation. Fertil Steril. 1992;58(1):19–23.
27. Morley LC, Simpson N, Tang T. Human chorionic gonadotrophin (hCG) for preventing miscarriagc. Cochranc Databasc Syst Rcv. 2013;(1):CD008611.
28. Van der Linden M, Buckingham K, Farquhar C, Kremer JA, Metwally M. Luteal phase support for assisted reproduction cycles. Cochrane Database Syst Rev. 2011;(10):CD009154.
29. Baker VL, Jones CA, Doody K, Foulk R, Yee B, Adamson GD, et al. A randomized, controlled trial comparing the efficacy and safety of aqueous subcutaneous progesterone with vaginal progesterone for luteal phase support of in vitro fertilization. Hum Reprod. 2014;29(10):2212–20.
30. Biberoglu EH, Tanrikulu F, Erdem M, Erdem A, Biberoglu KO. Luteal phase support in intrauterine insemination cycles: a prospective randomized study of 300 mg versus 600 mg intravaginal progesterone tablet. Gynecol Endocrinol. 2016;32(1):55–7.
31. O'Brien JM, Adair CD, Lewis DF, et al. Progesterone vaginal gel for the reduction of recurrent preterm birth: primary results from a randomized double blind placebo- controlled trial. Ultrasound Obstet Gynecol. 2007;30(5):687–96.
32. Meis PJ, Klebanoff M, Thom E, et al. Prevention of recurrent preterm delivery by 17 alpha-hydroxyprogesterone caproate. N Engl J Med. 2003;348:2379–85.
33. Lockwood G, Griesinger G, Cometti B, et al. 13 European Centers. Subcutaneous progesterone versus vaginal progesterone gel for luteal phase support in in vitro fertilization: a noninferiority randomized controlled study. Fertil Steril. 2014;101:112–9.

Cervical Cerclage: Does It Help? 25

Bindiya Gupta and Garima Vats

25.1 Introduction

Cervical insufficiency arises from a woman's inability to support a full-term pregnancy due to a functional or structural defect of the cervix resulting in membrane prolapse, premature rupture of the membranes, midtrimester pregnancy loss, or preterm birth [1].

Cervical cerclage or placement of suture at cervicoisthmic junction to prevent pregnancy loss and preterm labor was first performed in 1902 and is a common and established intervention for many years. However, till date, there are many unanswered questions regarding its efficacy especially in the prevention of pregnancy losses, selection criteria, route of surgery, timing of cerclage, etc. Evidence to support decisions is scarce due to the absence of recent adequately powered randomized controlled trials (RCT) or prospective studies. In this chapter the current evidence regarding the use of cerclage in recurrent pregnancy loss will be reviewed.

25.2 Cerclage for Previous Midtrimester Pregnancy Loss

Both midtrimester loss (MTL) and preterm labor (PTL) are known to have a similar origin and common causative factors. The former is defined as loss between 12 and 24 weeks, while preterm labor is after period of viability, i.e., after 24 weeks [2]. Out of all the known etiologies of midtrimester losses, cervical weakness is seen in 8%, while congenital uterine anomalies are present in 4% [3]. The cause remains unknown in 50–60% of women.

B. Gupta (✉) • G. Vats
Obstetrics and Gynecology, University College of Medical Sciences and GTB Hospital, Delhi, India
e-mail: dr_bindiya_gupta@yahoo.co.in; gvats.dr@gmail.com

S. Mehta, B. Gupta (eds.), *Recurrent Pregnancy Loss*,
https://doi.org/10.1007/978-981-10-7338-0_25

True cervical weakness is a diagnosis of exclusion, and according to the the Cervical Incompetence Prevention Randomized Cerclage Trial (CIPRACT) inclusion criterion, it was defined as "the initial, painless, progressive dilatation of the uterine cervix, where PTD seems inevitable without interference after excluding other causes such as uterine anomaly, fibroids, or infection, and only when singleton pregnancies are involved" [4]. The os will be open, and there is an expulsion of live fetus with intact membranes. True cervical insufficiency is estimated to complicate 0.1–1.0% of all pregnancies [5]. The passage of a size 9 Hegar dilator through the cervix without resistance, in the nonpregnant state, is predictive of cervical incompetence.

The length of the cervix is inversely related to the risk of adverse obstetric outcome. Cervical length of less than 25 mm has been found in most populations to have the best predictive accuracy for MTL/PTD and may be the most reliable threshold to define a high-risk population [6].

25.3 Indications of Cerclage

Current indications and timing for cerclage are summarized as follows [7–9]:

1. History-indicated cerclage: In cases of multiple (>2–3) prior second-trimester losses or preterm births, cerclage can be offered between 12 and 14 weeks of gestation. Women with a history of spontaneous second-trimester loss or preterm delivery who have not undergone a history-indicated cerclage may be offered serial sonographic surveillance in the current pregnancy.
2. Ultrasound-indicated cerclage: In cases of short cervical length (< 25 mm) by transvaginal ultrasound and history of second-trimester loss, cerclage can be done between 16 and 23 weeks. A large randomized study concluded that in the absence of a previous MTL/PTD, ultrasound-indicated cerclage is not beneficial in women who have an incidental finding of a short cervix of <15 mm [10]. Conversely, a meta-analysis of four randomized controlled trials showed that women with a previous MTL/PTD and a cervical length of less than 25 mm may benefit after insertion of cerclage [11]. There is no benefit of cerclage in a woman with an incidental finding of a short cervix by ultrasound examination but no prior risk factors for preterm birth.
3. Physical examination-indicated cerclage: In cases with dilated cervix on manual or speculum examination, emergent cerclage can be done between 16 and 23 weeks. Cerclage may be effective up to 4 cm of cervical dilatation [12].

Figure 25.1 shows the flowchart for cerclage indications in RPL.

The contraindications to cerclage are active preterm labor, clinical evidence of chorioamnionitis, continuing vaginal bleeding, PPROM, lethal fetal defect, or fetal death [9].

Prior to placement of a cerclage, it is essential to confirm the viability of the pregnancy by ultrasound, exclude malformations or risk of aneuploidy, and perform first-trimester

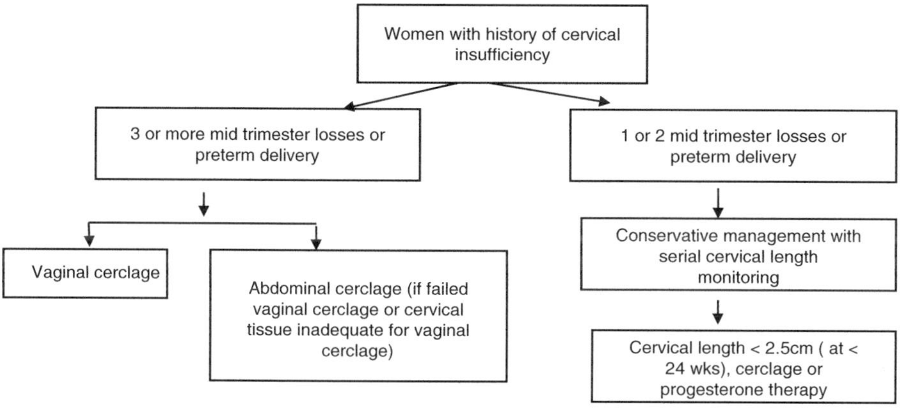

Fig. 25.1 Flowchart showing indication and timing of cerclage in RPL

biochemical screening. Urinalysis for culture and sensitivity and vaginal cultures for bacterial vaginosis should be taken, and any infections found should be treated.

25.4 Methods of Cerclage

25.4.1 Vaginal

1. **McDonald**: A purse-string suture is placed in 4–6 bites circumferentially around the cervix, just distal to the vesicocervical reflection and just distal to the vaginal-rectal reflection posteriorly (Fig. 25.1) [13]. About 1 cm space should be left between consecutive sutures, and each suture should be deep enough into the cervical stroma, but endocervical canal should be avoided to prevent membrane rupture. The suture should be placed as high as feasible, at least 2 cm or more above the external os [14]. The authors take the first bite and secure the knot posteriorly as this is the most likely site of suture displacement and to prevent bladder irritation by an anterior knot. The ends are left long enough (2–3 cm) to allow easy identification and removal.
2. **Shirodkar**: The technique is similar to McDonald, but the purse-string suture is placed following bladder mobilization, to allow insertion above the level of the cardinal ligaments. The dissection and suture placement and removal take a longer time than the McDonald technique. However, the two techniques have never been compared in an RCT. Data from various cohort studies have shown equal efficacy with both techniques. Hence, the US Preventive Services Task Force recommends that McDonald technique is preferred over Shirodkar because of its easier placement and removal and its proven comparative effectiveness (recommendation B; level, moderate). The most commonly used sutures are Mersilene 5 mm tape and large caliber nonabsorbable monofilament (e.g., Prolene, Ethicon, Inc.), but the suture choice depends on operator preference [7].

3. **Double cerclage**: There are two types of double cerclage. One involves the insertion of two cervical cerclages in an attempt to buttress the cervix more strongly. There is no added advantage of double cerclage except that a second stitch can be placed at the time of initial cerclage, only if the initial stitch is too low on the cervix, and gentle pulling on this first stitch may allow placing a second stitch much closer to the internal os, at least 2 cm above the external os (USPSTF recommendation B; level, moderate). In a recent randomized clinical trial of 33 singleton pregnancies suffering from recurrent second-trimester pregnancy loss due to cervical incompetence, the pregnancy success rate did not differ significantly between those who underwent double cerclage method or classic McDonald cerclage (100% vs. 85.7%; $P = 0.172$). However, those undergoing the double cerclage method had longer gestational duration (37.2 ± 2.6 vs. 34.3 ± 3.8 weeks; $P = 0.016$) [15].

   In the second type, a second occlusive suture is placed at the external os to retain the mucous plug and help the cervix maintain itself as a barrier to infection and is termed as cervical occlusion. A recent multicenter randomized trial which recruited 309 women to TVC with or without occlusion was stopped early because of slow recruitment and an interim analysis that showed no benefit associated with occlusion in terms of gestational age at delivery and admission to the neonatal intensive care unit [16].

25.4.2 Transabdominal Cerclage (TAC)

It is indicated in cases of amputated cervix, congenital short or absent cervix, marked cervical scarring, cervical defects, and previous failed vaginal cerclage. The inclusion criterion for an abdominal cerclage in a viable singleton pregnancy is that previous elective vaginal cerclage for the treatment of cervical weakness has failed, causing MTL, and completion of a full investigation protocol for MTL has been done and cervical length measurement >20 mm on transvaginal ultrasound [17]. In a recent retrospective cohort study, Sneider K showed that the recurrence rate of second-trimester loss was 28% due to cervical insufficiency without cerclage; prophylactic abdominal cerclage was associated with a greater reduction in recurrence of midtrimester loss compared to vaginal cerclage [adjusted OR 0.14; versus adjusted odds ratio (OR) 0.47] [18].

Placing the suture at the cervicoisthmic junction can be done via a laparotomy, laparoscopy, or robotic-assisted transabdominal cerclage (RoboTac). The bladder is dissected away from the uterus, and a ligature of tape or mesh is secured around the cervical isthmus and above the cardinal and uterosacral ligaments. The most dreaded complication is hemorrhage from the paracervical veins, and recently a needleless technique by using Mersilene tape after skeletonization of the uterine vessels and formation of window in the broad ligament has been described by both laparoscopic and robotic routes to minimize complications [19–21]. A recent multicenter retrospective cohort study evaluated the effectiveness of laparoscopic abdominal cerclage placement in the prevention of recurrent preterm birth. 71.4% delivered at 34 weeks of gestation, 8.6% experienced a second-trimester fetal loss, and total fetal survival rate was 90.0% [22]. Tulandi et al. reviewed laparoscopic versus abdominal cerclage by laparotomy in 678 pregnancies and demonstrated that there was no difference in the rates of third-trimester delivery and live birth rates between preconceptional abdominal cerclage via laparoscopy (71.4–83.3% and 90–100%, respectively) and laparotomy (97.3–100% and 100%, respectively) [23]. There was no difference in the live birth rates when abdominal cerclage was performed before or during pregnancy. Dawood F et al. compared preconceptional (PC) versus first-trimester (T1) abdominal cerclage and concluded that successful pregnancies >24 weeks occurred in 97% of PC TACs compared to 93% in the T1 group. Ninety percent in the PC group had a successful pregnancy >34 weeks compared to 74% in the T1 group. Hemorrhage >500 mL occurred in 50% of cases, and 5% had serious surgical complications in the T1 group versus none in the PC group [24]. The difficulties in second-trimester laparoscopic TAC or RoboTAC can be due to the larger uterine size, increased risk of trauma to the upper cervix, and cervical vasculature [25]. Hence, operator skill and comfort is important in deciding the method and timing of suture placement. Available evidence demonstrates that TAC should be limited preferably to non-pregnant patients. As with the open transabdominal approach, delivery has to be carried out by caesarean section.

25.5 Role of Cerclage in Uterine Anomalies

In patients with recurrent miscarriage, the reported frequency of uterine anomalies varies widely, from 1.8 to 37.6%, and the most frequent anomalies associated with RPL include bicornuate and septate uterus [26]. In a cohort study, Yassaee F et al., on women with uterine anomalies, concluded that cervical cerclage significantly reduces the rate of preterm delivery in bicornuate uterus, but it has no effect on the outcome of pregnancy in arcuate uterus [22].

The role of cerclage has not been studied in unicornuate uterus, but a study by Reichman et al. concluded that although unicornuate uterus is one of the causes of infertility and abortion, about 50% of the patients have term delivery [27]. Abramovici et al. reported a high percentage of (86.7%) term delivery with cervical cerclage in women with uterine anomaly [28].

25.6 Cerclage and First-Trimester Loss

Cerclage has hardly any role in first-trimester losses as cervical insufficiency or incompetence is rarely the cause of recurrent pregnancy losses in the first trimester. Women with an unclear history of incompetent cervix, including women with >3 first-trimester losses, Kelly S et al. concluded that early cerclage does not offer significant benefit over early transvaginal ultrasonography [29].

25.7 Cerclage Versus Progesterogen Supplementation

Progesterone has anti-inflammatory properties and thus prevents cervical ripening [30, 31]. Studies have been done to compare cerclage and progestogen supplementation in the prevention of preterm labor. There is no literature to support the use of progesterone in the prevention of midtrimester losses, and proposed treatment regimens are extrapolated from studies detailing previous preterm delivery or short cervical length. Progestogen can be prescribed in the form of a vaginal pessary or gel or as an intramuscular injection (17α–hydroxyprogesterone caproate). Vaginal progestogen was associated with a significant reduction in the rate of preterm birth before 28 weeks (5.1% vs. 10.3%) in women with a sonographically short cervix (<25 mm) in the second trimester [32]. A recent meta-analysis concluded that both vaginal progesterone and cerclage are equally efficacious in the prevention of preterm birth in women with a sonographic short cervix in the midtrimester, singleton gestation, and previous preterm birth. Selection of the optimal treatment depends on patient/clinician preferences and cost [33]. Another trial demonstrated no statistical significant difference after treatment with cerclage, vaginal progesterone, or cervical pessary in terms of perinatal losses, neonatal morbidity, and preterm births in women with cervical length <25 mm and previous history of preterm birth [34].

To conclude, cerclage has a role in management of women with history of midtrimester loss and short cervical length (<25 mm) on transvaginal sonography. There is a controversial role in uterine anomalies, and cerclage should not be offered in history of first-trimester losses. Although there is no data supporting the use of progestogens in RPL, results of trials on preterm labor can be extrapolated to justify its use.

Key Points

- History-indicated cerclage should be offered to women with three or more previous preterm births and/or second-trimester losses.
- With history of one or more spontaneous midtrimester losses or preterm births, cerclage can be done if cervical length is 25 mm or less on transvaginal scan.
- History- or ultrasound-indicated cerclage cannot be recommended in other high-risk groups such as women with müllerian anomalies, previous cervical surgery, recurrent first-trimester losses, or multiple dilatation and evacuation.
- Transabdominal cerclage is placed by either laparoscopy or through open laparotomy in congenital short or absent cervix, marked cervical scarring, cervical defects, and previous failed vaginal cerclage.
- Till date, evidence favors preconceptional transabdominal cerclage due to less complication rate as compared to first-trimester cerclage.
- Cerclage, vaginal progesterone, and cervical pessary have equal efficacy in terms of perinatal losses, neonatal morbidity, and preterm births in women with cervical length < 25 mm and previous history of preterm birth.

References

1. Shennan A, Jones B. The cervix and prematurity: aetiology, prediction and prevention. Semin Fetal Neonatal Med. 2004;9(6):471–9.
2. Flint S, Gibb DM. Recurrent second trimester miscarriage. Curr Opin Obstet Gynecol. 1996;8:449–53.
3. McNamee KM, Dawood F, Farquharson RG. Mid-trimester pregnancy loss. Obstet Gynecol Clin N A. 2014;41:87–102.
4. Althuisius SM, Dekker GA, Hummel P, Bekedam DJ, van Geijn HP. Final results of the Cervical Incompetence Prevention Randomized Cerclage Trial (CIPRACT): therapeutic cerclage with bed rest versus bed rest alone. Am J Obstet Gynecol. 2001;185(5):1106–12.
5. Ludmir J. Sonographic detection of cervical in- competence. Clin Obstet Gynecol. 1988;31:101–9.
6. Vidaeff AC, Ramin SM. Management strategies for the prevention of preterm birth: part II–update on cervical cerclage. Curr Opin Obstet Gynecol. 2009;21(6):485–90.
7. Berghella V, Ludmir J, Simonazzi G, Owen J. Transvaginal cervical cerclage: evidence for perioperative management strategies. Am J Obstet Gynecol. 2013;209(3):181–92.
8. Brown R, Gagnon R, Delisle MF, Bujold E, Basso M, Bos H, Cooper S, Crane J, Davies G, Gouin K, Menticoglou S. Cervical insufficiency and cervical cerclage. J Obstet Gynaecol Can. 2013;35(12):1115–27.
9. Royal College of Obstetricians and gynecologists. Cervical cerclage. Green top guideline No. 60. https://www.rcog.org.uk/globalassets/documents/guidelines/gtg_60.pdf. Accessed 3 Nov 2016.
10. Abbott D, To M, Shennan A. Cervical cerclage: a review of current evidence. Aust N Z J Obstet Gynaecol. 2012;52:220–3.
11. Berghella V, Odibo AO, To MS, et al. Cerclage for short cervix on ultrasonography: meta-analysis of trials using individual patient-level data. Obstet Gynecol. 2005;106:181–9.
12. Pereira L, Cotter A, Gomez R, et al. Expectant management compared with physical examination-indicated cerclage (EM-PEC) in selected women with a dilated cervix at 14(0/7)-25(6/7) weeks: results from the EM-PEC international cohort study. Am J Obstet Gynecol. 2007;197:483.e1–8.
13. Berghella V, Baxter J, Berghella M. In: Apuzzio JJ, Vintzileos AM, Iffy L, editors. Operative obstetrics. 3rd ed. London: Taylor and Francis; 2006.
14. Miroshnichenko G, Visintine JF, Suhag A, Gerson A, Berghella V. Is cerclage height associated with the incidence of preterm birth in women with a history-indicated cerclage? Am J Perinatol. 2011;28:83–6.
15. Zolghadri J, Younesi M, Asadi N, Khosravi D, Behdin S, Tavana Z, Ghaffarpasand F. Double versus single cervical cerclage for patients with recurrent pregnancy loss: a randomized clinical trial. J Obstet Gynaecol Res. 2014;40(2):375–80.
16. Brix N, Secher NJ, McCormack CD, et al. Randomised trial of cervical cerclage, with and without occlusion, for the prevention of preterm birth in women suspected of cervical insufficiency. Br J Obstet Gynaecol. 2013;120(5):613–20.
17. McNamee KM, Dawood F, Farquharson RG. Mid trimester pregnancy loss. Obstet Gynecol Clin N Am. 2014;41:87–102.
18. Sneider K, Christiansen OB, Sundtoft IB, Langhoff-Roos J. Recurrence of second trimester miscarriage and extreme preterm delivery at 16-27 weeks of gestation with a focus on cervical insufficiency and prophylactic cerclage. Acta Obstet Gynecol Scand. 2016;95(12):1383–90.
19. Menderes G, Clark LE, Azodi M. Needleless laparoscopic abdominal cerclage placement. J Minim Invasive Gynecol. 2015;22(3):321.
20. Mourad J, Burke YZ. Needleless robotic-assisted abdominal cerclage in pregnant and nonpregnant patients. J Minim Invasive Gynecol. 2016;23(3):298–9.
21. Summers JE, Kuper SG, Foster TL. Transabdominal cerclage. Clin Obstet Gynecol. 2016;59(2):295–301.

22. Burger NB, Einarsson JI, Brölmann HAM, et al. Preconceptional laparoscopic abdominal cerclage: a multicenter cohort study. Am J Obstet Gynecol. 2012;207:273.e1–12.
23. Tulandi T, Alghanaim N, Hakeem G, Tan X. Pre and post-conceptional abdominal cerclage by laparoscopy or laparotomy. J Minim Invasive Gynecol. 2014;21(6):987–93.
24. Dawood F, Farquharson RG. Transabdominal cerclage: preconceptual versus first trimester insertion. Eur J Obstet Gynecol Reprod Biol. 2016;199:27–31.
25. Menderes G, Clark M, Clark-Donat L, Azodi M. Robotic-assisted abdominal cerclage placement during pregnancy and its challenges. J Minim Invasive Gynecol. 2015;22(5):713–4.
26. Yassaee F, Mostafaee L. The role of cervical cerclage in pregnancy outcome in women with uterine anomaly. J Reprod Infertil. 2011;12(4):277–9.
27. Reichman D, Laufer MR, Robinson BK. Pregnancy outcomes in unicornuate uteri: a review. Fertil Steril. 2009;91(5):1886–94.
28. Abramovici H, Faktor JH, Pascal B. Congenital uterine malformations as indication for cervical suture (cerclage) in habitual abortion and premature delivery. Int J Fertil. 1983;28(3):161–4.
29. Kelly S, Pollock M, Maas B, Lefebvre C, Manley J, Sciscione A. Early transvaginal ultrasonography versus early cerclage in women with an unclear history of incompetent cervix. Am J Obstet Gynecol. 2001;184(6):1097–9.
30. Elovitz MA, Gonzalez J. Medroxyprogesterone acetate modulates the immune response in the uterus, cervix and placenta in a mouse model of preterm birth. J Matern Fetal Neonatal Med. 2008;21:223–30.
31. Xu H, Gonzalez JM, Ofori E, et al. Preventing cervical ripening: the primary mechanism by which progestational agents prevent preterm birth? Am J Obstet Gynecol. 2008;198:314.e1–8.
32. Hassan SS, Romero R, Vidyadhari D, Fusey S, Baxter JK, Khandelwal M, et al. Vaginal progesterone reduces the rate of preterm birth in women with a sonographic short cervix: a multicenter, randomized, double-blind, placebo-controlled trial. Ultrasound Obstet Gynecol. 2011;38:18–31.
33. Conde-Agudelo A, Romero R, Nicolaides K, Chaiworapongsa T, O'Brien JM, Cetingoz E, et al. Vaginal progesterone vs. cervical cerclage for the prevention of preterm birth in women with a sonographic short cervix, previous preterm birth, and singleton gestation: a systematic review and indirect comparison meta-analysis. Am J Obstet Gynecol. 2013;208(1):42.e1–42.e18.
34. Alfirevic Z, Owen J, Carreras Moratonas E, Sharp AN, Szychowski JM, Goya M. Vaginal progesterone, cerclage or cervical pessary for preventing preterm birth in asymptomatic singleton pregnant women with a history of preterm birth and a sonographic short cervix. Ultrasound Obstet Gynecol. 2013;41(2):146–51.

Immunotherapy for Recurrent Miscarriages

26

Mala Srivastava and Ankita Srivastava

26.1 Introduction

Recurrent miscarriage (RM) can be subdivided into primary RM in which there is no history of previous birth and secondary RM in which abortion occurs after a live or still birth [1, 2].

Immunological disturbances have been suggested to play an important role in RM [3–8] more so in secondary than primary RM [9–12]. The causative factors may be rejection reaction against male antigens or specific HLA antigen alleles [13].

26.2 Immunotherapy

The developing fetus contains tissue-specific differentiation antigens which are inherited paternally, and there is maternal reaction to these antigens. A weak immune response to these antigens or unusually strong responses can cause miscarriage. So, both immune-stimulating and immunosuppressive therapies have been proposed.

26.2.1 Intravenous Immunoglobulins

Intravenous immunoglobulin (IVIg) is made from plasma of normal blood donors. It acts mainly by modifying natural killer cells, cytokines, and autoantibodies and so can be used in the management of disorders caused by immunological

M. Srivastava (✉)
Gynae Robotic Surgeon, Institute of Obstetrics and Gynaecology, Sir Ganga Ram Hospital, New Delhi, India
e-mail: malasrivastava2001@yahoo.co.in

A. Srivastava
Lok Nayak Jai Prakash Hospital, New Delhi, India

S. Mehta, B. Gupta (eds.), *Recurrent Pregnancy Loss*,
https://doi.org/10.1007/978-981-10-7338-0_26

abnormalities. It has been tested in RM patients in many placebo-controlled trials [14–24].

Mechanism of action of intravenous Ig:

- It increases autoantibody clearance.
- It decreases autoantibody production.
- It causes inactivation of complement.
- T-cell suppressor function is increased.
- T-cell adhesion to the extracellular matrix is decreased.
- It causes downregulation of TH1 cytokine synthesis.

Intervention protocols of IVIg:

Dosage: 24 g (200 mL) if woman weighs <75 kg before pregnancy.
36 g (300 mL) if woman weighs ≥75 kg.

The dose is given over 3–4 h on an outpatient basis.

Vitals charting is done during the infusion, and other side effects (headache, skin rash, nausea, or chills) are noted and treated. More serious adverse effects include anaphylaxis (particularly in patients with IgA deficiency).

Subsequent dosage: three infusions at 3–5 days interval and three more infusions at 12–15 days interval. If hCG level measured at second infusion has decreased significantly, further doses are not given.

Meta-analyses of studies done on treatment of women with RM have been contradictory, but it has been recommended that IVIg should not be used in RM as it does not provide any benefit over placebo in all RM patients [21, 25–28]. All the women included in these studies had uterine abnormalities excluded by hysterosalpingography, hysteroscopy, or hydrosonography. Each couple had karyotyping done by conventional G-banding technique. Serum homocysteine levels, creatinine, and total IgA were measured, and infection with HIV and hepatitis was ruled out. IgG anticardiolipin antibodies and lupus anticoagulant were also measured in all women. A detailed history regarding pregnancy outcomes was also recorded.

According to the Cochrane review of immunotherapy for recurrent pregnancy loss, use of IVIg therapy did not change pregnancy outcome in such patients. It does improve pregnancy rates in the set of patients with autoimmune-mediated pregnancy loss [29]. The disadvantages of IVIg therapy include its high cost, it being an invasive procedure and decreased patient compliance due to multiple intravenous infusions which are required over the course of pregnancy.

26.2.2 Progesterone

Progesterone has long been known to be absolutely indispensable for the establishment of the receptive endometrium but is now being recognized as possibly also contributing immunologically to the sustenance of pregnancy by interacting with the maternal immune system. Almost 40 years ago, Stites referred to progesterone as "nature's immunosuppressant" based on studies that demonstrated immunosuppressive properties of progesterone [30]. Progesterone acts as an immunomodulator by:

- Suppressing the activation and proliferation of lymphocytes
- Decreasing the oxidative burst of monocytes
- Prolonging the survival of allografts when administered locally [31, 32]

An interesting observation pertinent to the immunology of pregnancy comes from a study by Kruse et al. who found that recurrent miscarriage patients with higher serum progesterone levels had lower Th1/Th2 cytokine ratios suggesting that progesterone levels modulate cytokine production patterns [33]. Progesterone has also been shown by Piccinni and colleagues to preferentially support the development of human T cells producing Th2 cytokines in vitro [34]. They suggested that Th2 cytokines may promote allograft tolerance and fetal survival.

Hill and colleagues reported that progesterone inhibits the production of Th1 cytokines by trophoblast antigen-activated peripheral blood cells from women with unexplained RSM [35].

Dydrogesterone (Duphaston®), which is an orally administered progestogen, has been evaluated in various studies. As it is similar to endogenous progesterone structurally, so it mimics the pharmacological effects also, but it is significantly more potent than natural progesterone, with a high affinity for the progesterone receptor [36].

Schindler et al. found that peripheral blood mononuclear cells (PBMC) from women with a history of unexplained RSM stimulated with a mitogen in the presence of dydrogesterone or progesterone produce significantly lower levels of the Th1 (pro-inflammatory) cytokines IFN-γ and TNF-α. On the other hand, levels of IL-4 and IL-6, both Th2 cytokines, are significantly elevated in the presence of dydrogesterone or progesterone [37]. In addition to the direct effects of progestogens on cytokine profiles, these hormones appear to mediate their cytokine-modulating effects via a protein called progesterone-induced blocking factor (PIBF) discovered by Szekeres-Bartho and coworkers about three decades ago [38]. Animal studies support important roles for PIBF in the maintenance of pregnancy; fetal wastage induced by the transfer of NK cells is corrected by the administration of PIBF [39].

A recent Cochrane review concluded that progesterone supplementation was effective in the treatment of recurrent, but not isolated, spontaneous pregnancy loss [29]. The review makes no recommendation on doses, timings of initiation, nor route of progesterone administration. Progesterone can be given both intramuscularly and intravaginally, but vaginal administration has the advantage of higher intrauterine concentration.

26.2.3 Leukocyte Immunization/Lymphocyte Immunization Therapy (LIT)

Recurrent miscarriage (REMIS) study which is one of the largest prospective, randomized trial evaluating the efficacy of leukocyte immunization in patients with unexplained recurrent pregnancy loss included over 90 patients per treatment arm. It concluded that LIT has no role in the management of unexplained recurrent pregnancy loss [40].

In LIT procedure, white blood cells from the prospective father are injected into the skin of the mother to sensitize the maternal immune system for pregnancy and help in the development of immunologic tolerance in her.

26.2.3.1 Mechanism of Action

T regulatory cells which were discovered by immunologist Shimon Sakaguchi have the ability to turn off an immune response started by conventional immune cells and thereby help to avoid autoimmunity [41].

Following ovulation, T regulatory cells increase and multiply further after contact with embryonic tissues and are then retained in placental tissues. A failure to increase the number of these regulatory cells can lead to miscarriage. LIT helps by increasing the number and distribution of T regulatory cells and augmenting tolerance.

26.2.3.2 Intervention Protocol

In LIT, the lymphocytes from the prospective father are collected and separated from the other blood constituents and injected into the mother. CD200 which is a marker found on fresh lymphocytes collected from the father helps in making the introduction of the collected lymphocytes to the immune system of the mother a friendly one [42]. The CD200 marker is lost when cells are refrigerated for storage. The cells are injected into the skin, a site which is guarded by dendritic cells, and not in the muscle or the vein. When properly conducted, LIT offers significant assistance to patients suffering recurrent pregnancy loss and unexplained infertility.

Risks associated with LIT:

- Graft-versus-host disease.
- Fetal growth restriction.
- Autoimmune complications.
- Fetal thrombocytopenia: alloimmunization to platelets which are present in the paternal leukocyte preparation leads to fetal thrombocytopenia.

Due to the risks involved, the routine use of this therapy for recurrent abortion cannot be clinically justified at this time. The procedure should be performed only as part of an appropriately controlled trial using informed consent.

26.2.4 Intralipid Infusion

The wide range of demonstrated effects of lipid preparations include reduced natural killer cell activity, reduced monocytes pro-inflammatory cytokine production, and increased susceptibility to infection led investigators to hypothesize as early as 1994 that lipid infusion might promote an immune environment that would favor pregnancy maintenance. Despite this paucity of data, intralipid infusion is being administrated to recurrent pregnancy loss patients with increasing frequency. The existing data do not support this practice. At this time intralipid infusion in recurrent pregnancy loss patients should only be administered under an institutional review board – approved protocol in a study setting.

26.2.5 TNF-α Inhibition

The development of antagonist of TNF-a in the form of blocking antibodies (adalimumab, infliximab) and inhibitory recombinant proteins has allowed for successful treatment of several autoimmune disorders, including rheumatoid arthritis, psoriasis, and Crohn's disease. Their use, however, has not been associated with universally positive outcomes and may worsen some disorders, including multiple sclerosis. These products are associated with rare but worrisome side effects, like liver failure, aplastic anemia, interstitial lung disease, and anaphylaxis. The safety of these compounds in pregnancy has not been appropriately studied, and preliminary reports associating exposure to TNF-a inhibitors during early pregnancy leading to fetal anomalies are concerning. As with intralipid therapy, use of TNF-a inhibition for the treatment of recurrent pregnancy loss should only be administered under a research setting.

26.2.6 Other Therapies

Plasmapheresis has been tried in couples with RPL but has not been shown to have beneficial effects. Other immunoregulating therapies theoretically useful in treating recurrent pregnancy loss include the use of cyclosporine, pentoxifylline, and nifedipine, although maternal and fetal risks with these agents preclude their clinical use.

26.3 Evidence Regarding Immunotherapy

Systematic reviews have consistently found no beneficial effect of immunotherapy for treatment of RPL [26, 29, 42, 43]. The general findings are illustrated by the examples discussed below.

A systematic review of 20 trials of high quality showed that immunotherapy did not result in a statistically significant improvement in live births compared to untreated controls [29]. Four types of immunotherapy were evaluated: paternal cell immunization (odd ratio [OR] 1.23, 95% CI 0.89–1.70; 12 studies including 641 participants), third-party donor cell immunization (OR 1.39, 95% CI 0.68–2.82; 3 studies including 156 participants), trophoblast membrane infusion (OR 0.40, 95% CI 0.11–1.45; 1 study including 37 participants), and intravenous immune globulin (OR 0.98, 95% CI 0.61–1.58; 8 studies including 303 participants).

Another systematic review evaluated three randomized and two cohort trials of immunotherapy treatment specifically in patients who failed IVF; a total of 373 patients were involved in these trials [31]. Patients treated with IVIG showed a consistently higher live birth rate than untreated controls; this benefit was statistically significant when the trial results were pooled in meta-analysis. However, there were many differences among these trials, such as the preparations used, the timing of the intervention (preconception, postconception, both), and dosage, as well as the immunological abnormalities of the patients. In addition, some controls received heparin and aspirin, while others did not receive any therapy. Thus, appropriate use of this therapy remains unclear.

Treatment of unexplained RPL with low-dose aspirin plus prednisone has been tried, but the pregnancy outcomes for treated and control patients were similar. Also, the incidence of maternal diabetes and hypertension increased among those treated with prednisolone and aspirin.

Conclusion

Immunotherapy as a treatment modality in unexplained recurrent pregnancy loss is still under investigation, and no consistent beneficial effect of this therapy has been found. Immunotherapy has not been found to alter pregnancy outcome in this group of women and is therefore not recommended routinely.

Key Points

- Immunological disturbances have been suggested to play an important role in RM, more so in secondary RM than primary RM.
- Meta-analysis has concluded that intravenous immunoglobulins do not provide any benefit over placebo in all RM patients.
- Progesterone also exhibits immune-modulatory effects by inhibiting Th1 cells and causes a shift from Th1- to Th2-type responses.
- LIT, though a promising immunotherapy, is still not routinely recommended as it poses a significant risk to both the woman and her fetus.
- Intralipid infusion and TNF-α inhibitors are to be used only in research settings.

References

1. Jauniaux E, Farquharson RG, Christiansen OB, Exalto N. Evidence based guidelines for the investigation and medical treatment of recurrent miscarriage. Hum Reprod. 2006;21:2216–22.
2. Shapira E, Ratzon R, Shoham-Vardi I, Serjienko R, Mazor M, Bashiri A. Primary versus secondary recurrent pregnancy loss—epidemiological characteristics, etiology, and next pregnancy outcome. J Perinat Med. 2012;40:389–96.

3. Hill JA, Polgar K, Anderson DJ. T-helper 1-type immunity to trophoblast in women with recurrent spontaneous abortion. JAMA. 1995;273:1933–6.
4. Quack KC, Vassiliadou N, Pudney J, Anderson DJ, Hill JA. Leukocyte activation in the decidua of chromosomally normal and abnormal fetuses from women with recurrent abortion. Hum Reprod. 2001;16:949–55.
5. Kruse C, Rosgaard A, Steffensen R, Varming K, Jensenius JC, Christiansen OB. Low serum level of mannan-binding lectin is a determinant for pregnancy outcome in women with recurrent spontaneous abortion. Am J Obstet Gynecol. 2002;187:1313–20.
6. Hiby SE, Regan L, Lo W, Farrell L, Carrington M, Moffett A. Association of maternal killer-cell immunoglobulin-like receptors and parental HLA-C genotypes with recurrent miscarriage. Hum Reprod. 2008;23:972–6.
7. King K, Smith S, Chapman M, Sacks G. Detailed analysis of peripheral blood natural killer (NK) cells in women with recurrent miscarriage. Hum Reprod. 2010;25:52–8.
8. Thangaratinam S, Tan A, Knox E, Kilby MD, Franklyn J, Coomarasamy A. Association between thyroid autoantibodies and miscarriage and preterm birth: meta-analysis of evidence. BMJ. 2011;342:d2616.
9. Piosik ZM, Goegebeur Y, Klitkou L, Steffensen R, Christiansen OB. Plasma TNF-a levels are higher in early pregnancy in patients with secondary compared with primary recurrent miscarriage. Am J Reprod Immunol. 2013;70:347–58.
10. Kruse C, Steffensen R, Varming K, Christiansen OB. A study of HLADR and –DQ alleles in 588 patients and 562 controls confirms that HLA-DRB1*03 is associated with recurrent miscarriage. Hum Reprod. 2004;19:1215–21.
11. Nielsen HS, Steffensen R, Varming K, van Halteren AG, Spierings E, Ryder LP, et al. Association of HY-restricting HLA class II alleles with pregnancy outcome in patients with recurrent miscarriage subsequent to a firstborn boy. Hum Mol Genet. 2009;18:1684–91.
12. Christiansen OB, Kolte AM, Dahl M, Larsen EC, Steffensen R, Nielsen HS, et al. Maternal homozygocity for a 14 base pair insertion in exon 8 of the HLA-G gene and carriage of HLA class II alleles restricting HY immunity predispose to unexplained secondary recurrent miscarriage and low birth weight in children born to these patients. Hum Immunol. 2012;73: 699–705.
13. Nielsen HS, Wu F, Aghai Z, Steffensen R, van Halteren AG, Spierings E, et al. H-Y antibody titers are increased in unexplained secondary recurrent miscarriage patients and associated with low male:female ratio in subsequent live births. Hum Reprod. 2010;25:2745–52.
14. The German RSA/IVIG Group. Intravenous immunoglobulin in the prevention of recurrent miscarriage. BJOG. 1994;101:1072–7.
15. Coulam C, Krysa L, Stern J, Bustillo M. Intravenous immunoglobulin for treatment of recurrent pregnancy loss. Am J Reprod Immunol. 1995;34:333–7.
16. Christiansen OB, Mathiesen O, Husth M, Rasmussen KL, Ingerslev HJ, Lauritsen JG, et al. Placebo-controlled trial of treatment of unexplained secondary recurrent spontaneous abortions and recurrent late spontaneous abortions with i.v. immunoglobulin. Hum Reprod. 1995;10:2690–5.
17. Perino A, Vassiliadis A, Vucetich A, Colacurci N, Cignitti M, Semprini AE. Short-term therapy for recurrent abortion using intravenous immunoglobulins: results of a double-blind placebo-controlled Italian study. Hum Reprod. 1997;12:2388–92.
18. Stephenson MD, Dreher K, Houlihan E, Wu V. Prevention of unexplained recurrent spontaneous abortion using intravenous immunoglobulin: a prospective, randomized, double-blinded, placebo-controlled trial. Am J Reprod Immunol. 1998;39:82–8.
19. Jablonowska B, Selbing A, Palfi M, Ernerudh J, Kjellberg S, Lindton B. Prevention of recurrent spontaneous abortion by intravenous immunoglobulin: a double-blind placebo-controlled study. Hum Reprod. 1999;14:838–41.
20. Christiansen OB, Pedersen B, Rosgaard A, Husth M. A randomized double-blind, placebo-controlled trial of intravenous immunoglobulin in the prevention of recurrent miscarriage: evidence for a therapeutic effect in women with secondary recurrent miscarriage. Hum Reprod. 2002;17:809–16.

21. Stephenson MD, Kutteh WH, Purkiss S, Librach C, Schultz P, Houlihan E, et al. Intravenous immunoglobulin and idiopathic secondary recurrent miscarriage: a multicentred randomized placebo-controlled trial. Hum Reprod. 2010;25:2203–9.
22. Schwab I, Nimmerjahn F. Intravenous immunoglobulin therapy: how does IgG modulate the immune system? Nat Rev Immunol. 2013;13:176–89.
23. Trinath J, Hegde P, Sharma M, Maddur MS, Rabin M, Vallat JM, et al. Intravenous immunoglobulin expands regulating T cells via induction of cyclooxygenase-2-dependent prostaglandin E2 in human dendritic cells. Blood. 2013;122:1419–27.
24. Negi V-S, Elluru S, Siberil S, Graff-Dubois S, Mouthon L, Kazatchkine MD, et al. Intravenous immunoglobulin: an update on the clinical use and mechanisms of action. J Clin Immunol. 2007;27:233–45.
25. Porter TF, LaCoursiere Y, Scott JR. Immunotherapy for recurrent miscarriage. Cochrane Database Syst Rev. 2006;2:Art. No. CD000112.
26. Hutton B, Sharma R, Fergusson D, Tinmouth A, Hebert P, Jamieson J, et al. Use of intravenous immunoglobulin for treatment of recurrent miscarriage: a systematic review. BJOG. 2007;114:134–42.
27. Ata B, Tan SL, Shehata F, Holzer H, Buckett W. A systematic review of intravenous immunoglobulin for treatment of unexplained recurrent miscarriage. Fertil Steril. 2011;95:1080–5.
28. Clark DA. Intravenous immunoglobulin and idiopathic recurrent miscarriage: methodological problems (letter to the Editor). Hum Reprod. 2011;26:2586–7.
29. Wong LF, Porter TF, Scott JR. Immunotherapy for recurrent miscarriage. Cochrane Database Syst Rev. 2014;(10):CD000112.
30. Siiteri PK, Febres F, Clemens LE, Chang RJ, Gondos B, Stites D. Progesterone and maintenance of pregnancy: is progesterone nature's immunosuppressant? Ann NY Acad Sci. 1977;286:384–97.
31. Hansen PJ, Bazer FW, Segerson EC. Skin graft survival in the uterine lumen of ewes treated with progesterone. Am J Reprod Immunol Microbiol. 1986;12:48–54.
32. Stites DP, Bugbee S, Siiteri PK. Differential actions of progesterone and cortisol on lymphocyte and monocyte interaction during lymphocyte activation—relevance to immunosuppression in pregnancy. J Reprod Immunol. 1993;5:215–28.
33. Kruse C, Varming K, Christiansen OB. Prospective, serial investigations of in-vitro lymphocyte cytokine production, CD62L expression and proliferative response to microbial antigens in women with recurrent miscarriage. Hum Reprod. 2003;18:2465–72.
34. Piccinni MP. T cells in normal pregnancy and recurrent pregnancy loss. Reprod Biomed Online. 2006;13:840–4.
35. Choi BC, Polgar K, Xiao L, Hill JA. Progesterone inhibits in vitro embryotoxic Th1 cytokine production to trophoblast in women with recurrent pregnancy loss. Hum Reprod. 2000;15(Suppl 1):46–59.
36. Schindler A. Dydrogesterone: A unique progestogen. Maturitas. 2009;65(Suppl 1):S1.
37. Raghupathy R, Al Mutawa E, Szekeres-Bartho J. Modulation of cytokine production by dydrogesterone in lymphocytes from women with recurrent abortion. BJOG. 2005;112:1096–101.
38. Szekeres-Bartho J, Kilar F, Falkay G, Csernus V, Torok A, Pacsa AS. Progesterone-treated lymphocytes of healthy pregnant women release a factor inhibiting cytotoxicity and prostaglandin synthesis. Am J Reprod Immunol Microbiol. 1985;9:15–8.
39. Szekeres-Bartho J, Polgar B. PIBF: the double edged sword. Pregnancy and tumor. Am J Reprod Immunol. 2010;64:77–86.s.
40. Karrison TG, Ober C. Recurrent miscarriage (REMIS) study: how should data from women who do not pregnant be handled? Control Clin Trials. 1998;19(5):430–9.
41. Sakaguchi S. Regulatory T cells: key controllers of immunologic self-tolerance. Cell. 2000;101(5):455–8.

42. Clark DA, Coulam CB, Stricker RB. Is intravenous immunoglobulins (IVIG) efficacious in early pregnancy failure? A critical review and meta-analysis for patients who fail in vitro fertilization and embryo transfer (IVF). J Assist Reprod Genet. 2006;23:1.
43. Egerup P, Lindschou J, Gluud C, et al. The effects of intravenous immunoglobulins in women with recurrent miscarriages: a systematic review of randomised trials with meta-analyses and trial sequential analyses including individual patient data. PLoS One. 2015;10:e0141588.

Preimplantation Genetic Diagnosis to Improve Pregnancy Outcome

27

Sumita Mehta and Nidhi Arora

27.1 Introduction

Prenatal testing by amniocentesis (16–18 weeks) and chorionic villus sampling (11–13 weeks) was used to be the method to detect genetic anomalies in the developing fetus before the advent of preimplantation genetic diagnosis in the 1980s. The recent advances in molecular biology and cytogenetic technology have paved way for genetic diagnosis at the oocyte and the embryo level. Preimplantation genetic diagnosis is a technique to determine genetic aberrations including single gene disorders, aneuploidy, and chromosomal abnormalities in an oocyte/embryo. Here, the embryos are first developed in vitro and are then screened for possible genetic alterations, and only genetically normal embryos are implanted in the uterus [1]. PGD was first introduced in England (late 1980s) in families with high risk for offspring affected by an X-linked disease, and only the unaffected female embryos were selected and transplanted [2]. After that, the role and application of PGD in other genetic conditions have increased manifold. It gives couples a chance of having a genetically normal offspring and avoids the emotional trauma caused by termination of pregnancy. PGD is currently also used for sex selection, HLA compatibility, to diagnose hereditary cancer syndromes like BRCA1 and BRCA2. Its another recent use is in the treatment of infertility. The embryos during IVF/ICSI cycle can be screened for chromosomal imbalance before implantation. This embryo testing with cytogenetic techniques for de novo aneuploidies is called as preimplantation genetic screening (PGS).

S. Mehta (✉)
Obstetrics and Gynecology, Babu Jagjiwan Ram Memorial Hospital, Delhi, India
e-mail: sumitadr@gmail.com

N. Arora
Apollo Center of Fetal Medicine, Indraprastha Apollo Hospital, New Delhi, India
e-mail: drnidhiarora84@gmail.com

S. Mehta, B. Gupta (eds.), *Recurrent Pregnancy Loss*,
https://doi.org/10.1007/978-981-10-7338-0_27

The process of PGD consists of obtaining embryos by IVF with intracytoplasmic sperm injection (ICSI), biopsy them on day 3 at six- to eight-cell stage or doing trophectoderm biopsy at day 5 or 6, and performing genetic analysis by fluorescent in situ hybridization (FISH) [3] for cytogenetic diagnosis or polymerase chain reaction (PCR) [1, 4, 5]. Comparative genomic hybridization (CGH) [6, 7] and microarray [8] are also used for molecular diagnosis to improve accuracy.

There are high rates of unbalanced gametes in individuals with translocations. They have implied or reduced gametogenesis [9, 10], produce high rates of unbalanced embryos [11], and are therefore at risk of pregnancy loss and infertility [12]. While conceiving naturally, these individuals experience spontaneous loss or miscarriage in most pregnancies [11]. The risk of recurrent miscarriages due to translocation with the use of PGD has been reported to decrease from almost 90 to 15% [11, 13, 14].

In this chapter, we will review the current evidence available on use of PGD and also its role in improving the outcomes of pregnancies affected by genetic disorders as well as in patients of recurrent pregnancy losses (RPL).

27.2 IVF and PGD

Assisted reproductive technology (ART) should be used whenever preimplantation genetic diagnosis is planned even in the absence of infertility. Embryos are retrieved by IVF with ICSI to minimize any paternal contamination by the sperm attached to the zona pellucida by directly obtaining the cell.

27.3 Obtaining Cells for PGD

Access to gamete DNA is required before transplantation that occurs at day 6 of conception. Three different methods (Table 27.1) can be used—(1) polar body biopsy (assesses oocyte), (2) blastomere aspiration at day 3 (six- to eight-cell stage embryo), and (3) trophectoderm biopsy/blastocyst stage biopsy (day 5–6) – and a new one known as morula stage biopsy.

27.3.1 Polar Body Biopsy

Polar body biopsy is obtained from the female gametes (egg) by making a slit in the zona pellucida with mechanical method (by using needles) or by using laser. The polar body is then retrieved from the egg using a biopsy pipette. This approach has been studied by Verlinsky et al. [15]. They have used both the first polar body and second polar body to improve the accuracy of the test. They were able to correctly identify genetic derangements in 98% (157 of 160) of oocytes tested [16] by using polar body analysis.

Table 27.1 Advantages and disadvantages of types of embryo biopsy

Stage of biopsy	Polar body (oocyte)	Cleavage stage/ day 3	Blastocyst stage/day 5 or 6
Advantages	Single cell is obtained Enough time for genetic analysis Best for maternal origin of genetic abnormality	Less number of cells required Time available for testing Used for all indications of PGD	Few cells to be tested 10–30 trophectoderm cells available Less mosaicism No harm to the inner cell mass Self-selection of embryos Used for all indications No problem of allele dropout and amplification failures
Disadvantages	Single cell biopsy High number of cells to be tested Consecutive stepwise biopsy Not for paternal genetic abnormalities	1–2 cells obtained Maximum degree of mosaicism Increased allele dropout Damage to the inner cells	Time limitation for genetic testing Very few embryos mature to this stage

27.3.2 Cleavage Stage Biopsy/Blastomere Biopsy

It is done at day 3 when the embryo is at the six- to eight-cell stage of development. Blastomeres are obtained with the help of biopsy pipette by opening the zona pellucida by either Tyrode's drilling, mechanical dissection, or laser dissection. The other methods that can be used for blastomere aspiration are extrusion (driving out the cells by making a hole in embryo) or fine needle aspiration. The main disadvantages of this methodology as described in Table 27.1 are that only up to two cells can be obtained and the possible worse outcome of embryo development as reported in different studies. Although this is the most frequently used biopsy method and allows for analysis of single genes as well as chromosomes, the cells obtained by this method exhibit chromosomal mosaicism (presence of cells with different karyotypes in the same embryo). This is seen at maximum levels on day 3 of embryo development. As there are different cell lines in this stage of embryos, aneuploidy testing becomes markedly affected.

27.3.3 Trophectoderm Biopsy (Embryo at Blastocyst Stage)

This is done at day 5 or 6 postfertilization. It is considered an important breakthrough in IVF and PGD. Up to 10–30 trophectoderm cells can be obtained with no damage to the inner cell mass. The blastocyst stage begins on day 5 post egg retrieval. It possesses an inner cell mass and an outer trophectoderm. The zona pellucida is penetrated, and cells are obtained using a fine needle biopsy pipette. The genetic analysis is done by fluorescent in situ hybridization (FISH), comparative genomic hybridization (CGH), or polymerase chain reaction (PCR) that will be discussed later in the chapter. The technical limitations that are faced by blastomere biopsy with single cell PCR analysis like high amplification failure and allele drop-out do not occur with the trophectoderm biopsy as more cells (10–30) can be used for testing. Another advantage of this method is that at this stage, there is less degree of mosaicism; however, only 50% of the embryos reach this stage, and in few patients, the blastocyst does not form. With recent evidence, the cleavage stage biopsy causes more damage to the embryo than blastocyst biopsy, thereby leading to poorer outcomes.

With the additional time required for culture beyond the eight-cell stage, there is some natural selection against the aneuploid embryos and the embryos that are unable to survive. Almost up to one third of embryos with chromosomal aberrations are selected against between three and five. The main disadvantage of this technique is that approximately 36% of embryos mature to this stage and this also gives less time for prenatal testing, as embryos need to be transferred by fifth or sixth day [17].

27.3.4 Morula Stage Biopsy

Morula is a stage of postfertilization zygote development consisting of about 12–15 cells. In human, morula is usually formed in the first week (day 4) after fertilization. One of the cells is obtained from the morula after opening the zone pellucida layer mechanically or by laser, and the DNA is sent for prenatal genetic evaluation. Human embryo is then implanted on day 5 or day 6 after evaluation. It has been reported safe with pregnancy rate comparable to IVF without pre-genetic screenings (32.8 vs. 34%). The other advantage is that it gives enough time for genetic screening comparable to blastocyst screening in which the cell is obtained on day 5.

27.4 Genetic Analysis of Cells

27.4.1 Fluorescent In Situ Hybridization (FISH)

FISH is a genetic technique that is used for aneuploidy screening, identification of chromosomal abnormalities, and for sex determination in X-linked disorders [3]. Target-specific DNA probes labeled using different fluorochromes/haptens are used to identify the copy number of specific loci and to detect imbalance seen with meiotic segregation of chromosomal rearrangements which comprises deletions, duplications, aneuploidy, and translocations. The type and number of probes which are used depend upon the indication. As an example; only two probes are required for X-linked defects (one for X and one for Y chromosome). For aneuploidy screening, either 5-color FISH or 9- or 12-color FISH probes are used. In five-color FISH, chromosomes 13, 18, 19, 21, and X and Y aneuploidy are tested. The nine-color FISH additionally tests for aneuploidy of chromosomes 15, 16, 17, and 22. Currently,

FISH is used for aneuploidy screening and translocations in both PGD and PGS. It gives immediate results with the help of fluorescent microscopy. The detection rate varies between 60 and 80% depending upon the number of probes used. The main disadvantages with this technique are that it can only identify up to ten chromosomes due to the limited availability of probes. It also cannot identify short sequence mutations, genomic imprinting with uniparental disomies, and some inversions. The error rate is close to 10% [18].

27.4.2 Polymerase Chain Reaction (PCR)

The major problem encountered with earlier cytogenetic techniques was the amount of DNA available for screening. Therefore, amplification techniques like PCR were introduced to overcome this problem. It was first used for X-linked disorders for sex identification of the embryo and selected transfer. It has become a lot complex with recent advancements. The various types include nested PCR, multiplex PCR, and fluorescent PCR. The current recommendation is to perform multiplex PCR coupled with blastocyst biopsy for detection of monogenic defects.

Major challenges to a single cell PCR include:

1. Amplification failure
2. Allele dropout (ADO)
3. Contamination—maternal/paternal

Maternal contamination can be checked by polymorphic markers, whereas paternal contamination is avoided by single sperm fertilization as in ICSI. When the amplification failure is affecting just one parental alleles present in a single cell, it is called an allele dropout. It can be seen if any allele does not amplify and results in misdiagnosis. Methods like direct mutation testing and linkage analysis have been adopted to overcome this. Multiplex PCR decreases the ADOs by amplification of the DNA fragment carrying the mutation along with amplification of linked polymorphisms, and thereby misdiagnosis is prevented. The benefits of trophectoderm stage along with frozen embryo transfer are improved genotyping with higher implantation and reduced amplification failures and allele dropouts.

27.4.3 Comparative Genomic Hybridization (CGH)

CGH enables analyzing all 24 chromosomes. It can be done as metaphase CGH or array CGH. Because metaphase CGH is time-consuming, results are usually not available before the embryo must be transferred. Therefore, embryos are usually cryopreserved following the biopsy. Those that test normal can be used in future cycles. However, cryopreservation is not ideal, as not all embryos will survive the freezing and thawing procedures, and developmental potential of surviving embryos may be reduced.

Use of microarray chips for CGH (i.e., array CGH) has several advantages over metaphase CGH. Array CGH has the ability of testing only embryos that matured to the blastocyst stage, and so they have high chances of being normal chromosomally. Multiple cells are available for analysis, and there is rapid turnaround time (usually within a few hours) so that cryopreservation is not needed for embryo transfer. It can perform a full chromosome analysis and identify copy number variants up to 5–10 kbp levels of DNA. Array is also to pick structural variations with 200 bp resolution and identify microdeletions and duplications. However; the array CGH is not able to detect polyploidies, inversions, balanced translocations, inversions, point mutations, and mosaicism up to 20%. Also, it adds more to the cost of the couple than previous technologies.

27.4.4 Single Nucleotide Polymorphism Arrays/SNP Array

Single nucleotide polymorphisms are identified after marking the DNA by fluorescent molecules. The intensity signals are then picked up and assessed by computer software. It is capable of performing high-resolution analysis with as minimum as 5 kbp spacing. It has the main advantage of giving results for balanced translocations and inversions. Whole genome sequence analysis is done. However, again, it cannot be performed on fresh embryo due to the increased time required for the testing which is around 72 hours and is also expensive to perform.

27.5 Indications for PGD

Primary candidates for PGD include:

1. History of X-linked disorders in maternal or paternal family
2. Couples affected by chromosome translocations that lead to recurrent miscarriages and have problems with implantation
3. History of physical or mental problems in offspring/siblings (which is due to chromosomal derangements in either parent)
4. Autosomal recessive disorders (both parents carrying the affected gene) with 25% probability of having diseased offspring
5. Either parent carrying the autosomal dominant gene (that has 50% probability of having diseased offspring)

PGD can be recommended in three types of genetic disorders:

1. Sex-linked defects
2. Monogenic disorders (Table 27.2)
3. Chromosomal defects [19] (Table 27.3)

Table 27.2 Single gene disorders for which PGD is currently available

Monogenic disorders
• Autosomal dominant polycystic kidney disease
• Autosomal recessive polycystic kidney disease
• Becker muscular dystrophy
• Beta thalassemia
• Congenital adrenal hyperplasia (gene CYP21A2)
• Cystic fibrosis
• Charcot-Marie-tooth type 1A
• Duchenne muscular dystrophy
• Familial amyloid polyneuropathy
• Fragile X syndrome
• Hemophilia A (F8)
• Hemophilia B (F9)
• Huntington's disease
• Tuberous sclerosis
• Marfan syndrome
• Neurofibromatosis type 1
• Multiple endocrine neoplasia, type 2A
• Myotonic dystrophy (Steinert)
• RhD incompatibility
• Spinal muscular atrophy
• X-linked adrenoleukodystrophy

27.5.1 Sex-Linked Disorders

X-linked disorders are transmitted to offspring by a carrier mother. If the father is affected and the mother is normal (not a carrier), there is a 100% chance that all daughters will become carriers of that particular diseased gene. However, the sons would not be affected at all. The females can be affected only when both parents are carriers of the gene. The carrier mother has a 50% chance of having an affected son and a 50% chance of having carrier daughter. PGD has been done for disorders like Duchenne muscular dystrophy (DMD) and hemophilia A and B (Table 27.3).

27.5.2 Monogenic Disorders (Table 27.1)

These are the defects within a single gene of a chromosome. The couples with disorders like beta thalassemia, congenital adrenal hyperplasia, sickle cell anemia, etc. can be offered PGD. The genetic defect is detected by using molecular techniques like PCR amplification of DNA from single cell. Genetic mutations like BRCA1 which does not cause a specific disease but is associated with many other diseases can also be picked up by PGD.

Table 27.3 Few examples of conditions for which preimplantation genetic diagnosis (PGD) is available

1.	Chromosomal defects (monosomy or trisomy of chromosomes)
2.	Inheritable cancers
	– BRCA1 mutations
	– Familial adenomatous polyposis coli
	– Von Hippel-Lindau disease
	– Retinoblastoma
	– Neurofibromatosis (NF-1 and NF-2)
	– Familial posterior fossa brain tumor
	– P 53 mutations
3.	Autosomal dominant conditions
	– Myotonic dystrophy
	– Huntington's disease
	– Neurofibromatosis
4.	Autosomal recessive conditions
	– Cystic fibrosis
	– B thalassemia
	– Sickle cell disease
	– Tay-Sachs disease
	– Spinal muscular dystrophy
	– Gaucher's disease
	– OTC deficiency
	– Phenylketonuria
5.	X-linked autosomal dominant conditions
	– Rett disease
	– Incontinentia pigmenti
	– Pseudohypoparathyrodism
	– Vitamin D-resistant rickets
6.	X-linked autosomal recessive conditions
	– Fragile X syndrome
	– Neuromuscular dystrophies
	– Hemophilia A disease

27.5.3 Chromosomal Disorders

These comprise chromosomal rearrangements like translocations (both balanced and Robertsonian), inversions, and deletions. These can be tested using FISH, PCR, and array.

27.6 Genetic Abnormalities and Recurrent Pregnancy Loss

Genetic abnormalities in the growing fetus mainly the fetal aneuploidy have been shown to be the leading cause of pregnancy loss in the first 10 weeks of gestation. Around 50–60% of pregnancy losses are reported due to cytogenetic aberrations, the most common being trisomy, polyploidy, and monosomy X [20, 21]. The most important cause of aneuploidy is because of errors during the first meiosis of oocyte. Spermatic abnormalities have also been reported in patients with recurrent pregnancy loss; however, paternal meiotic errors contributed to just 7% of fetal trisomies [22].

Till date little is known about the underlying mechanisms leading to increased fetal aneuploidies with advanced maternal age. One hypothesis is that with advancing maternal age, there is a paucity of oocyte at optimum stage of maturation. In general having one trisomic fetus increases the risk of heterotrisomy which means occurrence of different type of trisomy in subsequent pregnancies leading to repeated miscarriages [23, 24].

27.7 Types of Genetic Abnormalities in RPL

27.7.1 Balanced Translocations

Chromosomal rearrangement, mainly a balanced translocation, has been reported in about 4% of couple experiencing recurrent miscarriage [25, 26]. Balanced translocation (60% reciprocal and 40% Robertsonian) is seen with higher frequency in females than males (2:1). The parent carrying the translocation is phenotypically normal; however, due to meiotic segregation, there is an increased chance of chromosomal deletions and duplications in developing embryo that results in a miscarriage or an abnormally affected offspring [26]. Frequency of Robertsonian translocation is 0.1% in general population, 1.1% in couples with recurrent fetal loss, and 2–3% in infertile men [27, 28]. t(13;14) (q10;q10) is the most common Robertsonian translocation affecting chromosomes 13 and 14 and contributes to almost 75% of all Robertsonian translocations [29].

In a retrospective study looking at the rate of chromosomal abnormalities in recurrent pregnancy losses in an Indian population, the rate of chromosomal rearrangements was found in 3.5% of total population [30]. Translocations were seen in about 1.5% of total population out of which reciprocal translocations accounted for about 0.9%, and Robertsonian translocations were seen in about 0.6%. The same study reported about 1.6% cases with heteromorphic variants like inversions, etc. in their chromosomes. Female to male ratio was 2:1 for being a reciprocal translocation carrier when compared with 1.6:1 in Robertsonian translocation carriers. These findings are comparable to results with other studies [25–27]. The reproductive risk due to these chromosomal translocations depends on the type of rearrangement and whether it is carried by the female or the male partner. It has been seen that the risk increases if translocation is in the mother [26]. Translocation in the homologous chromosome always leads to abnormal offspring.

27.7.2 Inversions

An inversion is a rearrangement involving two breaks of the chromosomes followed by rotation of the segment 180° with the reinsertion. It is of two types: paracentric and pericentric. Chromosomal inversions have also been considered as causes of RPL. A pericentric inversion is one that involves the centromere. However, if it involves the long arm (q) or short arm (p), without interfering with the centromere, it is called paracentric. Usually inversions do not change the overall amount of genetic material, but some parts can be lost. These are mostly viable and show no adverse phenotype. But, when there is a cross-over at the time of meiosis, unbalanced gametes are produced. The chance that the resulting offspring is affected depends upon the site of inversion and amount of genetic material involved. It is also determined by the sex of the heterozygous carrier. Even small inversions can finally lead to large deletions or duplications and can be lethal resulting in miscarriages. On the contrary, survival is more often seen when large portions are involved. If the carrier of a pericentric inversion is female, the risk of having abnormal offspring increases (male/female, 5%:7%). On the other hand, the paracentric inversions are considered lethal [31]. Inversions have been found on all 22 autosomes and both sex chromosomes. They were most commonly observed on chromosome arms 6p, 7q, and 11q and least commonly observed on chromosome arms 2p, 2q, 3q, 4q, and 6q.

27.7.3 Recurrent Aneuploidy

Half of all sporadic miscarriages are due to fetal aneuploidy [32]. Few studies suggest that if there is aneuploidy detected after first pregnancy loss, the chance of recurrence of aneuploidy is 50–70% in subsequent pregnancy [33, 34]. Several PGD-based studies have reported aneuploidy as a cause of fetal loss in greater than 50% of embryos tested from patients with recurrent miscarriage [35, 36]. This view has been questioned in recent studies where the authors adjusted the karyotypic results of fetus for maternal age, and the relationship between aneuploidy and RPL was comparable to the control population [21, 37]. The rate of aneuploidy, mostly the trisomies, increases with increasing maternal age leading to recurrent fetal losses. However, Sullivan et al. in a retrospective study reported lower incidence of aneuploidy in abortuses of patients with RPL compared to the control population arguing less contribution of recurrent aneuploidy in RPL [37]. Nevertheless, it is essential to check karyotype of abortus to rule out aneuploidy as the cause.

27.8 Role of Preimplantation Genetic Diagnosis in RPL

PGD is being used worldwide in various centers to improve the live birth rates. According to the European Society of Human Reproduction and Embryology (ESHRE) PGD consortium, more than 6000 cycles of PGD have been performed worldwide [38–40].

In one of the earlier studies, Otani et al. reported significantly reduced losses and increased viable pregnancy rates using PGD in couples with repeated pregnancy losses attributed to translocation abnormalities [39]. They concluded that IVF-PGD offers a quicker alternative to conceive a live and unaffected progeny when compared to a spontaneous pregnancy, especially in couples with RPL attributed to chromosomal translocations with no previous living issues. Other authors have reported divergent views on the role of PGD in RPL [41, 42]. In another study by Fischer et al. significantly reduced pregnancy loss in translocation carriers with history of recurrent miscarriages was reported [43]. They reported less time to get pregnant in such population. The average time to conceive in their study was about 3–4 months compared to the average time ranging from 2 to 9 years reported by other studies.

In a more recent study, Ikuma et al. reported no significant difference in live birth rate when PGD was compared to spontaneous conception without PGD [44]. The cumulative live births in the former group were 67% while that of 65.4% in the latter group. However, PGD did reduce the miscarriage rate significantly. The mean time duration in months from counselling to achieve a live birth was also similar (12.4 vs. 11.4).

However, a systemic review (from MEDLINE, EMBASE, Cochrane database) by Franssen et al. reported a divergent view arguing insufficient data to support PGD in increasing the number of live births in couples with chromosomal aberrations [45].

Most prior studies have used FISH to detect chromosomal anomalies compared to CGH. FISH can analyse only 9 or 10 chromosomes out of the total 23 pairs, while CGH allows every chromosome in the cell to be studied for an anomaly. Fiorentino et al. [46] in their study reported a live birth rate of 50% and miscarriage rate of 0% in couples with RPL due to translocation. However, more studies are required to support this improvement in live birth and miscarriage rates with CGD-based PGD. The recent shift to blastocyst biopsy from the cleavage stage biopsy can be an important contributing factor in improving live birth rates in PGD/PGS in randomized controlled trials [47, 48]. In contrast, the live birth rate in patients with advancing maternal age has been reported with PGD while using of the cleavage stage biopsy as well as FISH [49].

Most randomized controlled trials have reported improved live births with FISH or comprehensive chromosome screening-based PGS/PGD [47–50]. However, in these studies only young women with low FISH were included. The number of oocytes removed was also high. The number of IVF failures and number of previous miscarriages were restricted to only one. In a way, it can be concluded that PGD/PGS is an acceptable approach to choose best embryos in couples with predictable good outcome. It can improve the timing of live birth by a couple of months only when compared to similar patients who opt for spontaneous conception. It might not prove good for couples with predictable poor outcome to begin with.

27.9 Outcomes

PGD is being frequently used currently in many centers worldwide. Since this is a growing technique, the experience is different depending upon the years of practice in a particular center. The European Society of Human Reproduction and Embryology (ESHRE) PGD consortium was established in 1997 to collect

PGD-related data. A total of 13 data collections have been done so far, last published for 2010 [51]. In the 13th data collection, 62 centers reported data for 5780 cycles with oocyte retrieval (OR), with follow-up details on 1503 pregnancies and 1152 babies born. A total of 1071 OR were reported for chromosomal abnormalities, 108 OR for sexing for X-linked diseases, 1574 for monogenic diseases, 2979 for PGS, and 48 for social sexing [51].

27.10 Limitations of PGD

27.10.1 Misdiagnosis by PGD

The ESHRE PGD consortium summarizes the number of cases of misdiagnosis in each annual data collection. There was no case of misdiagnosis reported in the data X and data XI. However, three cases of misdiagnosis have been reported in both data XII and data XIII. All of the cases reported in data XII were after FISH-based PGD, whereas in data XIII, one case was after PCR-based PGD (fragile X syndrome diagnosed by prenatal testing), and two cases were after FISH-based PGS (both trisomy 21). One of them was diagnosed prenatally and terminated, whereas the other was diagnosed after birth [51, 52]. The causes of misdiagnosis can be human errors like confusion in the embryo or cell number, wrong embryo transfer, or a wrong diagnostic procedure. Other problems like maternal and paternal contamination, allele dropout, and chromosome mosaicism can also result in misdiagnosis. Good quality control and external quality assessment methods can help in decreasing the errors. The couples opting for PGD or PGS should be encouraged to undergo invasive prenatal diagnostic procedures to confirm the results of PGD due to the inherent technical limitations of preimplantation screening procedures.

27.10.2 Multiple Pregnancy and Prematurity

Many authors have reported multiple pregnancies (twins and triplets) and preterm delivery as early as 26 weeks of gestation with IVF-PGD [41, 42, 46]. As for IVF, the protocol of single embryo transfer must be opted for in cases of PGD to avoid higher-order pregnancy which thereby leads to premature births.

27.10.3 Other Complications

Bay et al. (2016) [53] studied the obstetric and neonatal outcomes in PGD pregnancies from 1999 to 2013. Compared with spontaneously conceived pregnancies, these pregnancies were reported with increased risk of placenta previa, cesarean section, prematurity, and prolonged stay in nursery for such infants. These adverse outcomes were similar to IVF/ICSI pregnancies. However, when sub-analyses were done, these complications were seen in children born by PGD indicated for single gene disorders and were comparable to the children of parents with similar disorders who conceived naturally. However, the incidence of placenta previa was significantly higher in PGD pregnancies. Similarly, Strom et al. [54] reported reassuring outcomes in 102 pregnancies conceived after PGD with polar body retrieval. The authors concluded no significant increased risk of obstetric and neonatal complications other than placenta previa and cesarean section.

Conclusion

To conclude couples with recurrent pregnancy loss or those who are carriers of chromosomal aberrations must be counselled by a genetic counsellor/geneticist. They should be explained about the advantages and disadvantages of all existing alternatives for preimplantation and prenatal diagnosis. They should be explained that PGD can be opted to decrease the chances of transmitting the existing genetic abnormality to the future offspring. It can improve the live birth rates and also decrease the miscarriage rates in couples with recurrent pregnancy loss due to cytogenetic and molecular abnormalities.

Key Points

- PGD can decrease the chance of conceiving a child with genetic defect carried by either (dominant) or both (recessive) partners if that defect can be identified by tests on single cell or multiple trophectoderm cells.
- Blastocyst biopsy is better than cleavage stage biopsy and has no harmful effect on the embryo and must be considered as the preferred method when available.
- PGD of monogenic disorders has good results if trophectoderm biopsy is done followed by testing with multiplex PCR.
- PGD and IVF work hand in hand, so couples should be informed about the cost of the procedure.
- Before performing the PGS/PGD, couples should meet the genetic counselor and understand the merits and restrictions of the procedures.

References

1. Sermon K. Current concepts in preimplantation genetic diagnosis (PGD): a molecular biologist's view. Hum Reprod Update. 2002;8:1–10.
2. Handyside A, Kontogianni E, Hardy K, Winston R. Pregnancies from biopsied human preimplantation embryos sexed by Y-specific DNA amplification. Nature. 1990;344:768–70.
3. Wilton L. Preimplantation genetic diagnosis for aneuploidy screening in early human embryos: a review. Prenat Diagn. 2002;22:312–8.
4. Syvänen A-C. From gels to chips: "Minisequencing" primer extension for analysis of point mutations and single nucleotide polymorphisms. Hum Mutat. 1999;13:1–10.
5. Pierce K, Rice J, Aquiles Sanchez J, Brenner C, Wangh L. Real-time PCR using molecular beacons for accurate detection of the Y-chromosome in single human blastomeres. Mol Hum Reprod. 2000;6:1155–64.
6. Voullaire L, Slater H, Williamson R, Wilton L. Chromosome analysis of blastomeres from human embryos by using CGH. Hum Genet. 2000;105:210–7.

7. Wells D, Delhanty J. Comprehensive chromosomal analysis of human preimplantation embryos using whole genome amplification and single cell comparative genomic hybridisation. Mol Hum Reprod. 2000;6:1055–62.
8. Kurg A, Tonisson N, Georgiou I, Shumaker J, Tollett J, Metspalu A. Arrayed primer extension: solid-phase four-color DNA resequencing and mutation detection technology. Genet Test. 2000;4:1–7.
9. Estop AM, Van Kirk V, Cieply K. Segregation analysis of four translocations, t(2;18), t(3;15), t(5;7) and t(10;12), by sperm chromosome studies and review of the literature. Cytogenet Cell Genet. 1996;70:80–7.
10. Oliver-Bonet M, Benet J, Sun F, Navarro J, Abad C, Liehr T, et al. Meiotic studies in two human reciprocal translocations and their association with spermatogenic failure. Hum Reprod. 2005;20:683–8.
11. Munne S, Sandalinas M, Escudero T, Fung J, Gianaroli L, Cohen J. Outcome of preimplantation genetic diagnosis of translocations. Fertil Steril. 2000;73:1209–18.
12. Chandley AC. Genetic contribution to male infertility. Hum Reprod Suppl. 1998;3:76–83.
13. Gianaroli L, Magli C, Fiorentino F, Baldi M, Ferraretti AP. Clinical value of preimplantation genetic diagnosis. Placenta. 2003;24:S77–83.
14. Otani T, Roche M, Mizuikea M, Colls P, Escudero T, Munne S. Preimplantation genetic diagnosis significantly improves the pregnancy outcome of translocation carriers with a history of recurrent miscarriage and failing to produce a live birth. Reprod Biomed Online. 2006;13:879–94.
15. Verlinsky Y, Rechitsky S, Evsikov S, et al. Preconception and preimplantation diagnosis for cystic fibrosis. Prenat Diagn. 1992;12:103–10.
16. Rechitsky S, Strom C, Verlinsky O, et al. Accuracy of preimplantation diagnosis of single-gene disorders by polar body analysis of oocytes. J Assist Reprod Genet. 1999;16:192–8.
17. Veiga A, Sandalinas M, Benkhalifa M, et al. Laser blastocyst biopsy for preimplantation diagnosis in the human. Zygote. 1997;5:351–4.
18. Pehlivan T, Rubio C, Rodrigo L, et al. Impact of preimplantation genetic diagnosis on IVF outcome in implantation failure patients. Reprod Biomed Online. 2002;6:232–7.
19. Sermon K, Steirteghem AV, Liebaers I. Preimplantation genetic diagnosis. Lancet. 2004;363:1633–41.
20. Stirrat GM. Recurrent miscarriage. Lancet. 1990;336:673–5.
21. Stephenson MD, Awartani KA, Robinson WP. Cytogenetic analysis of miscarriages from couples with recurrent miscarriage: a case control study. Hum Reprod. 2002;17(2):446–51.
22. Kalousek DK, Pantzar T, Tsai M, Paradice B. Early spontaneous abortion: morphologic and karyotypic findings in 3912 cases. Birth Defects Orig Artic Ser. 1993;29:53–61.
23. Fritz B, Hallermann C, Olert J, et al. Cytogenetic analyses of culture failures by comparative genomic hybridisation (CGH)– re-evaluation of chromosome aberration rates in early spontaneous abortions. Eur J Hum Genet. 2001;9:539–47.
24. Warburton D, Dallaire L, Thangavelu M, Ross L, Levin B, Kline J. Trisomy recurrence: a reconsideration based on North American data. Am J Hum Genet. 2004;75:376–85.
25. De Braekeleer M, Dao TN. Cytogenetic studies in couples experiencing repeated pregnancy losses. Hum Reprod. 1990;5:519–28.
26. Daniel A, Hook EB, Wulf G. Risks of unbalanced progeny at amniocentesis to carriers of chromosome rearrangements: data from United States and Canadian laboratories. Am J Med Genet. 1989;33(1):14–53.
27. Therman E, Susman B, Denniston C. The nonrandom participation of human acrocentric chromosomes in Robertsonian translocations. Ann Hum Genet. 1989;53:49–65.
28. Fryns JP, Van Buggenhout G. Structural chromosome rearrangements in couples with recurrent fetal wastage. Eur J Obstet Gynecol. 1998;30:171–6.
29. Nussbaum R, McInnes R, Willard H. Principles of clinical cytogenetics. In: Thompson & Thompson genetics in medicine. Philadelphia: WB Saunders; 2007. p. 75–6.

30. Sheth FJ, Liehr T, Kumari P, Akinde R, Sheth HJ, Sheth JJ. Chromosomal abnormalities in couples with repeated fetal loss: an Indian retrospective study. Indian J Hum Genet. 2013;19(4):415–22.
31. Porter FT, Scott RJ. Evidence-based care of recurrent miscarriage. Best Pract Res Clin Obstet Gynaecol. 2005;19(1):85–101.
32. Sanchez JM, Franzi L, Collia F, et al. Cytogenetic study of spontaneous abortions by transabdominal villus sampling and direct analysis of villi. Prenat Diagn. 1999;19(7):601–3.
33. Stern JJ, Dorfmann AD, Gutierrez-Najar AJ, et al. Frequency of abnormal karyotypes among abortuses from women with and without a history of recurrent spontaneous abortion. Fertil Steril. 1996;65(2):250–3.
34. Daniely M, Aviram-Goldring A, Barkai G, Goldman B. Detection of chromosomal aberration in fetuses arising from recurrent spontaneous abortion by comparative genomic hybridization. Hum Reprod. 1998;13:805–9.
35. Simon C, Rubio C, Vidal F, et al. Increased chromosome abnormalities in human preimplantation embryos after in-vitro fertilization in patients with recurrent miscarriage. Reprod Fertil Dev. 1998;10:87–92.
36. Vidal F, Gimenez C, Rubrio C, et al. FISH preimplantation diagnosis of chromosome aneuploidy in recurrent pregnancy wastage. J Assist Reprod Genet. 1998;15:310–3.
37. Sullivan AE, Silver RM, LaCoursiere DY, et al. Recurrent fetal aneuploidy and recurrent miscarriage. Obstet Gynecol. 2004;104(4):784–8.
38. Munne S, Scott R, Sable D, Cohen J. First pregnancies after preconception diagnosis of translocations of maternal origin. Fertil Steril. 1998;69:675–81. PMID: 9548157.
39. Otani T, Roche M, Mizuike M, Colls P, Escudero L, Munne S. Preimplantation genetic diagnosis significantly improves the pregnancy outcome of translocation carriers with a history of recurrent miscarriage and unsuccessful pregnancies. Reprod Biomed Online. 2006;13:869–74. PMID: 17169213.
40. Harper JC, Wilton L, Traeger-Synodinos J, Goossens V, Moutou C, SenGupta SB, et al. The ESHRE PGD Consortium. 10 years of data collection. Hum Reprod Update. 2012;3: 234–47.
41. Lim C, Jun J, Min D, Lee H, Kim J, Koong M, et al. Efficacy and clinical outcome of preimplantation genetic diagnosis using FISH for couples of reciprocal and Robertsonian translocations: the Korean experience. Prenat Diagn. 2004;24:556–61. PMID: 15300749.
42. Feyereisen E, Steffann J, Romana S, Lelorc'h M, Ray P, Kerbrat V, et al. Five years' experience of preimplantation genetic diagnosis in the Parisian Center: outcome of the 441 started cycles. Fertil Steril. 2007;87:60–73. PMID: 17074325.
43. Fischer J, Colls P, Escuredo T, Munne S. Preimplantation genetic diagnosis (PGD) improves pregnancy outcome for translocation carriers with a history of recurrent losses. Fertil Steril. 2010;94:283–9. https://doi.org/10.1016/j.fertnstert.2009.02.060. PMID: 20034626.
44. Ikuma S, Sato T, Sugiura-Ogasawara M, Nagayoshi M, et al. Preimplantation genetic diagnosis and natural conception: a comparison of live birth rates in patients with recurrent pregnancy loss associated with translocation. PLoS One. 2015;10(6):e0129958.
45. Franssen MT, Musters AM, Van der Veen F, et al. Reproductive outcome after PGD in couples with recurrent miscarriage carrying a structural chromosome abnormality: a systematic review. Hum Reprod Update. 2011;17(4):467–75.
46. Fiorentino F, Spizzichino L, Bono S, Biricik A, Kokkali G, Rienzi L, et al. PGD for reciprocal and Robertsonian translocations using array comparative genomic hybridization. Hum Reprod. 2011;26:1925–35. https://doi.org/10.1093/humrep/der082. PMID: 21489979.
47. Scott RT Jr, Upham KM, Forman EJ, Hong KH, Scott KL, Taylor D, et al. Blastocyst biopsy with comprehensive chromosome screening and fresh embryo transfer significantly increases in vitro fertilization implantation and delivery rates: a randomized controlled trial. Fertil Steril. 2013;100:697–703. https://doi.org/10.1016/j.fertnstert.2013.04.035. PMID: 23731996.

48. Mastenbroek S, Twisk M, van der Veen F, Repping S. Preimplantation genetic screening: a systematic review and meta-analysis of RCTs. Hum Reprod Update. 2011;17:454–66. https://doi.org/10.1093/humupd/dmr003. PMID: 21531751.
49. Rubio C, Bellver J, Rodrigo L, Bosch E, Mercader A, Vidal C, et al. Preimplantation genetic screening using fluorescence in situ hybridization in patients with repetitive implantation failure and advanced maternal age: two randomized trials. Fertil Steril. 2013;99:1400–7. https://doi.org/10.1016/j.fertnstert.2012.11.041. PMID: 23260857.
50. Forman EJ, Hong KH, Franasiak JM, Scott RT Jr. Obstetrical and neonatal outcomes from the BEST Trial: single embryo transfer with aneuploidy screening improves outcomes after in vitro fertilization without compromising delivery rates. Am J Obstet Gynecol. 2014;210:157.e1–6. https://doi.org/10.1016/j.ajog.2013.10.016. PMID: 24145186.
51. Rycke De M, Belvia F, Goossens V, et al. ESHRE PGD Consortium data collection XIII: cycles from January to December 2010 with pregnancy follow-up to October 2011. Hum Reprod. 2015;30(8):1763–89.
52. Moutou C, Goossens V, Coonen E, et al. ESHRE PGD Consortium data collection XII: cycles from January to December 2009 with pregnancy follow-up to October 2010. Hum Reprod. 2014;29(5):880–903.
53. Bay B, Ingerslev JH, Lemmen GJ, Degn B, Rasmussen AI, Kesmodel SU. Preimplantation genetic diagnosis: a national multicenter obstetric and neonatal follow-up study. Fertil Steril. 2016;106(6):1363–1369.e1.
54. Strom CM, Strom S, Levine E, Ginsberg N, Barton J, Verlinsky Y. Obstetric outcomes in 102 pregnancies after preimplantation genetic diagnosis. Am J Obstet Gynecol. 2000;182:1629–32.

Termination of Failed Pregnancy: Surgical Versus Medical Methods

28

Anshul Grover

28.1 Introduction

Approximately 20% of pregnancies spontaneously result in miscarriage [1]. Recurrent pregnancy loss is associated with psychological stress for not only the woman but the whole family. Sympathetic handling of the situation and positive counseling are often required. Women should be allowed to choose the mode of management themselves after counseling, as this has shown to result in better mental health [2]. Women with previous history of pregnancy loss should be counseled to report to health facility in the event of complications such as pain or bleeding. Fetal well-being can be documented by offering transvaginal sonography (TVS) along with beta hCG if required. Transvaginal sonography is probably the single most important investigation for a woman with bleeding in early gestation [1, 3]. Using a 6.5 MHz transvaginal probe, a pregnancy can be visualized with almost 100% accuracy at 5.5 weeks of gestation [4].

28.2 Signs of Failed Pregnancy on Transvaginal Sonography [5]

- Crown-rump length >7 mm with no cardiac activity on TVS
- Mean sac diameter of >25 mm with no embryo on TVS
- Absence of embryo with heartbeat >2 weeks after a scan that showed a gestational sac without a yolk sac
- Absence of embryo with cardiac activity >11 days after a scan that showed a gestational sac with a yolk sac

A. Grover
Obstetrics and Gynecology, Babu Jagjiwan Ram Memorial Hospital, Delhi, India
e-mail: anshul_abc@yahoo.com

S. Mehta, B. Gupta (eds.), *Recurrent Pregnancy Loss*,
https://doi.org/10.1007/978-981-10-7338-0_28

Suspicious finding on TVS demands further evaluation, especially in women with recurrent pregnancy loss who are mentally stressed. A diagnosis of pregnancy loss using one ultrasound cannot be 100% accurate [1]. Repeated ultrasound to document nonviable pregnancy is justified.

Diagnoses of nonviable pregnancy once made should be managed keeping in mind the following principles:

- Sympathetic handling and proper counseling
- Decision regarding need for uterine evacuation
- Choice of method for evacuation

Possible options for mode of evacuation include:

- Expectant management
- Medical management
- Surgical management

Women with recurrent pregnancy loss may require more than one dilatation and curettage procedures. The obstetrician handling such cases should consider the risk of infection and chances of injury to cervix while managing them. Medical methods score better in terms of these complications but may not give 100% success. In women requiring chromosomal analysis of the products of conception to rule out genetic cause, surgical means of management are preferred.

Women who may require emergency surgical management [1]:

- Significant vaginal bleeding, affecting the hemodynamic parameters or resulting in hypovolemic shock
- Evidence of sepsis

Women with the following features should be offered surgical evacuation as first-line management, as per NICE guidelines 2012:

- Women with adverse and/or traumatic experiences associated with previous pregnancy like stillbirth, miscarriage, or antepartum hemorrhage
- Women with increased risk from the effects of hemorrhage like hemoglobinopathies or unable to have blood transfusion
- Women with evidence of infection

After weighing all pros and cons and counseling regarding the procedure and its complications, the final decision for mode of evacuation should be left to the patient and her family.

28.3 Management of First Trimester Pregnancy Loss

28.3.1 Expectant Management

Expectant management should be used as the first line of management for the initial 7–14 days for women with confirmed diagnosis of nonviable intrauterine pregnancy [1]. Women choosing expectant management should be explained that complete resolution of pregnancy may take several weeks. She may experience bleeding for up to 2 weeks followed by spotting.

In a meta-analysis conducted by Sotiriadus et al., in women with first trimester miscarriage, the success rate of expectant management was 39% only as compared to surgical or medical methods. The efficacy of expectant management was better with incomplete abortion [6]. In a randomized controlled trial conducted by Wieringa de Waraid M et al. on 122 patients, expectant management at 6 weeks had a success rate of 47% as compared to 95% for surgical evacuation. The study also concluded that a waiting period of 7 days after diagnosing pregnancy loss may avoid surgical intervention in 37% of women without any adverse effects [2]. Waiting for 7 days has the advantage that some women may start bleeding spontaneously and some may abort completely. This also softens the cervix and reduces the risk of cervical injury during dilatation [2]. The MIST trial conducted in the United Kingdom concluded that the risk of unplanned hospital admissions is highest with expectant management [7]. The woman with recurrent pregnancy loss and her family may require time to assimilate this news before opting for medical or surgical treatment. This lag period may be beneficial as the process of abortion may begin spontaneously.

Women opting for expectant management should be counseled that they must report to health facility if there is:

- No spontaneous bleeding by 14 days
- Bleeding or pain continues beyond 14 days
- Experience heavy bleeding (soaking more than two pads completely in 1 h)
- A urine pregnancy test is to be repeated after 3 weeks. If negative, nothing is to be done, but if positive patient should be asked to return to health facility for individualized care.

28.3.2 Medical Management

Medical management is an effective and safe alternative to expectant and surgical management in women with recurrent pregnancy loss. It is more definite than expectant management and also avoids the need for anesthesia and surgery. The procedure is more acceptable as it ensures privacy to the women and also gives her a feeling of being in control of the whole situation. However, in some it may be detrimental psychologically, as the onset of bleeding and abdominal cramps may be a reminder of failed pregnancy. Thus the decision for mode of evacuation should lie with the woman. The drug which is acceptable and found effective for this procedure is prostaglandin E1 analogue, misoprostol. It is a uterotonic, which results in uterine contractions to expel the products of conception. In addition to the above property, it also causes softening of the uterine cervix and its dilatation. This drug can be used vaginally, orally, and sublingually [8, 9]. Based on international trials in areas with limited resources, WHO has recommended a single-dose 600 μg of oral misoprostol for management of incomplete abortion and a single dose of 800 μg given vaginally for medical management of an embryonic pregnancy or fetal demise [10]. NICE guidelines (2015) for management of miscarriage also recommend the above drug in the same dosage [1].

Adverse effects of the drug are mainly gastrointestinal and depend on the route of administration. Most common side effect is diarrhea, which is more frequently associated with oral administration, followed by sublingual. Fever is also seen in some women following administration of misoprostol.

The success of medical management should be determined by expulsion of the gestational sac and not the endometrial thickness on TVS [11, 12]. In the largest multicenter RCT, comparison of medical versus surgical management for women with early pregnancy failure (EPF) was made. It was concluded that the overall success with the use of 800 μg of misoprostol was 84% as compared to 97% with surgical management. The success depended on the type of EPF and not the gestational age. Ninety-three percent success rate was observed with incomplete/inevitable abortion, 88% with embryonic demise, and 81% for anembryonic pregnancy. No difference was observed in hemorrhage or endometritis in either of the groups [11]. In a study by Crenin M.D. et al. and Neilson J.P. et al., it was observed that patients who had cramping and bleeding symptoms suggestive of incomplete or inevitable abortion had better success rates [13, 14].

All women opting for medical management should be counseled that they will experience bleeding which will be heavier for initial 3–4 days and will last for longer duration, approximately 1–2 weeks. In the event of heavy bleeding, the women should report to health facility and may require surgical management (vacuum evacuation). She may experience abdominal cramps during the process of expulsion, which respond well to antispasmodics. If she does not respond to drugs, evaluate her for infection. The symptoms of nausea and vomiting may occur which resolve in 2–6 h. High-grade fever more than 100.4 °F, persisting for several hours, may require evaluation for infection.

Women are advised to follow up for bimanual examination and transvaginal ultrasound after 7–14 days.

- Documentation of gestational sac on scan, 2 weeks after intake of medication, is defined as incomplete abortion. This has an incidence of 2–3% and requires surgical intervention.

- Presence of blood clots and decidua may also be interpreted as incomplete abortion. In the absence of heavy bleeding, it can be managed medically by repeating tablet misoprostol 600 μg orally in single dose.
  The woman needs to be counseled regarding delay in normal menstrual cycle by 3–6 weeks.

28.3.3 Surgical Management

Surgical methods for evacuation of pregnancy loss in first trimester can be traced back to the nineteenth century, with the discovery of the sharp curette [15]. Surgical methods have the advantage of completeness of procedure, high success rate (100% in most cases), and reduced blood loss. It is readily accepted by those women who wish to avoid the labor discomfort associated with medical management. The procedure has the advantage that it can be planned according to patient's preference. It is a short procedure, mostly completed in less than 30 min. The duration of hospital stay is short, and loss of working days is few. Although this procedure is widely accepted, it requires technical expertise. When performed by experienced surgeons, it is associated with low complication rates, approximately less than 3% [16]. It is the procedure of choice in women where products of conception are to be sent for chromosomal analysis. In such cases, medical methods are not acceptable as the products get lost in the toilet. Immediate complications include trauma to the cervix, perforation of the uterus, and endometritis, while long-term complications are formation of uterine synechia, hypomenorrhea, and infertility. Anesthetic complications are transient.

Moodliar S et al. conducted a study in 2005 which included 94 women with first trimester abortion. It was concluded that success rate was 100% in the surgical arm [17]. Sotiriadis A et al. in a retrospective meta-analysis published in 2005 concluded that medical management had only two-thirds chance to induce complete evacuation compared to surgical management, but it was better than expectant management which had a success rate of only 39% [6]. In a study by Shuaib and Alharazi et al. in 2012, it was concluded that though 78.8% of patients preferred medical termination as compared to 52.7% for surgical management because it was noninvasive, safe, and assured more privacy, satisfaction and success following surgical methods were higher at the end of the procedure [18].

Surgical methods available for evacuation for first trimester pregnancy loss are:

- Electric vacuum aspiration (EVA) under local or general anesthesia
- Manual vacuum aspiration (MVA) under local anesthesia
- Both EVA and MVA are acceptable procedures, but MVA has been found to be superior in respect to the duration, amount of blood loss, postoperative pain, and cost [16, 19, 20]. Success rate of MVA ranges from 95 to 97%, while for EVA it ranges from 97 to 98% [19].

Procedure

All women undergoing surgical management should give verbal and written consent for the procedure after other possible treatments have been explained. The complications and follow-up after treatment should also be discussed with the patient.

Preoperative antibiotic cover for gram negative and anaerobes may be given in under-resourced settings to avoid infection.

28.3.4 Electric Manual Evacuation

This procedure is performed under paracervical block using 2% xylocaine or general anesthesia. The patient is clinically examined, and assessment of the uterine size and cervical dilatation is made. The size of the uterus does not always correspond to the gestational age in missed abortion and mostly is smaller in size. The assessment helps to decide the size of the suction cannula required for the procedure and the dilatation of the cervix required. For example, an 8-week-sized uterus would require an 8-mm-sized suction cannula and cervical dilatation up to 8 number Hegar's dilator for easy and successful completion of procedure. After gradual dilatation of the cervix, suction is performed using suction cannula with a suction pressure up to 0.7 kg/cm^2. Once the pressure is generated, the cannula is rotated by 360° at the fundus in a clockwise and anticlockwise direction. As a precaution to avoid perforation, the cannula is placed in the uterine cavity just short of the fundus. Completeness of the procedure is judged by appearance of bubbles in the cannula or suction tubing and grating sensation. A check curettage is done to remove any adherent contents and to complete the procedure. Repeated curettage is to be avoided to prevent damage to the decidua basalis which can lead to formation of intrauterine adhesions and perforation of the uterus [21].

Ultrasound-guided surgical evacuation is recommended in patients where previous evacuations have failed or there is difficulty in dilatation of the cervix [22].

28.3.5 Manual Vacuum Aspiration

This procedure is recommended by the WHO over the sharp curettage method especially in low-resourced settings. The manual vacuum aspirator kit comprises of a specially designed 60 cm^3 handheld plastic aspirator, a plunger handle, and a collar stop. The kit also includes sterile flexible set of Karman's cannula of sizes 6 mm, 8 mm, 10 mm, and 12 mm, along with their adaptors.

- This procedure is cost-effective and can be performed in office settings rather than operation theater. It is also less traumatic in the event of a complication like perforation. The most important advantage of this procedure is the fact that tissue can be retrieved for evaluation in a sterile manner.

- Post-procedure advice given to the patient includes:
- Irregular spotting or bleeding for up to 2 weeks
- Abdominal cramps similar to menstrual cramps for 1–2 days
- The patient should be told to consult the health facility in the following events:
- Heavy bleeding
- Soaking more than two big pads in 1 h
- Bleeding heavily for more than 12 h
- Severe abdominal pain
- Fever more than 100.4 °F for more than 4 h
- Vomiting for 4–6 h
- Sudden abdominal swelling or rapid heart rate

28.3.6 Combined Medical and Surgical Management

A woman opting for surgical evacuation is given the advantage of medical ripening of the cervix using a single-dose 400 μg of misoprostol. As recommended by the NICE guidelines 2011, misoprostol can be administered vaginally 3 h prior or sublingually 2–3 h prior to the procedure to achieve cervical softening and dilatation. Cervical preparation with overnight osmotic dilators like laminaria tent has been found to be more effective than vaginal misoprostol although less preferable [23]. This reduces the need for mechanical dilatation of the cervix thus avoiding cervical injury. It also initiates the process of expulsion of the products, thus reducing the time duration of the surgical procedure.

28.4 Management of Second Trimester Pregnancy Loss

About 1–5% of all pregnancies are lost between 13 and 19 weeks of gestation and 0.3% of pregnancies between 20 and 27 weeks of gestation end as stillbirths [24]. The rate of pregnancy loss decreases as the gestational age advances. The use of ultrasound in early pregnancy, either as routine evaluation or following bleeding, results in detection of failed pregnancies at early gestations.

Once diagnosed, the woman is counseled and given the options of various managements.

28.4.1 Expectant Management

Approximately 85% of women with intrauterine fetal demise spontaneously go into labor and delivery within 3 weeks [24]. Expectant management is not advocated in women with evidence of excessive bleeding, infection, unstable vitals, preeclampsia, gestational trophoblastic disease, deranged coagulation profile, or closed cervix with intact membranes [25].

28.4.2 Medical Management

Medical induction of labor in the second trimester is a safe and effective alternative to dilatation and evacuation. The procedure does not require technical expertise as in surgical dilatation and evacuation. It also has the advantage of collection of the products for genetic and histopathological analysis [26].

Use of misoprostol with or without mifepristone appears to be safe and effective, but it still has not been approved by FDA for use of termination of pregnancy. Gomez Ponce de Leon and Wing in a review of 14 studies on use of misoprostol for termination of pregnancy for fetal demise in second and third trimester inferred that misoprostol is highly effective in inducing delivery after 24–48 h of administration [27]. The optimal dose, schedule, and route of administration are still under review. The data reviewed include use of 200 μg of misoprostol in repeated doses within 24 h. The review describes shortest induction to delivery interval in regimens which repeated the doses every 4–6 h [28, 29]. The review by Gomez Ponce de Leon [27] recommended use of 200 μg vaginal misoprostol every 6–12 h for a total of four doses for fetal demise from 13 to 17 weeks. The dose may be increased to 400 μg if 200 μg fails to induce uterine contractions. The maximum dose should not exceed 1600 μg in 24 h.

In cases of fetal demise from 18 to 26 weeks, the recommendation is of 100 μg every 6–12 h for a total of four doses. The dose may be doubled to 200 μg if it fails to induce contractions. The maximum dose should not exceed 800 μg. Hou et al. in a systematic review concluded the misoprostol has a shorter induction-delivery interval and higher success compared to extra-amniotic instillation of ethacridine lactate but has more gastrointestinal side effects [30].

Earlier oxytocin in concentrated doses was used for inducing labor in women with fetal demise, but it does not have a good success rate due to paucity of myometrial oxytocin receptors in early gestation [31]. Prostaglandins E2 in high doses were used earlier to initiate contractions, but associated gastrointestinal side effects put them in disrepute. Other modalities available for induction of labor are cervical dilatation using laminaria tent or Foley's catheter followed by oxytocin infusion.

28.4.3 Surgical Management

Dilatation and evacuation is recommended for women with failed pregnancies with prior cervical preparation but only up to 16 weeks of pregnancy. Women are at high risk for cervical injury or uterine perforation such as women with cervical anomalies, previous surgery, or adolescents. Prior cervical preparation reduces the need for mechanical dilatation and therefore cervical injury and uterine perforation. Cervical preparation using overnight osmotic dilators like laminaria tent is found to be more effective and associated with less bleeding than vaginal misoprostol insertion, although misoprostol insertion is more comfortable [23].

The procedure may be performed under local or general anesthesia. Local anesthesia using paracervical block is preferred over general anesthesia as the latter is associated with risk of hemorrhage [1, 2] and higher cost. Local anesthesia is associated with faster recovery time and ability of provider to communicate with the woman.

To conclude, women with recurrent pregnancy loss are most satisfied when given the option to choose their management plan. Medical management is a safe and effective alternative to surgical and expectant management but falls short in providing tissue sample for evaluation. Considering the fact that these women may have already undergone more than one pregnancy loses, the obstetrician should weigh the pros and cons before counseling her regarding the treatment options.

Key Points

- Recurrent pregnancy loss is associated with psychological stress for not only the woman but her whole family.
- Possible management options for pregnancy loss are expectant, medical, or surgical.
- Expectant management should be used as the first line of management for the initial 7–14 days.
- Medical management is an effective and safe alternative to surgical management.
- Surgical management in experienced hands has a success rate of 100% with minimal side effects.

References

1. National Institute for Health and Clinical Excellence. NICE guidelines 154: ectopic pregnancy and miscarriage. London: Nice; 2012.
2. Wieringa de Ward M, Hartman EE, et al. Expectant management versus surgical evacuation in first trimester miscarriage: health related quality of life in randomized and non randomized patients. Hum Reprod. 2002;17(6):1638–42.
3. Australian Society for Ultrasound in Medicine. Guidelines for the performance of first trimester ultrasound. Sydney: ASUM; 2014.
4. Practical guide to high risk pregnancy and delivery, 3rd ed. Early pregnancy complications. Parikshit Dayal Tank. p 104–9.
5. Jeve Y, Rana R, Bhide A, et al. Accuracy of first trimester ultrasound in the diagnosis of early embryonic demise: a systemic review. Ultrasound Obstet Gynecol. 2011;38(5):489–96. https://doi.org/10.1002/uog.10108. Epub 2011 Oct 13.
6. Sotiriadis A, Makrydimas G, Papatheodorou S, et al. Expectant, medical, or surgical management of first- trimester miscarriage: a meta-analysis. Obstet Gynecol. 2005;105(5 Pt 1):1104–13.
7. Tinder J, Brocklehurst P, Porter R, et al. Management for miscarriage: expectant, medical or surgical?. Results of a randomized controlled trial (Miscarriage Treatment (MIST) trial). BMJ. 2006;332(7552):1235–40.
8. American College of Obstetricians and Gynecologists, authors. ACOG committee opinion no. 427. Misoprostol for postabortion care. Obstet Gynecol. 2009;113:465–8.
9. ACOG guidelines, early pregnancy loss, Number 150. May 2015.

10. Gemzell- Danielsson K, Jo PC, et al. Misoprostol to treat missed abortion in the first trimester. Int J Gynaecol Obstet. 2007;99(Suppl 2):S186–5.
11. Zhang J, Gilles JM, Barnhart K, et al. A comparison of medical management with misoprostol and surgical management for early pregnancy failure. National Institute of Child Health Human Development (NICHD) Management of early pregnancy failure trial. N Engl J Med. 2005;353:761–9.
12. Crenin MD, Harwood B, Guido RS, et al. Endometrial thickness after misoprostol use for early pregnancy failure. NICD Management of early pregnancy failure trial. Int J Gynecol Obstet. 2004;86:22–6.
13. Crenin MD, Huang X, et al. Factors related to successful misoprostol treatment for early pregnancy failure. Obstet Gynecol. 2006;107(4):901–7.
14. Neilson JP, Hickey M, Vazquez J. Medical treatment for early fetal death (less than 24 weeks). The Cochrane Library Issue 3. Chichester: Wiley; 2006.
15. Harris LH, Dalton VK, Johnson TRB. Surgical management of early pregnancy failure: history, politics and safe cost- effective care. Am J Obstet Gynecol. 2007;196:445e1–5.
16. Goldberg AB, Dean G, Kang M, et al. Manual versus electric vacuum aspiration for early first-trimester abortion: a controlled study of complication rates. Obstet Gynecol. 2004;103(1):101–7.
17. Moodiliar S, Bagratee JS, Moodley J. Medical vs surgical evacuation of first trimester spontaneous abortion. Int J Gynecol Obstet. 2005;91(1):21–6.
18. Shuaib AA, Abdelrahman HA. Medical versus surgical termination of the first trimester missed miscarriage. Alexandria J Med. 2013;49(1):13–6. https://doi.org/10.1016/j.ajme.2012.08.004.
19. Wen J, Cai QY, Deng F, et al. Manual versus electric vacuum aspiration for first-trimester abortion: a systematic review. BJOG. 2008;115:5–13.
20. Dalto VK, Harris L, Weisman CS, et al. Patient preferences, satisfaction, and resource use in office evacuation of early pregnancy failure. Obstet Gynecol. 2006;108:103–10.
21. Lindell G, Flam F. Management of uterine perforations in connection with legal abortions. Acta Obstet Gynecol Scand. 1995;74:373–5.
22. Acharya G, Morgan H, Paramanantham L, et al. A randomized controlled trial comparing surgical termination of pregnancy with or without continuous ultrasound guidance. Eur J Obstet Gynecol Reprod Biol. 2004;114:69–74.
23. Firozabadi RD, Sekhavat L, Tabatabaii A, et al. Laminaria tent versus misoprostol for cervical ripening before surgical process of missed abortion. Arch Gynecol Obstet. 2012;285(3):699–703.
24. Clinical Practice Guidelines: Management of second trimester miscarriage. Institute of Obstetricians and Gynaecologists. Royal College of Physicians of Ireland and Directorate of Strategy and Clinical Programs, Health Service Executive Guideline No 29, 2014.
25. Parasnis H, Raje B, Hinduja IN. Relevance of plasma fibrinogen estimation in obstetric complications. J Postgraduate Med. 1992;38(4):183–5.
26. Saraswat L, Ashok PW, Mathur M. Medical management of miscarriage. Obstet Gynaecol. 2014;16(2):79–85.
27. Gomez Ponse de Leon R, Wing DA. Misoprostol for termination of pregnancy with intrauterine fetal demise in the second and third trimester of pregnancy—a systemic review. Contraception. 2009;79:259–71.
28. Niromanesh S, Hashemi-Fesharaki M, Mosavi-Jarrhi A. Second trimester abortion using intravaginal misoprostol. Int J Gynaecol. 2013;101:70–3.
29. Chittarcharoen A, Herabutya Y, Punyavachira P. A randomized trial of oral and vaginal misoprostol to manage delivery in cases of fetal death. Obstet Gynecol. 2003;101(10):70–3.
30. Hou SP, Fang AH, Chen QF. Termination of second trimester pregnancy by mifepristone combined with misoprostol versus intra-amniotic injection of ethacridine lactate: a systemic review of Chinese trial. Contraception. 2011;84:214–23.
31. Fuchs AR, Helmer H, et al. Concentration of oxytocin receptors in the placenta and fetal membranes of cows during pregnancy and labor. Reprod Fertil. 1992;96:775–83.

29 Obesity and Its Association with Recurrent Pregnancy Loss

Anupama Bahadur and Jaya Chaturvedi

29.1 Introduction

Recurrent pregnancy loss (RPL) affects 5% of couples trying to achieve parenthood and is defined as two or more clinical pregnancy losses, <10 weeks size, documented on ultrasound or on histopathology [1].

RPL has a multifactorial background involving a complex interaction of multiple genetic and environmental factors. However, 40–50% are unexplained miscarriages [2]. Mounting retrospective evidence has explored the link between recurrent pregnancy loss and obesity in spontaneous conceptions and assisted reproduction as well as in women with a history of RPL [3–6]. Poor dietary choices and limited physical activity lead to development and sustenance of obesity. It negatively impacts the reproductive potential of a woman and is associated with several endocrine disorders like diabetes, hypertension, hypothyroidism, and PCOS.

Logistic regression has demonstrated that maternal obesity, Asian ethnicity, age, and also the number of previous miscarriages are independent risk factors for couples with unexplained recurrent miscarriages (OR 1.73 vs. 2.87 vs. 1.99 vs. 2.08, 95% CI 1.06–2.83 vs. 1.52–5.39 vs. 1.45–2.73 vs. 1.42–3.06). Maternal age is the strongest predictor and any increase in BMI acts independent of age. Obesity (BMI >30 kg/m^2) per se is an independent risk factor for further miscarriages in patients with RPL. In a study, Lo et al. demonstrated that maternal obesity is an independent high-risk factor for a future miscarriage in women with unexplained recurrent miscarriages, and when compared with women with normal BMI, obese women had a 73% increased risk of another miscarriage in their subsequent pregnancies [6].

In obese women there is an increased risk of euploid miscarriages resulting from suboptimal implantation due to endocrine changes, a detrimental effect on ovaries

A. Bahadur (✉) • J. Chaturvedi
Obstetrics and Gynecology, All India Institute of Medical Sciences, Rishikesh, Uttarakhand, India
e-mail: anupama.bahadur@gmail.com; Jaya_sunil@yahoo.com

S. Mehta, B. Gupta (eds.), *Recurrent Pregnancy Loss*,
https://doi.org/10.1007/978-981-10-7338-0_29

Table 29.1 WHO classification of body mass index (obesity)

Classification	Principal cutoff points BMI (kg/m^2)
Normal range	18.50–24.99
Overweight	**≥25.00**
Pre-obese	25.00–29.99
Obese	**≥30.00**
Obese class I	30.00–34.99
Obese class II	35.00–39.99
Obese class III	≥40.00

resulting in compromised oocyte quality thereby affecting embryo viability. Patients are classified according to World Health Organization (WHO) classification system as obese when the body mass index (BMI) >30 kg/m^2 (Table 29.1) [7]. BMI is routinely recorded at the first hospital visit using the formula: weight in kilograms/height in $meter^2$ (kg/m^2). Obese women in their reproductive age group face problems like menstrual disorders, infertility, and poor reproductive outcome. Clinically obese (BMI >30 kg/m^2) women have a small but significant risk of miscarriage in their subsequent pregnancies.

Obesity increases the risk of miscarriage not only in the general population but also in those undergoing assisted conception [8, 9]. In a case-control study, Lashen et al. showed significantly higher odds of recurrent miscarriages in obese women compared to their normal-weight controls (OR 3.51; 95% CI 1.03–12.01) [10]. Metwally et al. observed that in obese women (BMI >30 kg/m^2) with recurrent miscarriages, there is a small but significantly higher odd (OR 1.71; 95% CI 1.05–2.8) of a miscarriage in the subsequent pregnancy that could be best predicted by increased BMI and maternal age. Their observation was based on a retrospective study of 844 pregnancies in 491 women with recurrent miscarriages [4]. In a meta-analysis that included 16 studies, the authors concluded that women with a BMI >25 kg/m^2 had significantly higher odds for miscarriage irrespective of the mode of conception [5]. In a systematic review by Maheshwari et al., the authors concluded that women who were overweight (BMI >25 kg/m^2) had an increased risk of miscarriage (as high as 25–37%) and a lower likelihood of pregnancy after in vitro fertilization (IVF). These women on one hand require higher doses of gonadotropins but yield lesser number of oocytes during assisted reproductive technology [11].

29.2 Pathophysiology

Management of RPL in obese women is a formidable clinical challenge to the physicians because of the controversial issues pertaining to the pathophysiology of the disease. The pathophysiology of how obesity adversely impacts pregnancy is yet to be elucidated. There are several explanations to this. With a slight increase in BMI, there is a mild rise of leptin that has an important role in early maintenance of normal pregnancy development [12]. Probably leptin has a beneficial effect on the endometrial receptivity as it stimulates the expression matrix metalloproteinase by cytotrophoblast. It also modulates the function of T lymphocytes and other proto-oncogenes [13]. However, when BMI further increases to a state of moderate to severe obesity, there occurs a state of leptin resistance, which in turn causes insulin resistance. Insulin resistance is very common in obese women and contributes to miscarriages by diminishing the endometrial production of the adhesion factors, insulin-like growth factor-binding protein-1 and uterine $\alpha_v\beta_3$ integrin [14]. This is being hypothesized as the etiology of poor reproductive outcome and thereby miscarriage in these obese women.

Elevated levels of fatty acids are also associated with impaired oocyte maturation.

Reproductive success depends on the ability of the endometrium to distinguish between normal and abnormal embryos. It may be a plausible explanation that obesity adversely impacts the endometrial development and has detrimental effect on the ovaries, which affects oocyte quality and embryo development or both.

29.3 Polycystic Ovarian Syndrome

The local hormonal milieu is crucial in the attachment of the embryo and early pregnancy leading to the successful growth and development of the fetus. Common endocrinopathies (8–12%) are a frequent contributor to spontaneous and recurrent miscarriage [15]. Polycystic ovarian syndrome (PCOS) is the most prevalent endocrine disorder associated with menstrual irregularity and polycystic ovaries. Around 35–80% of women in their reproductive age group with polycystic ovaries are obese and have an increased risk of pregnancy loss due to several underlying contributing and interrelated factors like hyperandrogenism, hyperinsulinemia, insulin resistance, high levels of plasminogen activator inhibitor-1 factor, and poor endometrial receptivity. The high insulin level causes the ovaries to produce more testosterone, which in turn is detrimental to folliculogenesis and prevents normal ovulation. In women with PCOS, endocrine and metabolic abnormalities like hyperandrogenism, high luteinizing hormone (LH), and insulin resistance play a pivotal role in recurrent miscarriages by affecting the oocyte quality and fertilization and causing implantation failure. Obese women have altered secretion of hormones like leptin, adiponectin, and ghrelin that may adversely affect pregnancy. Probably insulin resistance is the key factor in explaining the association that exists between obesity, PCOS, and recurrent miscarriages. Recent studies have evaluated the presence of hypofibrinolysis with high levels of PAI-1 as a potential cause of recurrent miscarriages in women with PCOS. Elevated levels of PAI-1 may contribute individually or in combination with thrombosis and eventually may lead to RPL [16]. Management of PCOS with normalization of weight or metformin seems to reduce the risk of pregnancy loss [17].

29.4 Hyperinsulinemia and Hyperandrogenism

Hyperinsulinemia and hyperandrogenemia have a detrimental effect on the endometrial development and decrease the oocyte and embryo viability due to an indirect effect via the insulin pathways or via insulin-like growth factors. However, existing studies have reported conflicting results whether or not there is an association between high androgen levels of women with recurrent miscarriages. The controversy is mainly attributed to the variation in specific measurement of androgens with respect to the menstrual cycle. It is the free testosterone and free androgen index (FAI) levels that are considered most sensitive and should be assessed during the early follicular phase. In a large-scale study, the measurement of FAI in the early follicular phase has shown a significantly increased risk of miscarriage with FAI > 5 [18]. Further studies should be conducted to validate whether therapeutic intervention by reducing FAI improves pregnancy outcome in women with hyperandrogenemia and recurrent miscarriages.

29.5 Luteal Phase Defect (LPD)

Luteal phase defect (LPD) causing endometrial defects is probably due to decreased production of progesterone by the corpus luteum or poor response of the endometrium to progesterone that is available. Studies have shown no difference in the prevalence of LPD between patients with normal BMI versus those with a high BMI. Although the diagnostic criterion for luteal phase defect (LPD) remains controversial, treatment of patients with both recurrent pregnancy loss and LPD using progestogen in early pregnancy may seem beneficial.

For patients who are hypothyroid, thyroid hormone replacement therapy along with careful monitoring in the preconception and early pregnancy period is associated with improved outcome.

29.5.1 Obesity and Euploid Miscarriage

Obese women have an increased frequency of euploid miscarriage which further increases the risk of subsequent miscarriage. In a study by Boots et al., the frequency of a euploid miscarriage was 58% among obese women (BMI $\geq$30 kg/m^2) compared with 37% of nonobese women (BMI <30 kg/m^2) (relative risk 1.63, 95% CI 1.08–2.47) [19].

29.6 Management

The management of obese women with RPL is challenging. There is paucity in literature of good-quality evidence from randomized controlled trials on testing and treating women with endocrinological disorders and RPL. Clinically obese (BMI >30 kg/m^2) women have a small but significant risk of miscarriage in their subsequent pregnancies. They require counseling and psychological support in their early pregnancy so that their chances of a successful pregnancy outcome increase.

Women should be counseled on the benefits of weight loss and advised lifestyle modifications. With supportive care within the settings of a specialist recurrent pregnancy loss clinic, these obese women show an excellent prognosis for a future successful pregnancy outcome.

Lo et al. observed that women from Asian ethnicity had significantly higher risk of miscarriages as compared to their Caucasian counterparts [6]. Although the reasons for this remain unclear, the plausible explanation may be the association between BMI and body fat percentage, which has been seen to differ across ethnic groups. This implies that a single universal BMI cutoff point cannot be applied across different ethnic groups. The National Institute of Clinical Excellence (NICE) clinical guideline on obesity (CG43), which was published in 2006 and revised in 2015, has recommended a revised BMI cutoff point for overweight and obesity for the Asians which is based on their mortality and morbidity risks, i.e., $\geq$23 kg/m^2 as overweight (increased risk) and $\geq$27.5 kg/m^2 as obese (high risk) [20].

Motivated obese women should be encouraged to lose weight by cost-effective, noninvasive regimes like exercise and dietary modification. The advantages of losing weight are a decrease in body fat, reduction in truncal-abdominal fat together with improved metabolism, and hormonal balance. In PCOS women the aim is to reduce serum fasting glucose and insulin, improve insulin sensitivity and decrease PAI-1 activity, decrease testosterone levels, and increase sex hormone-binding globulin levels. This can be achieved by eating a diet that is rich in proteins and very low in calories. A holistic approach will help in normalizing hyperinsulinemia, improve insulin sensitivity, and bring down the androgen levels, and this will result in a favorable reproductive outcome by improving both the ovarian function and endometrial receptivity.

29.6.1 Role of Bariatric Surgery

Bariatric surgery results in a sustained long-term loss of up to 15–25% of body weight, as well as significant reduction comorbidities like diabetes, hypertension, and certain cancers. Studies have found improvements in sex hormone profiles and the resolution of PCOS following bariatric surgery, but there is a paucity of evidence on miscarriage rates following bariatric surgery [21].

Till date no study has looked into the effect of weight loss on preventing further miscarriages in patients with RPL.

Conclusion

Obesity in women of reproductive age is known for its association with poor reproductive outcomes. High BMI increases the risk for miscarriages by adversely affecting folliculogenesis in the ovary, impaired endometrial receptivity, and embryo development. Large, well-defined clinical trials are required, which focus on ethnicity and standardized classification for obesity and recurrent pregnancy loss that will be useful in providing concrete evidence in this challenging condition.

Key Points

- Clinically obese (BMI >30 kg/m^2) women have a small but significant risk of miscarriage in their subsequent pregnancies.
- Obesity is associated with euploid embryo, which may be contributed by multiple factors like polymorphisms of multiple susceptibility genes and lifestyle factors.
- Factors leading to increased risk of pregnancy are hyperandrogenism, hyperinsulinemia, insulin resistance, high levels of plasminogen activator inhibitor-1 factor, and poor endometrial receptivity.
- Management of RPL in obese women is a formidable clinical challenge to the physicians because of the controversial issues pertaining to the pathophysiology of the disease.
- Empirical treatment is the mainstay in idiopathic RPL. These patients should be counseled that they have a 70% chance of success without treatment in their subsequent pregnancies.
- Till date no study has looked into the effect of weight loss on preventing further miscarriages in patients with RPL.

References

1. Bashiri A, Ratzon R, Amar S, Serjienko R, Mazor M, Shoham-Vardi I. Two vs. three or more primary recurrent pregnancy losses—are there any differences in epidemiologic characteristics and index pregnancy outcome? J Perinat Med. 2012;40:365–71.
2. Stephenson MD. Frequency of factors associated with habitual abortion in 197 couples. Fertil Steril. 1996;66:24–9.
3. Boots C, Stephenson MD. Does obesity increase the rate of miscarriage in spontaneous conception: a systematic review. Semin Reprod Med. 2011;29:507–13.
4. Metwally M, Saravelos SH, Ledger WL, Li TC. Body mass index and risk of miscarriage in women with recurrent miscarriage. Fertil Steril. 2010;94:290–5.
5. Metwally M, Ong KJ, Ledger WL, Li TC. Does high body mass index increase the risk of miscarriage after spontaneous and assisted conception? A meta-analysis of the evidence. Fertil Steril. 2008;90:714–26.
6. Lo W, Rai R, Hameed A, Brailsford SR, Al-Ghamdi AA, Regan L. The effect of body mass index on the outcome of pregnancy in women with recurrent miscarriage. J Family Community Med. 2012;19:167–71.
7. World Health Organization. Obesity: preventing and managing the global epidemic. Report of a WHO consultation on obesity. Geneva: World Health Organization; 1999.
8. Veleva Z, Tiitinen A, Vilska S, Hyden-Granskog C, Tomas C, Martikainen H, et al. High and low BMI increase the risk of miscarriage after IVF/ICSI and FET. Hum Reprod. 2008;23:878–84.
9. Helgstrand S, Andersen AM. Maternal underweight and the risk of spontaneous abortion. Acta Obstet Gynecol Scand. 2005;84:1197–201.
10. Lashen H, Fear K, Sturdee DW. Obesity is associated with increased risk of first trimester and recurrent miscarriage: matched case control study. Hum Reprod. 2004;19:1644–6.
11. Maheshwari A, Stofberg L, Bhattacharya S. Effect of overweight and obesity on assisted reproductive technology: a systematic review. Hum Reprod Update. 2007;13(5):433–4.

12. Kolaczynski JW, Ohannesian JP, Considine RV, Marco CC, Caro JF. Response of leptin to short-term and prolonged overfeeding in humans. J Clin Endocrinol Metab. 1996;81:4162–5.
13. Sagawa N, Yura S, Itoh H, Kakui K, Takemura M, Nuamah MA, et al. Possible role of placental leptin in pregnancy: a review. Endocrine. 2002;19:65–71.
14. Moschos S, Chan JL, Mantzoros CS. Leptin and reproduction: a review. Fertil Steril. 2002;77:433–44.
15. Smith ML, Schust DJ. Endocrinology and recurrent early pregnancy loss. Semin Reprod Med. 2011;29:482–90.
16. Sun L, Lv H, Wei W, Zhang D, Guan Y. Angiotensin-converting enzyme D/I and plasminogen activator inhibitor-1 4G/5G gene polymorphisms are associated with increased risk of spontaneous abortions in polycystic ovarian syndrome. J Endocrinol Investig. 2010;33:77–82.
17. Ke RW. Endocrine basis for recurrent pregnancy loss. Obstet Gynecol Clin N Am. 2014;41(1):103–12.
18. Cocksedge KA, Saravelos SH, Wang Q, Tuckerman E, Laird SM, Li TC. Does free androgen index predict subsequent pregnancy outcome in women with recurrent miscarriage? Hum Reprod. 2008;23:797–802.
19. Boots CE, Bernardi LA, Stephenson MD. Frequency of euploid miscarriage is increased in obese women with recurrent early pregnancy loss. Fertil Steril. 2014;102:455–9.
20. NICE clinical guideline CG43: obesity: the prevention, identification, assessment and management of overweight and obesity in adults and children. UK: National Institute for Health and Clinical Excellence; 2006.
21. Malik SM, Traub ML. Defining the role of bariatric surgery in polycystic ovarian syndrome patients. World J Diabetes. 2012;3:71–9.

Minimally Invasive Surgery: Diagnostic and Therapeutic Role

30

Punita Bhardwaj, Tarun Das, Sanskriti Batra, and Shivaji Dhopte

30.1 Introduction

Recurrent pregnancy loss is a distressing situation causing a significant mental impact on the couple, especially women. The aetiology comprises of genetic, chromosomal, immunological, anatomic and endocrinological causes, with ~50% cases having no known definitive cause [1]. Anatomic abnormalities are usually associated with second-trimester losses. Along with pregnancy losses, these are also associated with adverse complications like infertility, preterm labour, malpresentation, antepartum haemorrhage, operative delivery, etc [2]. The structural anomalies contributing to habitual losses can be classified into congenital and acquired.

Congenital Mullerian malformations result from defective gene expression causing anomalous fusion and resorption in utero. Congenital anomalies as a cause for RM varies from 1.8 to 37.6% (versus ~7% in general population) with septate uterus being the most common cause [3, 4]. Bicornuate uteri has also been commonly implicated in recurrent losses.

Acquired abnormalities can be a sole or coexistent pathology in recurrent miscarriages. These develop after puberty due to excessive hormonal stimulus, infections like tuberculosis and physical trauma due to excessive curettage. Submucous fibroids and intrauterine synechiae are proven determinants of recurrent miscarriages. Cervical insufficiency also leads to premature painless cervical dilation causing recurrent mid-trimester losses.

Hysteroscopy and laparoscopy offer excellent treatment options to women having recurrent losses due to anatomical defects. This chapter provides a

P. Bhardwaj (✉) • T. Das • S. Batra • S. Dhopte
Obstetrics and Gynecology, Institute of Obstetrics and Gynecology, Sir Ganga Ram Hospital, New Delhi, India
e-mail: punitadoc@yahoo.com

S. Mehta, B. Gupta (eds.), *Recurrent Pregnancy Loss*,
https://doi.org/10.1007/978-981-10-7338-0_30

comprehensive overview of the anomalies, their impact on the fertility and recurrent miscarriages and a critical evaluation of the endoscopic surgical techniques available for correction.

30.2 Septate Uterus

Septate uterus which is the most common Mullerian anomaly consists of a septum, a muscular or fibrous wall that divides the inside of the uterus, creating two cavities. It is most amenable to hysteroscopic correction [5–7]. It is more common in patients with primary infertility or who have had repeated miscarriages.

30.2.1 Types of Septate Uterus

Partial—Septum begins at the fundus but does not reach the internal cervical os and divides the endometrial cavity only partially (Fig. 30.1).

Complete—In this the septum extends from the fundus of the uterus to the internal cervical os, or even to the external os, thus completely dividing the endometrial cavity into two (Fig. 30.2).

30.2.2 Impact of Septate Uterus on Fertility

The incidence of uterine septa is higher in infertile women as compared to the general population, suggesting a link with infertility [8–11]. It is often difficult to determine if the uterine septum is the sole reason as infertility can be multifactorial. One of the larger studies compared 153 women with all types of uterine anomalies to a control group of 27 women with no uterine anomaly [11]. Thirty-three women with

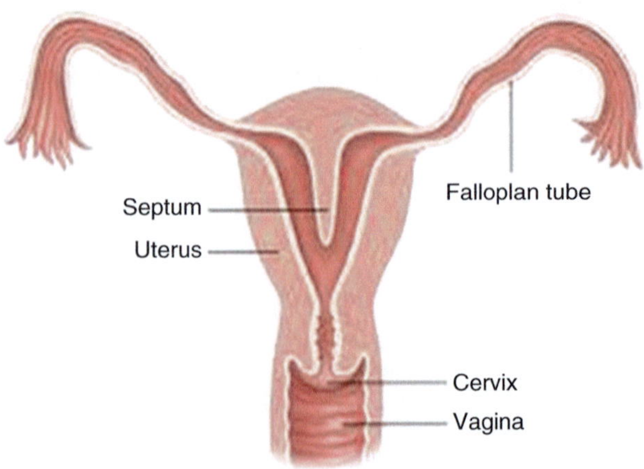

Fig. 30.1 Partial septum

Fig. 30.2 Complete septum

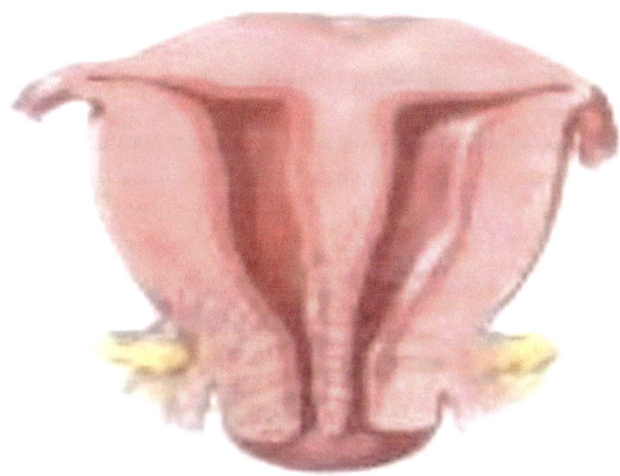

septate uterus had a higher incidence of infertility compared with controls (21.9% vs. 7.7%); however, this was not statistically significant.

One study evaluated 193 women who had primary infertility of at least 2 years. Following septum excision, the cumulative pregnancy probability was 10% in the first 6 months, 18.1% in the first 6–12 months and 23.3% after 18 months [12]. There are no RCTs with untreated controls assessing whether incision of uterine septum improves fertility. Several observational studies reported improved clinical pregnancy rates in women undergoing resection.

30.2.3 Role of Septum on Pregnancy Loss and Adverse Pregnancy Outcome

Although many women with a uterine septum have an uncomplicated reproductive history, studies suggest that a septate uterus is associated with a higher rate of miscarriage and preterm delivery when compared with controls. A study [13] evaluated 689 women with septate uterus and compared their reproductive outcomes with those in 15,060 women in the general pregnant population. The incidence of early miscarriage was 41.1% in patients with septate uterus compared with 12.1% in control. Late abortions and premature deliveries developed in 12.6% of patients with septate uterus compared with 6.9% in the general population. The most common cause is vascular compromise as the fibrous tissue of the septum compromises foetal development [5–7]. In later gestations, the septum can directly compromise available space for growth, leading to miscarriage, malpresentation, or preterm birth.

There is insufficient evidence to conclude that obstetric outcomes are different when comparing the length or width of uterine septa [12]. However, it is better to know the type and thickness to assess prognosis and potential benefit.

30.2.4 Preoperative Evaluation

The gold standard method for diagnosing Mullerian anomalies was direct visualisation of the uterus using laparoscopy and hysteroscopy. This helped to distinguish a septate from a bicornuate uterus. With improvement in radiology, diagnosis need not be surgical. Compared from hysteroscopy/laparoscopy, several studies indicate that the diagnostic accuracy of hysterosalpingography (HSG) ranges from 5.6 to 88% [14–17].

Some studies suggest that sonohysterography or saline infusion sonography (SIS) is superior to HSG. Three-dimensional (3-D) ultrasonography combined with saline infusion had 100% accuracy when compared with laparoscopy/hysteroscopy [18]. Only 3-D ultrasound has been found to be over 88% accurate for diagnosing uterine septa in two studies when compared with hysteroscopy/laparoscopy [18, 19]. MRI is only 70% accurate for the diagnosis of uterine septum [20].

The main differentiating features between bicornuate and septate uterus are shown in Table 30.1

30.2.4.1 Should Thin Endometrium Be Managed Preoperatively?

There is insufficient evidence for or against recommending danazol or GnRH agonists for thinning the endometrium prior to hysteroscopic septum incision as a routine [21].

30.2.5 Operative Technique

With the advent of less invasive hysteroscopic techniques, laparotomy for septum resection using Jones or modified Tompkins procedures has largely been abandoned.

Commonly used techniques include incision or resection of the septum utilising cold scissors, unipolar and bipolar cautery or laser (Figs. 30.3, 30.4, and 30.5).

Table 30.1 Bicornuate versus septate uterus

Bicornuate uterus	Septate uterus
• Fundal dimple—present	• Fundal dimple—absent
• <5-mm uterine wall above the line joining tips of the two cavities	• >5-mm uterine wall above the line joining tips of the two cavities
• Angle between two cavities >90°	• Angle between two cavities <90°
• Medial margins of uterine cavities–convex	• Medial margins of uterine cavities-straight

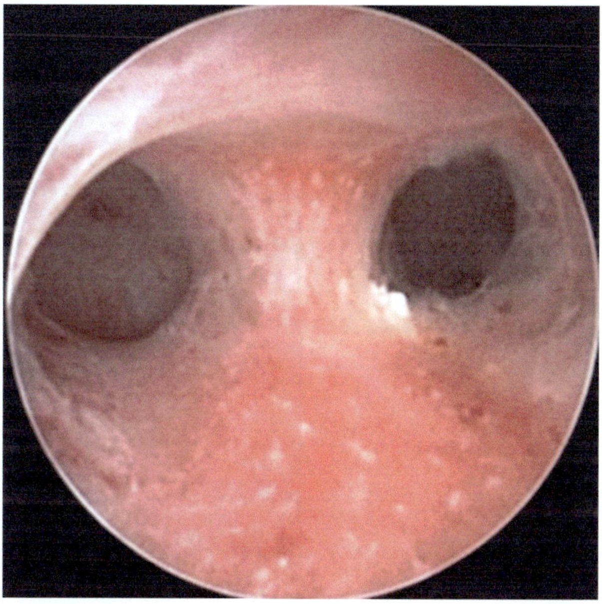

Fig. 30.3 Hysteroscopic view of uterine septum

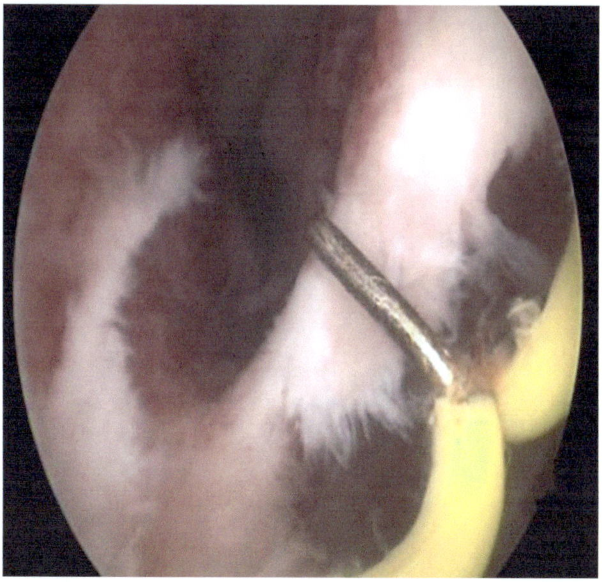

Fig. 30.4 Resection of septum using electrode

Use of distending media for the uterus is dependent on the incision technique or energy source [22].

Laparoscopy and, more recently, transabdominal ultrasound have been used concurrently with hysteroscopic incision to confirm uterine contour, decrease the risk of uterine perforation and assess complete excision of the septum and to rule out other anomalies [23].

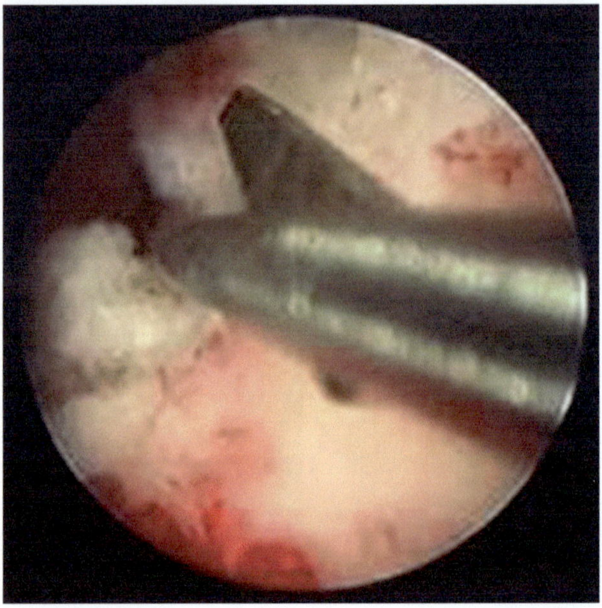

Fig. 30.5 Resection of septum using a scissor

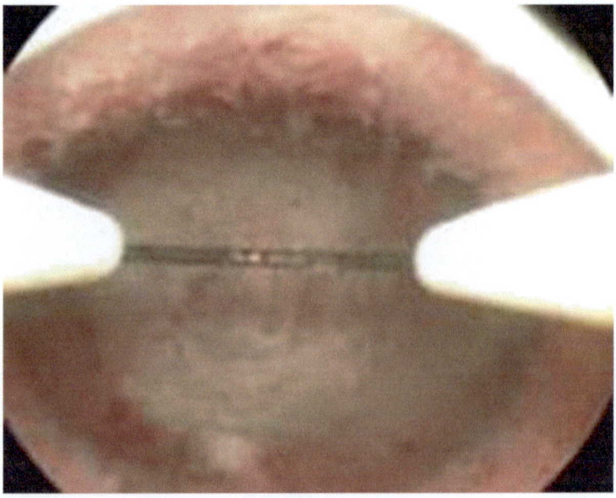

Fig. 30.6 Uterine cavity after septum resection

The septum is incised from the apex upwards while simultaneously working from side to side. The resection is continued upwards until the cavity is seen as single at the fundus and the hysteroscope can be moved freely without hitting residual septal tissue (Fig. 30.6). Slight retraction of anterior and posterior walls of the uterus occurs; therefore, slight undercorrection is permissible [24]. Studies have shown that reproductive outcomes do not change with small residual septa of less than 1 cm [25]. Repeat procedure can be done after 6 weeks if needed.

Differentiation between septal fibres and myometrial fibres determines the end point. Bleeding can be seen when myometrium is reached.

30.2.6 How Long Should a Woman Wait to Conceive After Surgical Correction of Septum?

Available evidence suggests that the uterine cavity is healed by 2 months postoperatively [26]. But there is insufficient evidence to advice a specific length of time before a woman should conceive.

30.3 Bicornuate Uterus

Bicornuate uterus which accounts for 25% of Mullerian duct anomalies results from lack of fusion of the Mullerian ducts and is diagnosed by the presence of an external indentation at the fundus exceeding 50% of the uterine wall thickness [27, 28] (Fig. 30.7). Women with bicornuate uterus abort more commonly in the second trimester as against women with septate uterus who commonly miscarry in the first trimester [29]. Almost 60% of women with this anomaly have a successful pregnancy without surgery, and metroplasty results in successful pregnancy outcomes in 65–85% of patients [30]. Laparoscopic metroplasty for the bicornuate uterus was reported for the first time in one patient in January 2006 with a successful outcome [31].

30.3.1 Types of Bicornuate Uterus

ESHRE has classified bicornuate uterus into three types depending on the degree of the deformity:

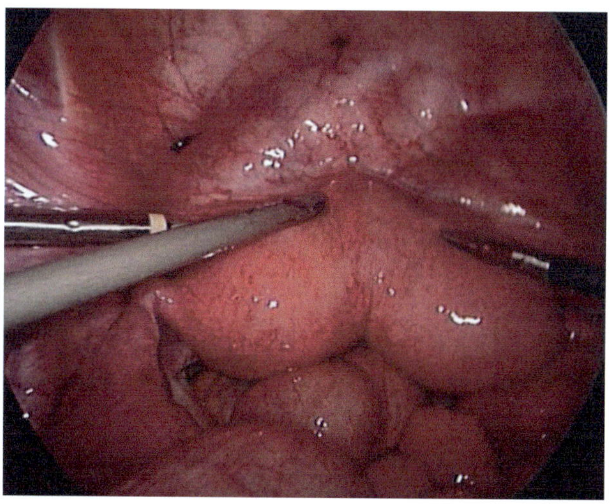

Fig. 30.7 Bicornuate uterus

1. *Partial bicorporeal uterus*: In this subtype, the fundal indentation partly divides the uterine corpus above the level of the cervix.
2. *Complete bicorporeal uterus*: In this deformity, the uterus is divided externally up to the level of the cervix.
3. *Bicorporeal septate uterus*: It is characterised by an absorption defect in addition to the main fusion defect, and the midline fundal indentation exceeds the uterine wall thickness by almost 150% [27].

30.3.2 Signs and Symptoms [32]

- Asymptomatic
- Dysmenorrhoea, abdominal pain and pelvic mass
- Recurrent abortion (15% to 25% of such women have uterine abnormalities)
- Infertility
- Preterm labour
- Pain or uterine rupture in early pregnancy
- Malpresentation (breech or transverse lie)
- Retained placenta

30.3.3 Preoperative Evaluation

Hysterosalpingography (Fig. 30.8): The sensitivity, specificity and overall accuracy of HSG in differentiating septate and bicornuate uterus are 77.4%, 60% and 75%, respectively [33].

3-D USG (Fig. 30.9): The 3-D ultrasound showed the highest diagnostic parameters, with sensitivity of 96.7%, specificity of 100%, PPV of 100% and negative predicative value of 83.3%, with overall accuracy of 97.2% [33].

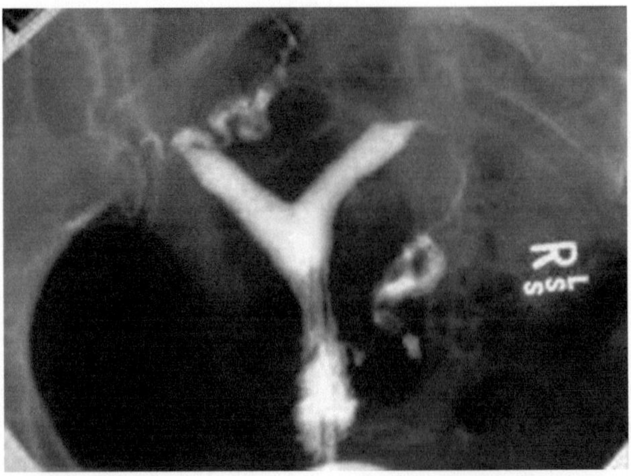

Fig. 30.8 Bicornuate uterus on HSG

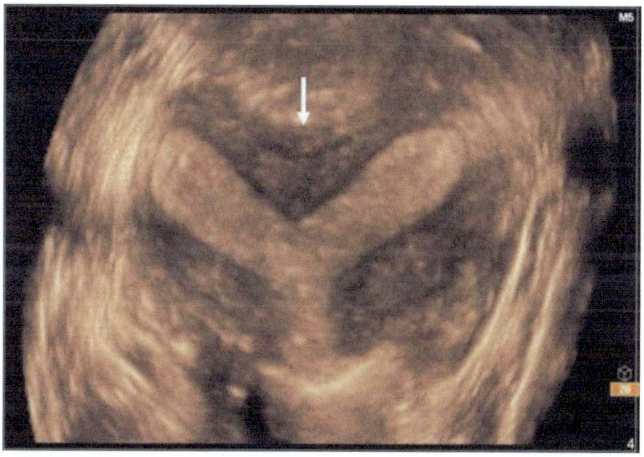

Fig. 30.9 3-D USG image of bicornuate uterus

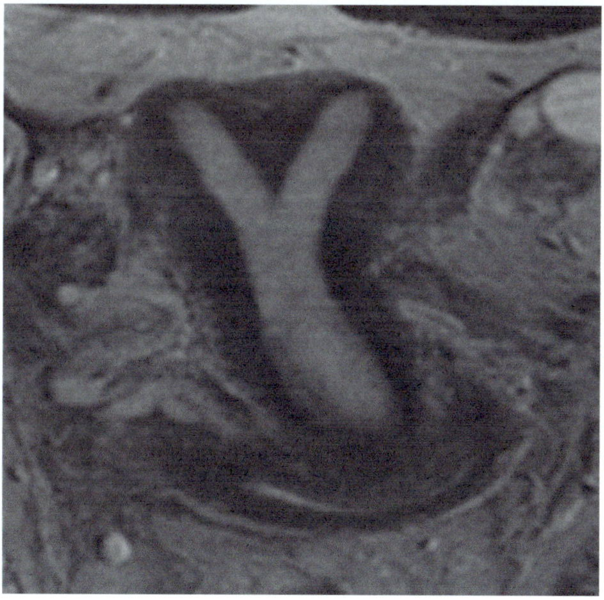

Fig. 30.10 MRI of bicornuate uterus

Magnetic Resonance Imaging (Fig. 30.10): MRI has a sensitivity of 93.5%, specificity of 80%, PPV of 96.6% and negative predicative value of 66.6%, with overall accuracy of 91.6% in diagnosing bicornuate uterus [33].

30.3.4 Operative Procedure

Abdominal metroplasty—open Strassman's operation
Laparoscopic metroplasty

30.3.4.1 Laparoscopic Metroplasty

Port placement is done after patient is placed in low lithotomy position. Vasopressin solution is infiltrated subserosally in the uterus. A deep incision through the myometrium, 2 cm medial to fallopian tube origin, is made extending from the superomedial aspect of each horn towards the medial aspect and the base of the horn. The endometrial cavity is now opened along this incision, and the vagina is packed to prevent leakage of gas. The myometrial edges are sutured with interrupted sutures using 1.0 Vicryl. Care is taken not to include the endometrium in these sutures. The serosa is then closed with no.1 Vicryl. And haemostasis is confirmed [28].

In another method, under laparoscopic monitoring uterine fundus is perforated transversally by needle electrode of hysteroscopy. The uterine cavity is connected with peritoneal cavity. And then using monopolar shovel, separate the fundus transversally and continuously. Transverse uterine incision is made to the both ends of uterine horn from 1 to 1.5 cm. No. 1-0 Vicryl is used to suture the superficial muscularis mucosa. Uterine wall is closed with interrupted suturing longitudinally [34] (Fig. 30.11).

Advantages of laparoscopic metroplasty include decreased prevalence of adhesion formation, reduced tissue handling and chances of drying, reduced blood loss during surgery and improved pregnancy outcome compared with abdominal approach [28].

30.3.4.2 Outcomes Following Laparoscopic Metroplasty

E Xia et al. [34] found improvement in the reproductive outcome after management of complete bicornuate uterus with hysteroscopy combined with laparoscopic metroplasty.

According to Kriplani et al. [35], uterine malformation is found in 6.7% of general population and 16.7% in women with RPL. There are only two case studies reported in literature of laparoscopic Strassman's metroplasty. Evidence shows an improvement in live birth rates from 3.7% to as high as 80% following abdominal metroplasty.

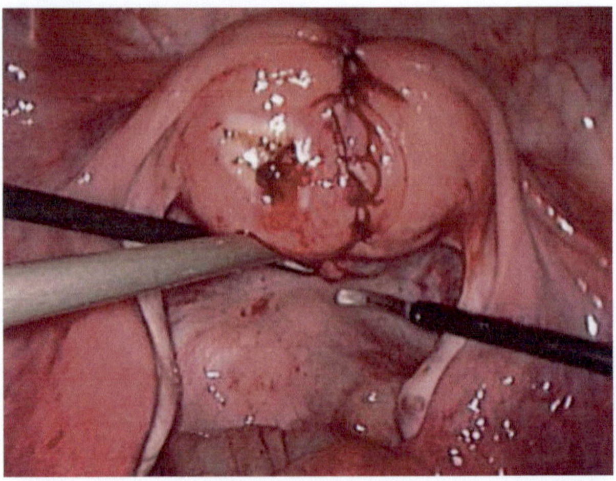

Fig. 30.11 Uterus after laparoscopic suturing

30.4 Endoscopic Cerclage in Cervical Incompetence

Cervical insufficiency is defined as recurrent painless cervical dilation that leads to three or more mid-trimester abortions in the absence of other causes. Cerclage helps to retain the cervical length and also forms the endocervical mucus plug which prevents ascending infection.

Cervical cerclage which was first performed in 1902 in women with a history of mid-trimester abortion can be done through vaginal or transabdominal, open or by minimal access surgery [36]. Cerclage can be applied during pregnancy or as an interval procedure irrespective of the fact whether the approach is open or laparoscopic.

There are many case reports describing cerclage placement with the da Vinci robotic system also [37–39].

30.4.1 Risk Factors for Cervical Insufficiency

- History of previous induced or spontaneous abortions
- Anomalies of the uterus
- Multiple gestation
- Previous preterm birth
- Prior cervical destructive surgery (i.e. trachelectomy, loop electrosurgical excision procedure [LEEP], laser conisation or cold-knife cone biopsy)
- In utero diethylstilbestrol (DES) exposure, though not so common now

30.4.2 Indications for Cerclage

Cerclage based on previous history: Cerclage is required in women with history of three or more second-trimester losses at 12–14 weeks gestation or preterm deliveries. Previous obstetric outcomes such as painless dilation of the cervix or other risk factors, such as cervical surgery, do not play a significant role in the decision to place a cerclage.

Women with significant history should have complete assessment with hysterography and cervical resistance index prior to placement of cerclage.

Ultrasound-indicated cerclage: Transvaginal ultrasound is recommended at 14–24 weeks of pregnancy in women with history of second-trimester losses or preterm delivery to see for cervical length.

If the cervical length is more than 25 mm even in the presence of cervical funnelling, cerclage is not indicated [40]. Funnelling as a part of cervical shortening has been confirmed in various studies, but its association with preterm birth is not clear [41, 42].

Rescue cerclage: This refers to application of cerclage in presence of dilated cervix with exposed foetal membranes in the vagina. It may be picked up during examination of the woman or on ultrasonography.

Rescue cerclage should be performed after evaluating the patient completely including the gestational age as the neonatal outcomes still remain poor.

Data on improvement in neonatal morbidity and mortality following rescue cerclage is limited. Insertion of a rescue cerclage helps to prolong pregnancy by another 4–5 weeks compared with expectant management or bed rest alone [36]. The chances of failure are high if the cervix is dilated >4 cm or the membranes are prolapsed till the external os.

30.4.3 Contraindications to Cerclage Insertion

- If the patient is already in preterm labour
- Chorioamnionitis
- Active vaginal bleeding
- Premature rupture of membranes
- Evidence of foetal compromise
- Foetal defect incompatible with life
- Intrauterine death of foetus

30.4.4 Preoperative Evaluation

1. An ultrasound scan in first trimester
2. Screening for aneuploidy to rule out lethal/major foetal abnormality
3. Maternal WBC count to rule out any infection

30.4.5 Operative Procedure

Transabdominal cerclage: Transabdominal cerclage is placing the suture at the cervicoisthmic junction via laparotomy, laparoscopically or robotically [43]. It can be considered in women with a previous failed transvaginal cerclage but is associated with increased maternal morbidity in this group of women.

Patient positioning and port placement: Laparoscopic placement of cerclage is done under general anaesthesia. The patient is placed in the modified dorsal lithotomy position, the bladder is catheterised and a uterine manipulator is inserted in non-pregnant patients. Generally, 10-mm port is placed at the umbilicus and 5-mm accessory trocars in the bilateral lower quadrants and left upper quadrant (Fig. 30.12).

- The vesicouterine peritoneum is dissected off the lower uterine segment using the Harmonic scalpel. This exposes the uterine vessels anteriorly on both sides.
- A 5-mm non-absorbable Mersilene polyester suture is introduced into the abdominal cavity.
- The needle is passed at the level of the internal cervical os poster-anteriorly medial to the uterine vessels. The needle is placed at a distance of 1.5 cm supe-

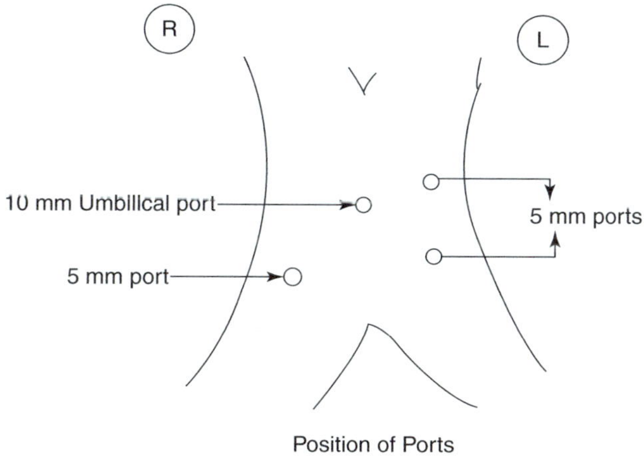

Fig. 30.12 Port placement

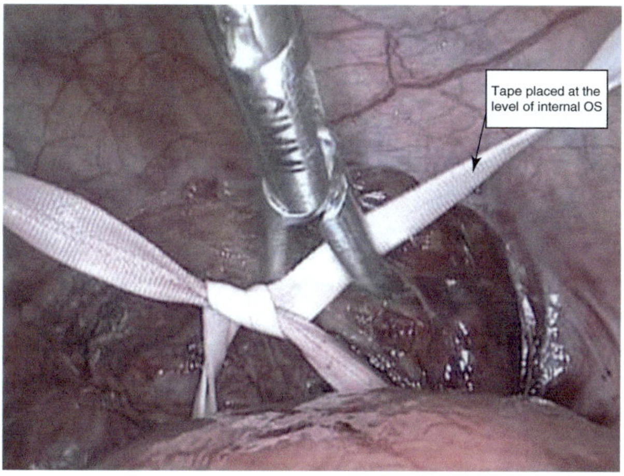

Fig. 30.13 Anterior placement of cervical cerclage

rior and 1 cm lateral to uterosacral ligament. The procedure is repeated on the other side also.

- After removing the needles, the Mersilene suture is tied around the cervix with six knots (Fig. 30.13).
- The vesicouterine peritoneum is then closed with running 2-0 suture over the laparoscopic cerclage.

30.4.5.1 Robotic Cerclage

Robot-assisted laparoscopic cerclage is another minimally invasive alternative to transvaginal or open transabdominal cerclage. 12-mm camera port is made through the umbilicus, with two ancillary 8-mm robotic ports and a 5-mm assistant port [44, 45].

One ¼-inch-width Mersilene tape is preloaded in the abdomen through the 12-mm port before docking and is parked on the right parietal peritoneum (Fig. 30.14). The rest of the procedure is the same as laparoscopic cerclage.

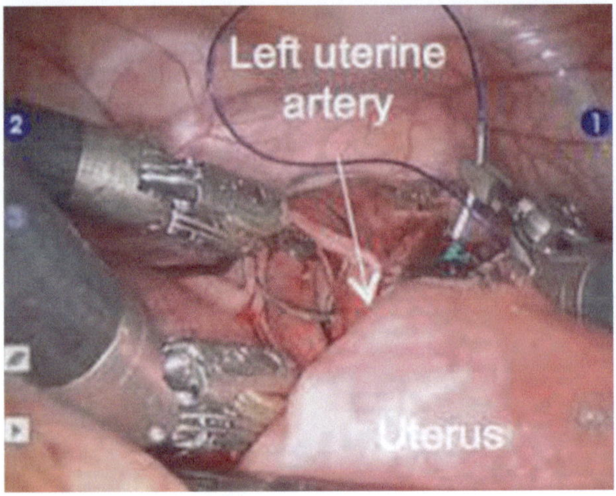

Fig. 30.14 Robotic cervical cerclage

30.4.6 Adjuvant Management

Bed rest, sexual abstinence, perioperative tocolysis and supplemental progesterone are not routinely recommended due to lack of convincing evidence; however, the decision should be individualised [40, 46].

30.4.7 Mode of Delivery

Caesarean section is required for all women with a transabdominal laparoscopic cerclage, and the abdominal suture may be left in place following the surgery. In case of delayed miscarriages and late intrauterine deaths, posterior colpotomy may be done; failing which laparotomy/hysterotomy/caesarean section may be required.

30.4.8 Disadvantages

It can lead to preterm delivery, premature rupture of membranes, haemorrhage, chorioamnionitis and injury to bowel or bladder.

30.4.9 Advantages [47]

- Best potential advantage is reuse in subsequent pregnancies
- Less failure rate: Live birth rates of 95% (19/20) and 83% (10/12) have been reported in 2 case series of 31 women (32 pregnancies) treated with laparoscopic cervical cerclage. The proportion of term deliveries was 70% and 67%, respectively. [43]

- Less chance of infection
- A minimal access approach has better surgical outcomes, is less expensive and is associated with low postoperative morbidity. According to two case series, complications in the form of uterine vessel injury have been reported as 33%, mean operating time varies between 50 and 60 minutes and mean blood loss was estimated to be less than 40 mL and less than 100 mL, respectively, in both the studies [43].

30.4.10 Outcomes Following Laparoscopic Cerclage Placement

Carter and associates [48] studied 12 women who underwent a laparoscopic cerclage placement between 2003 and 2008 and compared the data with retrospective study of seven women who had a transabdominal cerclage placed during the same time period. They found that both surgical approaches resulted in significantly improved foetal salvage rate (75% vs. 71%, respectively).

Whittle and colleagues [49] prospectively followed 65 patients who underwent laparoscopic cerclage between 2003 and 2008 and reported foetal salvage in 89% cases with mean gestational age of 35.8 ± 2.9 weeks. The complication rate was 10.7%; laparotomy had to be done in seven cases due to excessive bleeding or impaired surgical visibility; six patients developed chorioamnionitis. The authors concluded that the gestational age at delivery was independent of the timing of cerclage.

Burger and coworkers [50] undertook a review of literature comparing the outcomes of various routes of cerclage in which 31 eligible studies were selected. There were 135 patients in the laparoscopic group and 1116 patients in the transabdominal group which were analysed. Interval transabdominal approach had the highest foetal survival rate (94%), while the lowest rate (80.9%) was seen with laparoscopic cerclage placed during pregnancy. The rates of other complications like foetal loss, premature rupture of membranes and chorioamnionitis were similar between the groups. Laparoscopic cerclage was associated with reduced operative time, incidence of severe haemorrhage and hospital stay.

Laparoscopic cervical cerclage placement is an effective option for management of recurrent pregnancy loss. Laparoscopic approach has better obstetric and surgical outcomes, as suggested by several studies.

30.5 Submucous Fibroids

Uterine leiomyomas are the most common benign lesions seen in 20–25% of women in reproductive age group. They have been traditionally classified into submucosal, intramural and subserosal. The expanded FIGO classification [51] has a numbered system based on the position of fibroid.

The understanding of location of leiomyoma is important in view of the varied symptomatology. Most complications like abnormal uterine bleeding, dysmenorrhoea, infertility, pregnancy losses and complications during pregnancy leading to poor reproductive outcomes are seen with submucous fibroids and intramural fibroids with intracavitary component. This is so as they cause impaired gamete transport [52], impaired embryo implantation (low levels of HOXA 10,11 in the endometrium) [53], chronic endometrial inflammation, impaired endometrial blood supply, increased uterine contractility, glandular atrophy and impaired placentation and disruption [54].

30.5.1 Reproductive Outcomes with Submucous Fibroids

Infertility: Fibroids are found in 5–10% of infertile women, and the only abnormal finding in 1–2% of women presenting with infertility [55]. Submucous myomas and intramural myomas with intracavitary component have been implicated, and subserous fibroids are not found to be associated with infertility [56]. A meta-analysis comparing infertile women with or without myoma observed that submucosal and intramural fibroids with intracavitary component were associated with slightly decreased likelihood of pregnancy (RR 0.36, 95% CI 0.18–0.74) and increase in spontaneous abortions (RR 1.7, 95% CI 1.4–2.1) [57]. Myomectomy was seen to result in significant increase in conception rate with slight but not significant decrease in risk of miscarriage [54, 58].

Submucous fibroids also decrease the chances of success of IVF. According to a meta-analysis which included 19 studies, such fibroids decreased the live birth rate (RR 0.79) and clinical pregnancy rate (RR 0.85) [59].

30.5.1.1 Adverse Pregnancy Outcomes

Submucous fibroids are also seen to be associated with adverse pregnancy outcomes like first-trimester bleeding and miscarriage (0.6 OR, 95% CI 0.5–0.7), preterm labour (1.9 OR, CI 1.5–2.3), abruptio placentae (3.2 OR, 95% CI 2.6–4), placenta previa (2.3 OR, 95% CI 1.7–2.8), malpresentation (OR 2.9, 95% CI 2.6–3.2) and dysfunctional labour and caesarean delivery and PPH (OR 1.8, 95% CI 1.4–2.2) [60].

30.5.2 Diagnosis of Submucous Fibroids

1. Radiological investigations:
   - Transvaginal ultrasonography (TVS)
   - Saline infusion sonohysterography (SIS) and gel instillation Sonohysterography (GIS)
   - Magnetic resonance imaging (MRI)
   - HSG
2. Hysteroscopy

SIS and hysteroscopy are highly efficient and equivalent modalities for diagnosis and considered superior to TVS, as per high-quality evidence from Cochrane systematic review [61, 62].

Table 30.2 ESGE classification of submucous fibroids

Type of fibroid	Characteristics
Type 0	Fibroid is present totally within endometrial cavity. It does not have any myometrial extension
Type 1	Fibroid has less than 50% extension into the endometrial cavity
Type 2	Fibroid has more than 50% myometrial extension (sessile)

Table 30.3 Presurgical classification of submucous myoma

Score	Size	Topography	Extension of the base	Penetration	Lateral wall
0	<2	Low	<1/3	0	+1
1	2–5	Middle	1/3–2/3	<50%	
2	>5	Upper	>2/3	>50%	

0–4: Low complexity hysteroscopic myomectomy
5–6: High complexity hysteroscopic myomectomy. Can consider GnRH use or two-step hysteroscopic myomectomy
7–9: Hysteroscopic myomectomy not recommended; consider alternatives

30.5.3 Classification of Submucous Myomas

Two major classification systems [63, 64] of submucous fibroid are commonly used by clinicians to assess the treatment approach (Tables 30.2 and 30.3).

30.5.4 Hysteroscopic Myomectomy

The first reported hysteroscopic myomectomy was performed in 1976, by Neuwirth and Amin, using a urologic resectoscope, monopolar current and 32% dextran 70 distension medium [65]. Haleez in 1987 reported on the development of gynaecologic resectoscope [66]. There have been numerous advances in the instruments and techniques henceforth, and hysteroscopic myomectomy is considered as the standard minimally invasive surgical modality for treatment of submucous fibroids for abnormal uterine bleeding, infertility or pregnancy losses.

Various hysteroscopic techniques are:

1. Resectoscopic excision (TCRM)
2. Laser excision (Nd:YAG)
3. Laser ablation (Nd:YAG)
4. Morcellation by intrauterine morcellators (IUM)
5. Cold loop myomectomy: Mazzon's technique
6. Enucleation in toto: Litta's technique
   Lasmar's technique
7. Global endometrial ablation.
8. Others: Vapourising electrode
   Hydromassage technique, manual massage technique

30.5.5 Preoperative Assessment

Type of fibroid: Hysteroscopic myomectomy is preferred for Type 0,1 submucous fibroids (ESGE classification). Fibroids with >50% extension into the myometrium or with Lasmar's presurgical score ≥ 7 should be managed by other modalities [64]. For type 1 fibroids, the distance between the deepest extension of fibroid and serosa should be at least 5 mm, although there are no universally accepted limits of this thickness [67]. In some cases, type 2 fibroids require laparoscopic assistance. Depth of myometrial penetration correlates with volume of distension medium absorbed.

Fibroid size and number [68]: No exact guidelines are available, and this is largely guided by operator's surgical skills and knowledge of distension media. However, it is usually wise to counsel the patients about the probability of two-stage procedure and risks of perforation and fluid electrolyte imbalance in case of multiple myoma or myomas with size >4 cm.

Presence of other pelvic pathology: This helps to guide the route of surgery.

GnRH analogues [69]: GnRH agonists (11.75 mg i.m. thrice monthly) decrease the fibroid volume by ~40% and also help to correct preoperative anaemia. They lead to loss of tissue planes and are usually avoided by clinicians. The treatment is also associated with high costs and hypoestrogenic side effects. There have been no RCTs advocating or contradicting their use. However, some clinicians may prefer to use GnRH agonists in case of large fibroids for aforementioned reasons.

Serum progesterone receptor modulators (SPRMs) [70] like ulipristal acetate (5–10 mg/day for 3 months) and mifepristone have been shown to reduce fibroid volume; however, their use before hysteroscopic surgery and effect on outcome have not been studied so far.

Cervical preparation: Routine use of prostaglandins or mechanical dilators for cervical preparation before hysteroscopic surgery has not been conclusively proven in studies. A meta-analysis of six randomised controlled trials (RCTs) did not find definitive evidence to suggest their routine use. In a recent meta-analysis of 19 trials, women who had been treated with misoprostol required additional mechanical dilation much less than women treated with placebo or no intervention (odds ratio [OR] 0.08, 95% CI 0.04–0.16) or women treated with dinoprostone (OR 0.58, 95% CI 0.34–0.98 [71]. The complication rate was also less in the study group than those treated with placebo (OR 0.37, 95% CI 0.18–0.77) or those treated with dinoprostone (OR 0.32, 95% CI 0.12–0.83). Two hundred to four hundred micrograms of misoprostol can be given buccally or vaginally. The side effects are mild abdominal pain, vaginal bleeding and increased body temperature.

Intracervical vasopressin [72]: A well-designed RCT assessed the role of 20 mL diluted intracervical vasopressin (4 U in 80 mL) injected at 3 and 9 o'clock position of the cervix. It was shown to have significantly reduced the force of dilation with similar rates of cervical trauma. More studies are required on the use of vasopressin in this field.

30.5.6 Operative Procedure

30.5.6.1 Resectoscopic Excision by Wire Loop Electrode [73]

A resectoscope is an operating hysteroscope used to perform myomectomy under direct and constant visual control. It includes a telescope of outer diameter 3– 4 mm (0° straight or 12–30° fore oblique) and an internal and external sheath of 24–27 Fr outer diameter for continuous exchange of distension medium. It also has a working element for the attachment of electrosurgical and mechanical instruments. Electrosurgical system may be monopolar or bipolar with a U-shaped cutting loop electrode at the end. A nonconducting distension medium like 1.5% glycine or 5% sorbitol should be used with monopolar systems. Commonly used resectoscopes are Storz (26Fr, 0/12/30, monopolar and bipolar) (Fig. 30.15), Gynecare (27Fr, 12/30, bipolar), Olympus (0/12) and Wolf (30).

Transcervical resection of myoma (TCRM) is done by slicing, starting from the top and uniformly progressing to the base. The chips can be extracted out under visual control with a resectoscope, an ovum forceps or a curette. Some new resectoscopic instruments have an integrated chip aspirator (Wolf, Germany).

The operator should understand the difference between fibroid tissue and normal fasciculate myometrium to ensure adequate removal without increasing the risk of perforation and excess fluid absorption.

Shokeir T et al. [74] did a randomised controlled study in 2010, on the implications of submucous myoma on fertility. They included 215 women in the study and randomised them to undergo TCRM or diagnostic hysteroscopy with biopsy only. Conception rates in the treated group was 63% as compared to 28% in the group

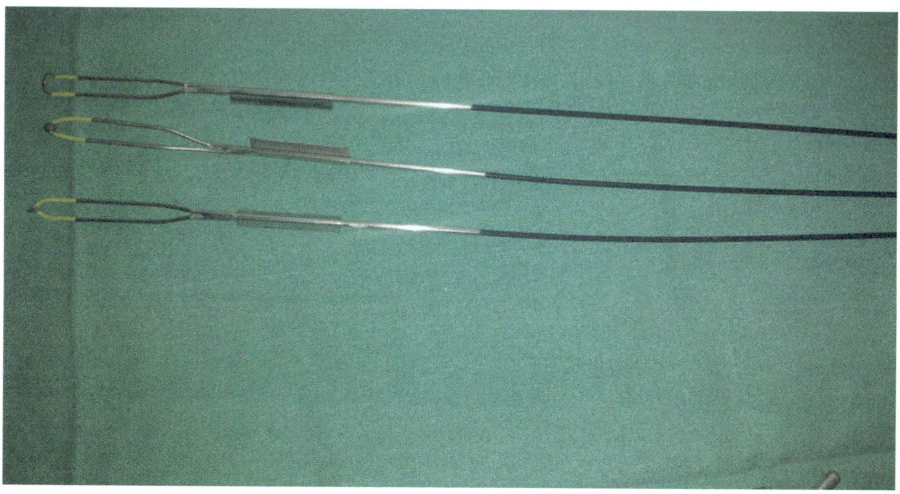

Fig. 30.15 Types of electrodes

who did not undergo any treatment. TCRM showed increase in fertility rates for type 0 and 1 myomas, but there was no difference in type 2 myomas.

Two-resectoscope technique: Hysteroscopic myomectomy using two resectoscopes was first described by Lin et al. in 2000 [75]. First a 7-mm resectoscope was used to cut the capsule of fibroid (to prevent sinking in) followed by its dissection from the muscular layer and shaving it off by using the 9-mm standard resectoscope.

30.5.6.2 Laser Excision/Ablation by Nd:YAG Laser [76]

Nd:YAG laser can also be used to coagulate the base of a pedunculated fibroid. Smaller fibroids ≤2 cm in diameter can also be ablated by coagulating the surface vessels and then repetitive dragging by touch technique till it is flattened. Disadvantages include complications like intrauterine infection, colicky pain, lack of specimen for pathologic evaluation and increased time and costs.

30.5.6.3 Vapourising Electrode [77]

The vapourising electrode is dragged along the surface in direction towards the operator, taking precaution that the electrode is not kept at a particular point for long. It operates at higher power density (120–220 W). The depth of vapourisation depends on duration of contact, resistance and power of generator. It is faster than resectoscopic surgery and has lesser blood loss. It should be avoided near cornua and isthmus due to thinner wall and increased risk of perforation. The disadvantages include lack of specimen for histopathological study and formation of gas bubbles which obscure the view. The bubbles get absorbed and dissipate quickly in blood. However, constant end tidal CO_2 monitoring is essential. It is recommended that a substantial portion of fibroid should be conserved for histology.

30.5.6.4 Morcellation by Intrauterine Morcellator

Hysteroscopic morcellator resolves the time-consuming process of chip extraction and enables tissue retrieval for histology. The first tissue removal system TRUCLEAR (Smith and Nephew, USA) was invented by Emanuel. Morcellator consists of two hollow metal tubes fitted into each other, and the inner tube is able to rotate within the outer one (Fig. 30.16). There is a control unit connected to handheld motor drive unit with morcellator. There is no electrocoagulation or lateral spread. Initial IUM consisted of 4-mm morcellator introduced into the uterus through 8–9-mm hysteroscope. Newer smaller diameter systems by Hologic (MYOSURE) and Storz are also available.

A retrospective comparison was conducted by Emanuel and Wamstekar [78] between this technique and conventional resectoscopy and found it faster than conventional, with a shorter learning curve.

It was developed by Mazzon [79] in 1995. The first step is excision of intracavitary component by slicing by repeated passages of monopolar cutting loop, till the level of plane of endometrial surface. In the second step, intramural component is enucleated by a blunt dissection cold loop, by inserting it between the fibroid and myometrium, using single tooth loop to hook and lacerate the connective tissue bridges. In the third step, the enucleated part is excised by usual excision methods.

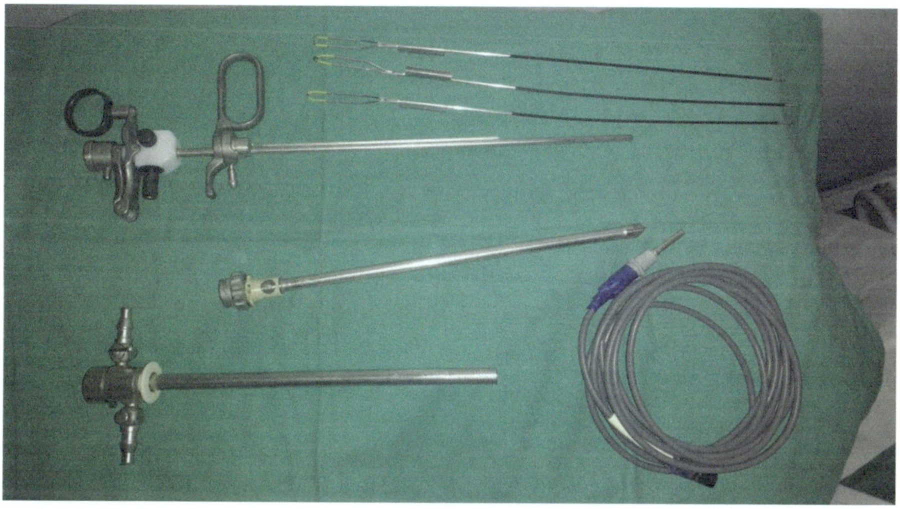

Fig. 30.16 Intrauterine morcellator

Advantages: The procedure is safe, preserves pseudocapsule, saves myometrial tissue, better healing, reduced complications, suitable for relatively large myomas and with safety margin <1 cm.

Disadvantage: Longer learning curve and experience.

30.5.6.5 Enucleation Methods

1. Litta's technique [80]: An electrode is used to give an elliptical incision on the endometrial mucosa, at the level of reflection on the uterine wall, and correct plane is entered, resecting the connecting bridges wherever required. The fibroid gets pushed into the cavity and can be then safely resected.
2. Lasmar's technique [81]: The endometrium is dissected around the fibroid using the electrode in the shape of L. The fibroid is mobilised and pushed to the cavity and bleeding vessels are coagulated.

30.5.6.6 Global Endometrial Ablation

Hydrothermal ablation system and microwave endometrial ablation are suitable for small fibroids and only in patients with AUB. This is not recommended for infertility patients.

30.5.7 Outcomes Following Hysteroscopic Myomectomy

Hysteroscopic myomectomy is a safe, efficient, minimally invasive surgery which can be offered to young women with submucous fibroids, who are trying to conceive. As per Cochrane review [82], 39% of women (95% CI 21–58%) will achieve a successful outcome following the hysteroscopic removal of the fibroids compared to 21% of women with fibroids having timed intercourse only.

30.6 Intrauterine Synechiae

It was first described by Heinrich Fritsch in 1894 and then further characterised by Asherman in 1948 wherein he described the radiologic appearance intrauterine adhesions at HSG. Asherman [83] in his study showed that if placental bits are retained for more than 24 h, adhesions develop in 40% of such women. It has been suggested that Asherman's syndrome potentially exists in a milder form in the asymptomatic eumenorrhoeic infertile woman [84].

Classically Asherman's syndrome is most commonly seen in secondary amenorrhoea following post abortion curettage though role of infection cannot be ruled out. There are no recommendations regarding the optimal treatment regimen for this condition, and treatment outcomes reported are generally poor [85–91].

30.6.1 Causes of Intrauterine Synechiae

1. Miscarriage or termination of pregnancy
2. Dilation and evacuation for retained products of conception
3. Prior surgery
4. Caesarean section
5. Childhood tuberculosis

30.6.2 Classification Systems

Many classification systems have been proposed. The European Society Hysteroscopic Staging and American Society for Reproductive Medicine classification have been described here (Table 30.4).

30.6.2.1 European Society Hysteroscopic Staging [92]

1. Thin or flimsy adhesions easily lysed with the tip of the scope.
2. Single firm adhesion not rupturable by the sheath of the hysteroscope. Bilateral tubal ostia are free.
3. Multiple firm adhesions or obscured single tubal ostia.
4. Extensive firm adhesions/agglutination of uterine walls/obscured bilateral ostia.

American Society for Reproductive Medicine (ASRM) [93] *system*: This is based on the amount of cavity obliterated, density of the adhesions and the menstrual pattern.

Table 30.4 ASRM classification of intrauterine synechiae

Feature	1 Score	2 Score	3 Score
Extent of cavity involved	<1/3	1/3–2/3	>2/3
Type of adhesions	Flimsy	Flimsy and dense	Dense
Menstrual pattern	Normal	Hypomenorrhoea/less bleeding	Amenorrhoea

30.6.2.2 Scores 1–4 (Mild Disease), 5–8 (Moderate Disease) and 9–12 (Severe Disease) (Figs. 30.17, 30.18, and 30.19)

Though successful pregnancies occur with small residual cavities, the risk of adverse obstetric outcomes is high in them. Tubal ostia patency is crucial for spontaneous pregnancies but can be overcome by in vitro fertilisation (IVF) when obstructed.

30.6.3 Preoperative Evaluation

Accurate preoperative evaluation is important to ensure the best operative outcomes.

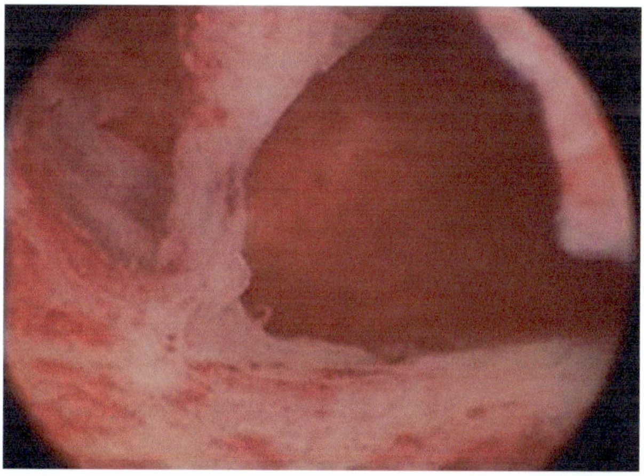

Fig. 30.17 Mild intrauterine synechiae

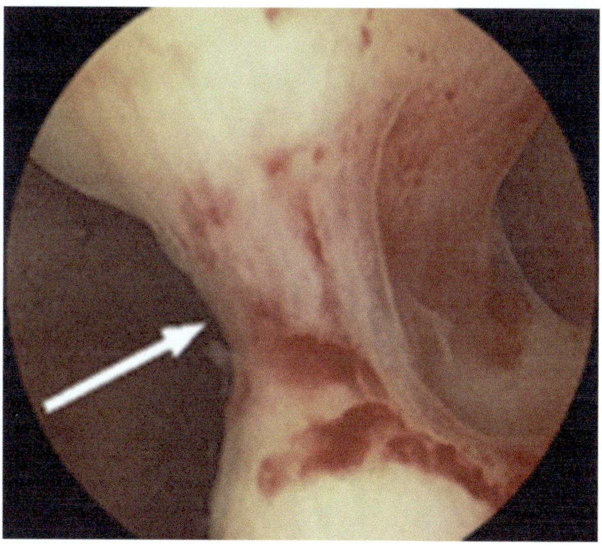

Fig. 30.18 Moderate intrauterine synechiae

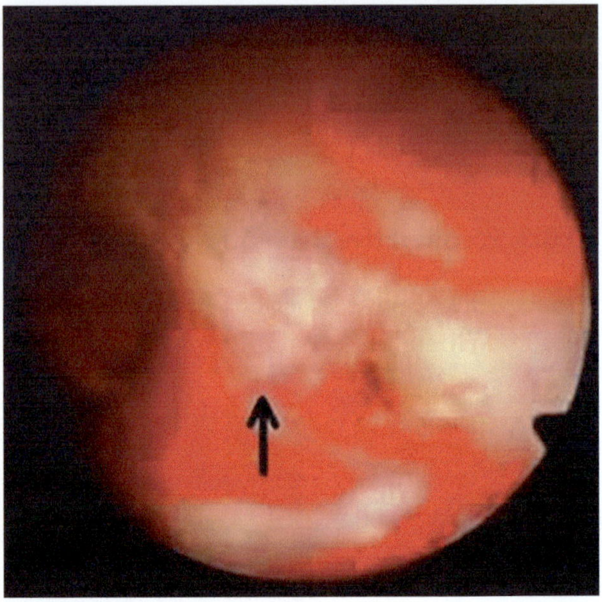

Fig. 30.19 Severe intrauterine synechiae

- 2-D sonohysterographic mapping
- 3-D coronal plane sonohysterographic mapping: Sonohysterography is best because it can assess cavity beyond the obstruction.
- USG pelvis—with particular attention to any signs of endometriosis on the ovaries. Uterus is evaluated for any signs of haematometra and thickness of endometrial stripe, presence of any irregularity or discontinuity of the stripe.

30.6.4 Operative Technique

- Simple localised flimsy avascular adhesions have been successfully treated by office hysteroscopy. Lysis of thick intrauterine adhesions are done under general anaesthesia.
- USG guidance can be used during this procedure to guide the operator in lysis of adhesions.
- The bladder is retrogradely filled up with saline, and an acoustic window is made before the procedure.
- During resection, continuous scan can be done in the mid-transverse and mid-sagittal planes. This enables resection in the midline and creation of false passage can be avoided.
- The dissection can be guided to islands of intact endometrium and also to the lateral limits of the scar. To prevent further adhesion formation, adhesiolysis is done using semiflexible microscissors without the use of intrauterine energy sources (Fig. 30.20).

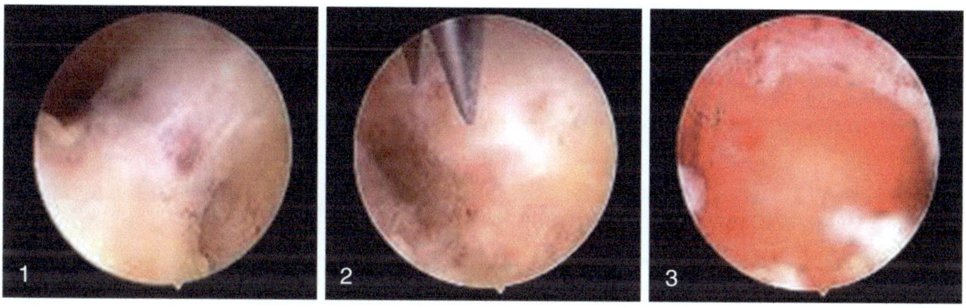

Fig. 30.20 Showing (1) intrauterine synechiae, (2) excision with cold hysteroscopic scissor, (3) uniform uterine cavity after excision of synechiae

30.6.5 Versa Point Bipolar System Versus Resectoscope [94]

Systems which utilise bipolar energy allow the use of saline as distending medium, decreasing the risk of fluid overload. Electrosurgery decreases bleeding by coagulation.

When dividing adhesions, however, the resectoscope loop may not be the appropriate electrode to use because it designed to resect rather than to selectively divide the adhesions centrally. Resectoscopic loop has been associated with formation of sacculations of the uterus, dehiscences and perforations. Resection has to be done carefully so as to prevent shaving off portions of the myometrium. This can be ensured by using knife or wires that can selectively be directed to the adhesions and divide them systematically. Energy sources may scatter energy and damage peripheral healthy endometrium. So specific electrodes and appropriate choice of cutting mode where possible, lowest effective power, and limited duration of exposure is used. In selected cases, concomitant laparoscopy or sonography may be useful. Thermal damage to surrounding organs with or without perforation is a risk.

30.6.6 Outcomes Following Hysteroscopic Synechiolysis

According to Thomson AJ et al. [95], using blunt and sharp dissection or electrosurgery, menstruation can be restored in >90% women and pregnancy rates of 50–60% can be achieved.

Deans R and Abott J [92] reported that none of the classification systems out of the seven which are described are validated. Medical management has no role in treatment of adhesions and hysteroscopy is the mainstay of both diagnosis and treatment. Special consideration should be given to prevention of recurrence.

In a study by Thomson AJ et al. [96], it has been noted out of the 60% of patients of Asherman's syndrome who were amenorrhoeic before treatment (13%

AFS Grade I, 43% AFS Grade II and 43% AFS Grade III), 96% had regular menses after surgery. The median number of procedures per patient was 1.5 (range, 1–6), and the mean length of the procedure was 42 min (range, 10–70 min). Fifty-three percent of women who attempted pregnancy after surgery were successful.

According to Cruz Orozco OP et al. [97], after evaluating the results of hysteroscopic adhesiolysis in Asherman's syndrome, they found that all 39 cases had normal menses after the first 3 months of surgery. The pregnancy rate after hysteroscopic treatment was 71.7% with a live birth rate of 28.2% of all cases (11/39). All were spontaneous conceptions, and a history of menstrual pattern before hysteroscopy was associated with perinatal success.

Roy K K et al. [98] in his study noted that of all the women included in the study, 64% patients had history of curettage on gravid uterus. After hysteroscopic adhesiolysis, the conception rate was 40.4%; it also varied with the severity of the disease being 58% in mild Asherman's syndrome, 30% in moderate and 33.3% in severe cases. The conception rate was much lower (10%) in women who did not resume their menses after surgery as compared to 44.3% in those who continued to have improved menstrual pattern. The live birth rate was 86.1% and miscarriage rate was 11.1%. The cumulative pregnancy rate was 97.2% and maximum patients conceived within 24 months. There was increased incidence (43.8%) of caesarean section, and four patients had PPH for adherent placenta.

Hysteroscopy is the gold standard for diagnosis and treatment of intrauterine synechia and can be used in restoring normal menstrual function and fertility for women with intrauterine adhesions.

30.7 Complications of Minimally Invasive Techniques

30.7.1 Operative Hysteroscopy

Operative hysteroscopy is associated with a complication rate of 0.8–2.6% [99].

30.7.1.1 Uterine Perforation

Small perforations can be managed conservatively by monitoring. Larger perforation can be managed by suturing. In case of injury caused by electrode, bowel needs to be checked by laparoscopy/laparotomy.

30.7.1.2 Excessive Bleeding

The most common reason is uterine perforation, which should be managed accordingly. Heavy bleeding may also occur if resection involves deep myometrial vessels. Cervical laceration (~1%) can also lead to bleeding. Electrocoagulation should be used judiciously. Preoperative misoprostol or intracervical vasopressin may be used for ease of cervical dilation. Intrauterine Foley catheter can be placed inside the cavity for a few hours. Uterine size should be well assessed and balloon should be inflated accordingly. Cervical laceration can be stitched by figure of eight suture.

30.7.1.3 **Fluid Overload** [100]

Amount of fluid absorbed depends on the patient characteristics, medical status, intrauterine pressure, depth of myometrial excision, surgical expertise, duration of surgery and type of distension medium used. Noncrystalloid media can cause serious imbalances, pulmonary oedema, cerebral oedema, cardiac failure and death. The distension media should hence be chosen wisely.

Prevention is the best management strategy. During the procedure, monitor saturation and input/output balance. If there is an overload of 1 L, monitor the patient for signs and symptoms of pulmonary oedema and send serial electrolyte level. But if the fluid deficit is more than 1.5 L, then the procedure needs to be abandoned.

With high-viscosity distending media, the maximum infused volume should not exceed 500 mL.

30.7.1.4 Uterine Synechiae

These can be managed by the following methods:

- Oestrogen therapy [96, 101]—Use of postoperative oestrogen therapy (oral 2.5 mg conjugated equine oestrogen with or without progestin for two or three cycles) can help to prevent development of synechiae.
- IUD [102] can be used. IUDs which contain copper are not recommended because of their inflammatory properties. An inert loop IUD (e.g. Lippes loop) can be used although it is no longer available in many areas.
- Intrauterine placement of Foley catheter [103]—Placing a Foley catheter for 24–48 h after surgery acts as a physical intrauterine barrier, thereby preventing intrauterine synechiae.
- Intrauterine auto-cross-linked hyaluronic acid gel [104]—Hyaluronic acid gel which is a natural component of the extracellular matrix and vitreous humour has anti-adhesive properties which depend on its molecular weight as well as concentration of the preparation.

30.7.1.5 Creation of false passage

Stop the procedure or do it under USG guidance. Preoperative oestrogen can be given to increase endometrial thickness.

30.7.1.6 Delayed Complication

- Amenorrhoea
- Hypomenorrhoea
- Recurrent synechia formation
- Infertility
- Early pregnancy loss
- Sepsis.

Role of antibiotics: Risk of infection with operative hysteroscopy has been found to be as low as 0.01–1.4% [105]. Routine use of antibiotics is not recommended for diagnostic or therapeutic hysteroscopy [106]. However, many surgeons use antibiotic therapy due to theoretical risk of secondary infection.

30.7.2 Laparoscopic/Robotic Surgery

The overall complication rate with laparoscopy ranges from 0.2 to 10.3% [107]. The general complications associated with minimal access surgeries are abdominal wall vascular injury (0.5%) [107], intestinal injury (0–0.5%) [107], bladder injury (0.02–8.3%) [108], ureteral injury (0.025–2%) [109], major vascular injuries (0.04–0.5%) [110], sepsis, etc. Entry-related injuries constitute 50% [107] of the injuries related to laparoscopic procedures. These can be prevented to a large extent by adhering to the correct surgical principles and techniques.

Mesh erosion: There have been reports of erosion of the Mersilene tape through the lower uterine segment [111]. Though it has been suggested that propylene mesh is a better alternative to the traditional Mersilene tape [49, 112], yet more studies are needed to confirm the effectiveness and safety of this approach. A Prolene suture can also be used instead of the Mersilene tape [113, 114].

Scar rupture: This has been reported after hysteroscopic septal resection, myomectomy and metroplasty. The incidence is 1–2.7% for hysteroscopic septal resection [115]. Congenital uterine anomalies, number and type of previous surgeries, intraoperative use of monopolar and uterine perforation are the factors associated with risk of rupture in subsequent pregnancy. Good endoscopic suturing skills, and optimal dead space obliteration can ensure a better scar formation, reducing the risk. However, there is no uniform follow-up protocol that reduces perinatal risk in these patients. The patients should be well counselled and informed about the signs and symptoms of rupture during pregnancy, i.e. pain and significant bleeding per vaginum. Patient should ideally have an elective LSCS at term, especially if the cavity was opened.

Morbid adherent placenta: Like caesarean section, uterine surgeries like synechiolysis, septal resection, myomectomy and metroplasty are also associated with risk of morbid adherent placenta, i.e. placenta accreta, increta and percreta, and one should take a detailed history to exclude positive past history. Ultrasound can be a diagnostic modality but MRI is superior to assess the extent of invasion. The pregnancy should be monitored at a tertiary care centre with a multidisciplinary team approach.

Key Points

- Septate uterus is associated with the worst reproductive outcome and is most amenable to hysteroscopic correction.
- Metroplasty for bicornuate uterus has been seen to result in successful pregnancy 65–85%. However, 59.5% of the patients can have a successful subsequent pregnancy without surgery also.

- Laparoscopic metroplasty is better than abdominal metroplasty as it helps in decreasing prevalence of adhesion formation, reducing tissue handling and reducing blood loss during surgery and improving pregnancy outcome.
- An ultrasound-indicated cerclage is not recommended even when funnelling is present in the absence of cervical shortening to 25 mm or less.
- Hysteroscopic myomectomy is preferred for Type 0,1 submucous fibroids (ESGE classification).
- Risk of infection with operative hysteroscopy has been found to be as low as 0.01–1.4%.
- SIS and hysteroscopy both are highly efficient modalities for diagnosis of intrauterine adhesions and are considered superior to TVS.
- Patient should be well counselled about the risk of scar rupture and morbidly adherent placenta, after synechiolysis, myomectomy and metroplasty.

References

1. Practice Committee of the American Society for Reproductive Medicine. Definitions of infertility and recurrent pregnancy loss: a committee opinion. Fertil Steril. 2013;99(1):63.
2. Chan YY, Jayaprakasan K, Tan A, Thornton JG, Coomarasamy A, Raine-Fenning NJ. Reproductive outcomes in women with congenital uterine anomalies: a systematic review. Ultrasound Obstet Gynecol. 2011;38(4):371–82.
3. Grimbizis GF, Camus M, Tarlatzis BC, Bontis JN, Devroey P. Clinical implications of uterine malformations and hysteroscopic treatment results. Hum Reprod Update. 2001;7:161–74. 43.
4. Salim R, Regan L, Woelfer B, Backos M, Jurkovic D. A comparative study of the morphology of congenital uterine anomalies in women with and without a history of recurrent first trimester miscarriage. Hum Reprod. 2003;18:162–6.
5. Homer HA, Li TC, Cooke ID. The septate uterus: a review of management and reproductive outcome. Fertil Steril. 2000;73:1–14.
6. Raga F, Bauset C, Remohi J, et al. Reproductive impact of congenital Müllerian anomalies. Hum Reprod. 1997;12:2277–81.
7. Salim R, Regan L, Woelfer B, et al. A comparative study of the morphology of congenital uterine anomalies in women with and without a history of recurrent first trimester miscarriage. Hum Reprod. 2003;18:162–6.
8. Assaf A, Serour G, Elkady A, el Agizy H. Endoscopic management of the intrauterine septum. Int J Gynaecol Obstet. 1990;32:43–51.
9. Braun P, Grau FV, Pons RM, Enguix DP. Is hysterosalpingography able to diagnose all uterine malformations correctly? A retrospective study. Eur J Radiol. 2005;53:274–9.
10. Saravelos SH, Cocksedge KA, Li TC. The pattern of pregnancy loss in women with congenital uterine anomalies and recurrent miscarriage. Reprod Biomed Online. 2010;20:416–22.
11. Sheth SS, Sonkawde R. Uterine septum misdiagnosed on hysterosalpingogram. Int J Gynaecol Obstet. 2000;69:261–3.
12. Ludwin A, Pityński K, Ludwin I, Banas T, Knafel A. Two- and three-dimensional ultrasonography and sonohysterography versus hysteroscopy with laparoscopy in the differential diagnosis of septate, bicornuate, and arcuate uteri. J Minim Invasive Gynecol. 2013;20:90–9.

13. Moini A, Mohammadi S, Hosseini R, Eslami B, Ahmadi F. Accuracy of 3-dimensional sonography for diagnosis and classification of congenital uterine anomalies. J Ultrasound Med. 2013;32:923–7.
14. Mueller GC, Hussain HK, Smith YR, Quint EH, Carlos RC, Johnson TD, et al. Müllerian duct anomalies: comparison of MRI diagnosis and clinical diagnosis. AJR Am J Roentgenol. 2007;189:1294–302.
15. Acién P. Reproductive performance of women with uterine malformations. Hum Reprod. 1993;8:122–6.
16. Tomaževič T, Ban-Frangež H, Virant-Klun I, Verdenik I, Požlep B, Vrtačnik-Bokal E. Septate, subseptate and arcuate uterus decrease pregnancy and live birth rates in IVF/ICSI. Reprod Biomed Online. 2010;21:700–5.
17. Raga F, Bauset C, Remohi J, Bonilla-Musoles F, Simón C, Pellicer A. Reproductive impact of congenital Müllerian anomalies. Hum Reprod. 1997;12:2277–81.
18. Shuiqing M, Xuming B, Jinghe L. Pregnancy and its outcome in women with malformed uterus. Chin Med Sci J. 2002;17:242–5.
19. Kupesic S, Kurjak A. Septate uterus: detection and prediction of obstetrical complications by different forms of ultrasonography. J Ultrasound Med. 1998;17:631–6.
20. Kupesić S, Kurjak A, Skenderovic S, Bjelos D. Screening for uterine abnormalities by three-dimensional ultrasound improves perinatal outcome. J Perinat Med. 2002;30:9–17.
21. Uterine septum: a guideline. Fertil Steril. 2016.
22. ACOG technology assessment in obstetrics and gynecology, number 4, August 2005: hysteroscopy. Obstet Gynecol 2005;106:439–42.
23. Karande VC, Gleicher N. Resection of uterine septum using gynaecoradiological techniques. Hum Reprod. 1999;14:1226–9.
24. Wang S, Shi X, Hua X, Gu X, Yang D. Hysteroscopic transcervical resection of uterine septum. JSLS. 2013;17(4):517–20.
25. Fedele L, Bianchi S, Marchini M, Mezzopane R, et al. Residual uterine septum of less than 1 cm after hysteroscopic metroplasty does not impair reproductive outcome. Hum Reprod. 1996;11:727–9.
26. Yang JH, Chen MJ, Chen CD, Chen SU, Ho HN, Yang YS. Optimal waiting period for subsequent fertility treatment after various hysteroscopic surgeries. Fertil Steril. 2013;99:2092–2096.e3.
27. Grimbizis GF, Gordts S, Di Spiezio Sardo A, Brucker S, De Angelis C, et al. The ESHRE/ESGE consensus on the classification of female genital tract congenital anomalies. Hum Reprod. 2013;28(8):2032–44.
28. Alborzi S, Asadi N, Zolghadri J, Alborzi S, Alborzi M. Laparoscopic metroplasty in bicornuate and didelphic uteri. Fertil Steril. 2009;92(1):352–5.
29. Woelfer B, Salim R, Banerjee S, Elson J, Regan L, Jurkovic D. Reproductive outcomes in women with congenital uterine anomalies detected by three-dimensional ultrasound screening. Obstet Gynecol. 2001;98:1099–103.
30. Sugiura-Ogasawara M, Ozaki Y, Katano K, Suzumori N, Mizutani E. Uterine anomaly and recurrent pregnancy loss. Semin Reprod Med. 2011;29(6):514–21.
31. Sinha R, Mahajan C, Hegde A, Shukla A. Laparoscopic metroplasty for bicornuate uterus. J Minim Invasive Gynecol. 2006;13:70–3.
32. Roger P. Smith MD. Chapter 120. Uterine anomalies: bicornuate, septate, and unicornuate uterus. In: Netter's obstetrics and gynecology; 2008. p. 300–2.
33. Dewan KA, Hefeda MM, ElKholy DG. Septate or bicornuate uterus: Accuracy of three-dimensional trans-vaginal ultrasonography and pelvic magnetic resonance imaging. Egypt J Radiol Nucl Med. 2014;45(3):987–95.
34. Xia E, Liu Y, Huang X, Zheng J, Yu D, Ma NM, Li Y, Qu J. Hysteroscopy combined with laparoscopic metroplasty for the treatment of complete bicornuate uterus—two cases report. J Minim Invasive Gynecol. 2010;17(6):S119.
35. Kriplani A, Kachhawa G, Wangdi T, Menon RP. Laparoscopic Strassman's metroplasty for bicornuate uterus. J Minim Invasive Gynecol. 2013;20(6):S186.

36. Ludmir J, Owen J and Berghella V. Chapter 28. Obstetrics: normal and problem pregnancies, 7th ed. 2016. p. 595–614.e1.
37. Wolfe L, DePasquale S, Adair CD, et al. Robotic assisted laparoscopic placement of transabdominal cerclage during pregnancy. Am J Perinatol. 2008;25:653–5.
38. Barmat L, Glaser G, Davis G, Craparo F. Da Vinci-assisted abdominal cerclage. Fertil Steril. 2007;88:1437.e1–3.
39. Fechner AJ, Alvarez M, Smith DH, Al-Khan A. Robotic-assisted laparoscopic cerclage in a pregnant patient. Am J Obstet Gynecol. 2009;200:e10–1.
40. Green-top Guideline No. 60. Cervical cerclage. May 2011.
41. To MS, Skentou C, Liao AW, Cacho A, Nicolaides KH. Cervical length and funneling at 23 weeks of gestation in the prediction of spontaneous early preterm delivery. Ultrasound Obstet Gynecol. 2001;18:200–3.
42. Benson RC, Durfee RB. Transabdominal cervico uterine cerclage during pregnancy for the treatment of cervical incompetency. Obstet Gynecol. 1965;25:145–55.
43. NICE Guideline. Laparoscopic cerclage for prevention of recurrent pregnancy loss due to cervical incompetence (IPG228).
44. Gungor M, Ozbasli E, Kahraman K, Genim C. Robotic cerclage performed for cervical insufficiency. J Minim Invasive Gynecol. 2014;21(6):S226.
45. Moawad GN, Abi Khalil ED, Samuel D. Robotic cerclage in advanced-stage endometriosis. J Minim Invasive Gynecol. 2016. pii: S1553-4650(16)30065-6.
46. Tusheva OA, Cohen SL, McElrath TF, Einarsson JI. Laparoscopic placement of cervical cerclage. Rev Obstet Gynecol. 2012;5(3–4):e158–65.
47. Owen J, Hankins G, Iams JD, Berghella V, Sheffield JS, PerezDelboy A, et al. Multicenter randomized trial of cerclage for preterm birth prevention in high-risk women with shortened midtrimester cervical length. Am J Obstet Gynecol. 2009;201:375.e1–8.
48. Carter JF, Soper DE, Goetzl LM, Van Dorsten JP. Abdominal cerclage for the treatment of recurrent cervical insufficiency: laparoscopy or laparotomy? Am J Obstet Gynecol. 2009;201:111.e1–4.
49. Whittle WL, Singh SS, Allen L, et al. Laparoscopic cervico-isthmic cerclage: surgical technique and obstetric outcomes. Am J Obstet Gynecol. 2009;201:364.e1–7.
50. Burger NB, Brölmann HA, Einarsson JI, et al. Effectiveness of abdominal cerclage placed via laparotomy or laparoscopy: systematic review. J Minim Invasive Gynecol. 2011;18:696–704.
51. Munro MG, Critchley HO, Broder MS, Fraser IS, FIGO Working Group on Menstrual Disorders. FIGO classification system (PALM-COEIN) for causes of abnormal uterine bleeding in nongravid women of reproductive age. Int J Gynaecol Obstet. 2011;113(1):3–13.
52. Orisaka M, Kurokawa T, Shukunami K, et al. A comparison of uterine peristalsis in women with normal uteri and uterine leiomyoma by cine magnetic resonance imaging. Eur J Obstet Gynecol Reprod Biol. 2007;135:111.
53. Rackow BW, Taylor HS. Submucosal uterine leiomyomas have a global effect on molecular determinants of endometrial receptivity. Fertil Steril. 2010;93:2027–34 (L).
54. Casini ML, Rossi F, Agostini R, Unfer V. Effects of the position of fibroids on fertility. Gynecol Endocrinol. 2006;22:106.
55. Buttram VC Jr, Reiter RC. Uterine leiomyomata: etiology, symptomatology, and management. Fertil Steril. 1981;36:433–45 (R).
56. Donnez J, Jadoul P. What are the implications of myomas on fertility? A need for a debate? Hum Reprod. 2002;17:1424–30 (III).
57. Pritts EA, Parker WH, Olive DL. Fibroids and infertility: an updated systematic review of the evidence. Fertil Steril. 2009;91:1215.
58. Bernard G, Darai E, Poncelet C, Benifla J-L, Madelenet P. Fertility after hysteroscopic myomectomy: effect of intramural fibroids associated. Eur J Obstetr Gynaecol Reprod Biol. 2000;88:85–90.
59. Sunkara SK, Khairy M, El. Toukhy T, et al. The effect of intramural fibroids without uterine cavity involvement on the outcome of IVF treatment: a systematic review and meta-analysis. Hum Reprod. 2010;25(2):418–29.

60. Klatsky PC, Tran ND, Caughey AB, et al. Fibroids and reproductive outcomes: a systematic literature review from conception to delivery. Am J Obstet Gynecol. 2008;198:357.
61. Cepni I, Ocal P, Erkan S, et al. Comparison of transvaginal sonography, saline infusion sonography and hysteroscopy in the evaluation of uterine cavity pathologies. *Aust N Z J Obstet Gynaecol*. 2005;45:30–5.
62. Nieuwenhuis LL, Hermans FJR, Bij de Vaate A, Leeflang MMG, Brölmann HAM, Mol BJ, Clark T, Huirne JAF. Three-dimensional saline infusion sonohysterography for the diagnosis of focal intracavitary lesions. Cochrane Database Syst Rev. 2014;(6): Art. No.: CD011126.
63. Wamsteker K, Emanuel MH, de Kruif JH. Transcervical hysteroscopic resection of submucous fibroids for abnormal uterine bleeding: results regarding the degree of intramural extension. Obstet Gynecol. 1993;82:736–40 (II-2).
64. Lasmar RB, Barrozo PR, Dias R, Oliveira MA. Submucous myomas: a new presurgical classification to evaluate the viability of hysteroscopic surgical treatment–preliminary report. J Minim Invasive Gynecol. 2005;12:308–11 (II-2).
65. Neuwirth RS, Amin HK. Excision of submucus fibroids with hysteroscopic control. Am J Obstet Gynecol. 1976;126:95–9.
66. Hallez JP. Single-stage total hysteroscopic myomectomies: indications, techniques, and results. Fertil Steril. 1995;63:703–8.
67. Emanuel MH. Hysteroscopy and the treatment of uterine fibroids. Best Pract Res Clin Obstet Gynaecol. 2015;29(7):920–9.
68. Hart R, Molnár BG, Magos A. Long term follow up of hysteroscopic myomectomy assessed by survival analysis. Br J Obstet Gynaecol. 1999;106:700.
69. Campo S, Campo V, Gambadauro P. Short-term and long-term results of resectoscopic myomectomy with and without pretreatment with GnRH analogs in premenopausal women. *Acta Obstet Gynecol Scand*. 2005;84:756–60.
70. Donnez J, Tatarchuk TF, Bouchard P, Puscasiu L, Zakharenko NF, Ivanova T, et al. Ulipristal acetate versus placebo for fibroid treatment before surgery. N Engl J Med. 2012;366:409–20.
71. Al-Fozan H, Firwana B, Al Kadri H, et al. Preoperative ripening of the cervix before operative hysteroscopy. Cochrane Database Syst Rev. 2015;(4):CD005998.
72. Phillips DR, Nathanson HG, Milim SJ, Haselkorn JS. The effect of dilute vasopressin solution on the force needed for cervical dilatation: a randomized controlled trial. Obstet Gynecol. 1997;89:507.
73. Sardo AD, Mazzon I, Bramante S, Bettocchi S, Bifulco G, Guida M, Nappi C. Hysteroscopic myomectomy: a comprehensive review of surgical techniques. Hum Reprod Update. 2008;14(2):101–19.
74. Shokeir T, El-Shafei M, Yousef H, Allam AF, Sadek E. Submucous myomas and their implications in the pregnancy rates of patients with otherwise unexplained primary infertility undergoing hysteroscopic myomectomy: a randomized matched control study. Fertil Steril. 2010;94(2):724–9.
75. Lin B, Akiba Y, Iwata Y. One-step hysteroscopic removal of sinking submucous fibroid in two infertile patients. Fertil Steril. 2000;74:1035–8.
76. Smets M, Nisolle M, Bassil S, Donnez J. Expansive benign lesions: treatment by laser. Eur J Obstet Gynecol Reprod Biol. 1996;65:101–5.
77. Glasser MH. Endometrial ablation and hysteroscopic myomectomy by electrosurgical vaporization. J Am Assoc Gynecol Laparosc. 1997;4:369–74.
78. Emanuel MH, Wamsteker K. The Intra Uterine Morcellator: a new hysteroscopic operating technique to remove intrauterine polyps and fibroids. J Minim Invasive Gynecol. 2005;12:62–6.
79. Mazzon I. Nuova tecnica per la miometomia isteroscopica: enucleazione con ansa fredda. In: Cittadini E, Perino A, Angiolillio M, Minelli L, editors. Testo-Atlante di Chirurgia Endoscopica Ginecologica. Palermo, Italy: COFESE Ed; 1995. cap XXXIIIb.
80. Litta P, Vasile C, Merlin F, Pozzan C, Sacco G, Gravila P, et al. A new technique of hysteroscopic myomectomy with enucleation in toto. J Am Assoc Gynecol Laparosc. 2003;10:263–70.

81. Lasmar RB, Barrozo PR. Histeroscopia: uma abordagem pràtica, vol. 1. Rio de Janeiro: Medsi; 2002. p. 121–42.
82. Bosteels J, Kasius J, Weyers S, Broekmans FJ, Mol BJ, D'Hooghe TM. Hysteroscopy for treating subfertility associated with suspected major uterine cavity abnormalities. Cochrane Database Syst Rev. 2015;(2): Art. No.: CD009461.
83. Westdorp IC, Ankum WM, Mol BW, Vonk J. Prevalence of Asherman's syndrome after secondary removal of placental remnants or a repeat curettage for incomplete abortion. Hum Reprod. 1998;13(12):3347–50.
84. Palter S, Coad J, Slayden O. Global endometrial dysfunction secondary to scarring cervix and lower uterine segment only: A new form of uterine infertility?—Clinical and non human primate model evidence. J Minim Invasive Gynecol. 2006;13:S52.
85. Capella-Allouc S, Morsad F, Rongieres-Bertrand C, et al. Hysteroscopic treatment of severe Asherman's syndrome and subsequent fertility. Hum Reprod. 1999;14:1230–3.
86. Fernandez H, Al-Najjar F, Chaureaud-Lambling A, et al. Fertility after treatment of Asherman's syndrome stage 3 and 4. J Minim Invasive Gynecol. 2006;13:398–402.
87. Ismajovich B, Lidor A, Confino E, David MP. Treatment of minimal and moderate intrauterine adhesions (Asherman's syndrome). J Reprod Med. 1985;30:769–72.
88. Katz Z, Ben-Arie A, Lurie S, Manor M, Insler V. Reproductive outcome following hysteroscopic adhesiolysis in Asherman's syndrome. Int J Fertile Menopausal Stud. 1996;41:462–5.
89. Klein SM, Garcia CR. Asherman's syndrome: a critique and current review. Fertil Steril. 1973;24:772–35.
90. March CM, Israel R. Intrauterine adhesions secondary to elective abortion. Hysteroscopic diagnosis and management. Obstet Gynecol. 1976;48:422–4.
91. March CM, Israel R, March AD. Hysteroscopic management of intrauterine adhesions. Am J Obstet Gynecol. 1978;130:653–7.
92. Deans R, Abbott J. Review of intrauterine adhesions. J Minim Invasive Gynecol. 2010;17(5):555–69.
93. The American Fertility Society classification of adnexal adhesions, distal tubal occlusion, tubal occlusion secondary to tubal ligation, tubal pregnancies, Mullerian anomalies and intrauterine adhesions. Fertil Steril. 1988;49:944.
94. Friedman A, DeFazio J, DeCherney A. Severe obstetric complications after aggressive treatment of Asherman syndrome. Obstet Gynecol. 1986;67:864–7.
95. Thomson AJ, Abbott JA, Deans R, Kingston A, Vancaillie TG. The management of intrauterine synechiae. Curr Opin Obstet Gynecol. 2009;21(4):335–41.
96. Thomson AJ, Abbott JA, Deans R, Kingston A, Vancaillie TG. Fluoroscopically guided synechiolysis for patients with Asherman's syndrome: menstrual and fertility outcomes. Fertil Steril. 2007;87(2):405–10.
97. Cruz Orozco OP, Castellanos Barrosog G, Gavino Gavino F, De la Jara Diaz J, Garcia Vargas J, Roque Sanchez AM. Future reproductive ability in post treatment Asherman's syndrome patients. Ginecol Obstet Mex. 2012;80(6):389–93.
98. Roy KK, Baruah J, Sharma JB, Kumar S, Kachawa G, Singh N. Reproductive outcome following hysteroscopic adhesiolysis in patients with infertility due to Asherman's syndrome. Arch Gynecol Obstet. 2010;281(2):355–61.
99. Jansen FW, Vredevoogd CB, van Ulzen K, et al. Complications of hysteroscopy: a prospective, multicenter study. Obstet Gynecol. 2000;96:266.
100. American Association of Gynecologic Laparoscopists (AAGL). Advancing Minimally Invasive Gynecology Worldwide. AAGL practice report: practice guidelines for the diagnosis and management of submucous leiomyomas. J Minim Invasive Gynecol. 2012;19(2):152.
101. Kodaman PH, Arici A. Intra-uterine adhesions and fertility outcome: how to optimize success? Curr Opin Obstet Gynecol. 2007;19:207–14.
102. Vesce F, Jorizzo G, Bianciotto A, Gotti G. Use of intrauterine device in the management of secondary amenorrhea. Fertil Steril. 2000;73:162–5.
103. Orhue AA, Aziken ME, Igbefon JO. A comparison of two adjunctive treatments for intrauterine adhesions following lysis. Int J Gynecol Obstet. 2003;82:49–56.

104. Tsapanos VS, Stathopoulou LP, Papathanassopoulou VS, Tzingounis VA. The role of Seprafilm bioresorbable membrane in the prevention and therapy of endometrial synechiae. J Biomed Mater Res. 2002;63:10–4.
105. Agostini A, Cravello L, Shojai R, Ronda I, Roger V, Blanc B. Postoperative infection and surgical hysteroscopy. Fertil Steril. 2002;77:766–8 (II-2).
106. American College of Obstetrics and Gynecology Practice Bulletin 74: antibiotic prophylaxis for gynecologic procedures. Obstet Gynecol. 2006;108:225–34.
107. Magrina JF. Complications of laparoscopic surgery. *Clin Obstet Gynecol*. 2002;45:469–80.
108. Ostrzenski A, Ostrzenska KM. Bladder injury during laparoscopic surgery. *Obstet Gynecol Surv*. 1998;53:175–80.
109. Ostrzenski A, Radolinski B, Ostrzenska KM. A review of laparoscopic ureteral injury in pelvic surgery. *Obstet Gynecol Surv*. 2003;58:794–9.
110. Munro MG. Laparoscopic access: complications, technologies, and techniques. *Curr Opin Obstet Gynecol*. 2002;14:365–74.
111. Marx PD. Transabdominal cervicoisthmic cerclage: a review. Obstet Gynecol Surv. 1989;44:518–22.
112. Rust OA, Atlas RO, Jones KJ, et al. A randomized trial of cerclage versus no cerclage among patients with ultrasonographically detected second-trimester preterm dilatation of the internal os. Am J Obstet Gynecol. 2000;183:830–5.
113. Fechner AJ, Alvarez M, Smith DH, Al-Khan A. Robotic-assisted laparoscopic cerclage in a pregnant patient. Am J Obstet Gynecol. 2009;200:e10–1.
114. Groom KM, Jones BA, Edmonds DK, Bennett PR. Preconception transabdominal cervicoisthmic cerclage. Am J Obstet Gynecol. 2004;191:230–4.
115. Propst AM, Liberman RF, Harlow BL, Ginsburg ES. Complications of hysteroscopic surgery: predicting patients at risk. Obstet Gynecol. 2000;96:517–20.

31 Non-Pharmacological Methods for Management of RPL

Namita Grover, Manpreet Singh, and Swati Verma

31.1 Introduction

Today fertility is recognized as a disease by WHO and recurrent pregnancy loss as disordered fertility. Agony of childlessness and tragic plight of such couples has to be dealt with great sensitivity by us. Much has been discussed in the earlier chapters regarding etiopathogenesis, investigations, and pharmacological management. This chapter will discuss about non-pharmacological methods of dealing with this vexing issue in this chapter.

31.2 Non-pharmacological Methods for Prevention of RPL

1. Lifestyle modifications.
2. Healthy diet.
3. Supplements/herbs that strengthen the reproductive organs and help promote successful pregnancy.
4. Maintain hormonal balance.
5. Treat infections.
6. Alternative medicine such as Chinese medicine and Ayurveda.

N. Grover (✉) • S. Verma
Department of Obstetrics and Gynaecology, ESIC Model Hospital, Industrial Area II, Chandigarh, India
e-mail: namitagrover1@gmail.com

M. Singh
Department of Anaesthesia and Intensive Care, Govt. Medical College and Hospital, Chandigarh, India

S. Mehta, B. Gupta (eds.), *Recurrent Pregnancy Loss*,
https://doi.org/10.1007/978-981-10-7338-0_31

7. Complementary measures such as femoral massage, acupressure, acupuncture, and essential oils.
8. Meditation, yoga, and relaxation techniques to keep stress-free. Adopt a positive attitude and stay motivated.

31.3 Lifestyle Modifications

31.3.1 Maternal Age

The risk of miscarriages increases with increasing age in the general population. A large study conducted on 634,272 Danish women concluded that miscarriage rates in women of age 31–35 years and 36–39 years were almost same (38–40%) but increased to 70% in women above 40 years [1].

31.3.2 Periodontal Infection and RPL

Periodontal disease is one of the most common chronic infections with a prevalence of 10–60%. Recently, attention has been focused on relationship between periodontal infection and late miscarriage. Oral hygiene maintenance should become a part of routine antenatal care [2].

Antiphospholipid antibody syndrome is linked to RPL. In this context it is of interest to note that antiphospholipid antibody syndrome has been reported to disappear when *H. pylori* is eradicated [3].

31.3.3 Addictions: Alcohol, Caffeine, and Smoking

Links between RPL and occupational and environmental exposures have been suggested, and smoking, alcohol, and caffeine intake are particularly important as they are modifiable in nature [4].

There are studies showing that moderate alcohol intake (>3 drinks/week) leads to increased risk of pregnancy loss [5].

Cigarette smoking leads to nicotine ingestion which decreases placental blood flow because of its vasoconstrictor activity. Also, carbon monoxide, which is released during smoking, depletes both fetal and maternal oxygen supply. Tobacco chewing and smoking is to be discouraged entirely [6]. In males, smoking causes high concentrations of ROS which produces hydrogen peroxide and results in DNA damage. Cadmium and lead derived from cigarette smoke also lead to DNA injury by inducing double-stranded DNA breaks in sperm DNA. Cotinine, its major metabolite, is detected in the seminal plasma of smokers. DNA fragmentation has been implicated as a cause of RPL [7].

Large cohort study done by Weng et al. including 1063 patients demonstrated that caffeine consumption had a dose-dependent increase in the risk of miscarriage.

Caffeine increases estrogen levels. Women drinking more than four to five cups of coffee a day produce 70% more estrogen in follicular phase. Risk of miscarriage increased two times with caffeine intake of 200 mg/day [8].

Caffeine, even in amounts as low as three to five cups of coffee per day, may increase the risk of spontaneous pregnancy loss with a dose-dependent response [9].

31.3.4 Weight

Obesity has been shown to be an independent risk factor for first trimester miscarriages. Association is strongest in BMI>40. Exercising daily for 30 min, 5 days a week, helps in improving insulin sensitivity and increasing metabolism [10].

On the other hand, prepregnancy underweight women are 72% more likely to have a miscarriage in the first trimester, according to a study from the London School of Hygiene & Tropical Medicine [11].

Obesity has also been linked with male factor infertility as it may lead to abnormal semen parameters mainly due to hormonal aberrations and negative lifestyle factors [7].

31.3.5 Homocysteine Levels and RPL

Homocysteine is a demethylated derivative of methionine, and increased levels of homocysteine can occur with dietary or vitamin deficiency or reduced enzyme activities.

High homocysteine levels put a normal pregnancy at risk. Studies show that homocysteine levels higher than 10–10.7 μmol/L increased a woman's chance of a miscarriage by 38%. Its level can be decreased by taking folic acid, vit B6 and vit B12 [12, 13].

31.3.6 Male Factor

Male partners with normal semen parameters could have underlying genetic abnormalities in sperm DNA that can lead to RPL. DNA fragmentation index (DFI) and fluorescence in situ hybridization (FISH) are helpful tests for evaluating sperm aneuploidy . DNA fragmentation has been shown to be a robust indicator of fertility potential and reproductive outcome. However, it is not routinely assessed in semen analysis according to World Health Organization guidelines [14, 15]. It is still debated whether DNA fragmentation should become a part of the routine analysis in fertility investigation [16]. It is also strongly associated with recurrent pregnancy loss [17]. The most common cause of DNA fragmentation in spermatozoa is reactive oxygen species (ROS) and oxidative stress [18]. This may be an area where treatment is warranted in subfertility or ahead of proceeding to assisted reproduction treatment.

31.3.7 BPA

Bisphenol A (BPA) is a chemical used to manufacture certain plastics and epoxy resins. When plastics containing it are heated or stressed in any way, they break down allowing the chemical to mix into the food or water it is in contact with. BPA resembles hormones like adrenaline, testosterone, and estrogen, and even their small amounts can cause major hormonal imbalances. BPA binds to estrogen-related receptor γ (gamma) which activates transcription. ERR γ is found in high concentration in placenta explaining BPA accumulation in the placenta [19]. BPA via epigenetic mechanism suppresses DNA methylation and can detrimentally affect T-cell subsets, B-cell functions, dendritic cell and macrophage function, oligospermia, and both physical and mental aspects of sexuality [20, 21].

31.3.8 Other Factors

Use of NSAIDS [22], too much high-impact exercise [23], and physical or psychological stress all increase the risk of miscarriage (Table 31.1).

Table 31.1 Modifiable lifestyle factors

Lifestyle factor	Results	Recommendations
Smoking	Strong correlation with % DFI, DFI markedly higher in infertile smokers	Cessation of smoking
POP/PCB	Positive correlation between exposure and % DFI	PCB accumulate in food chain: avoid fatty fish, particularly farmed
Organophosphorus	Marked increase in % DFI (>30%) in exposed workers	Avoid pesticide exposure
Lead	Increase in percentage of spermatozoa with DNA fragmentation	Avoid occupational exposure and smoking or exposure to cigarette smoke
Bisphenol A	Significant trend of increased DNA damage with increased urinary bisphenol A concentration	Avoid plastic packaging, tinned foods, heating or storing foods in plastic
Testicular heat	Increase in DNA fragmentation and impaired spermatogenesis, with 2–3 °C temperature increase	Avoid cycling with tight pants, avoid sauna use, avoid using laptop on closed legs
Mobile phone radiation	Studies suggest DNA fragmentation, increased ROS, and decreased antioxidants (CAT, SOD, GPX)	Do not store mobile phone in trouser pocket
Obesity	Positive correlation of body mass index and DNA fragmentation, higher incidence in obese males	Weight loss through diet and moderate exercise

DFI DNA fragmentation index, *PCB* polychlorinated biphenyls, *ROS* reactive oxygen species

31.4 Influence of Diet on Reproductive Outcome

Nutrition plays a big role in enhancing fertility potential. Hormonal balance in our body is largely governed by our diet. Antioxidants help in combating the free radicals and protect the ovum and sperms.

31.4.1 Vegetables, Fruits, and Nuts

Vegetables, fruits, and nuts provide us with a gamut of antioxidants and micro- and macronutrients. Vegetables that are red or green in color are high in vitamin C, orange have high vitamin A, and white vegetables tend to have sulfur. Hence, eat a variety of colors daily. It is advisable to use butter or coconut oil when cooking dark leafy greens. If hypothyroid, try to eat your greens steamed. Lentils and beans are high in proteins, essential vitamins, and minerals including zinc, iron, and biotin.

Fruits may be taken raw or in the form of a fertility smoothie. Avocados balance hormones and are a rich source of therapeutic fats. Figs boost semen quality. Olives are high in antioxidants helping cell repair and regeneration.

Nuts are a rich source of antioxidants, zinc, vitamin E, proteins, and essential fatty acids.

31.4.2 Multivitamins and Minerals

Vitamin D is essential in synthesis of estrogen and progesterone which in turn also affects ovulation and hormonal balance. Food sources are eggs, fatty fish, dairy, and cod liver oil, but we need exposure to sunlight for 25–30 min per day.

Vitamin E which is an antioxidant helps to improve sperm number and motility.

Vitamin C improves hormone levels and increases fertility in women with luteal phase defects. In males, it improves sperm quality and motility and protects them from DNA damage, thus helping to reduce the chance of miscarriage and chromosomal damage [24].

It is found in guava bell peppers, broccoli, cranberries, cabbage, potatoes, tomatoes, amla, and other citrus fruits.

Vitamin B_6 regulates blood sugars, alleviates PMS, and is helpful in women with luteal phase defect. It is found in tuna, banana, spinach, turnip, cauliflower, and asparagus. Vitamin B_{12} improves sperm quality and quantity. It improves endometrial thickness which helps in implantation, thereby decreasing the chances of miscarriage. It also helps in ovulation and is found in oysters, liver, fish eggs, fish, cheese, and eggs.

Folic acid/folate is very important for pregnancy. It helps in prevention of neural tube defects and congenital heart defects. Deficiency in folic acid increases the risk of preterm labor, fetal growth restriction, and low birth weight and increases the homocysteine levels in the blood. This can lead to recurrent abortions and pregnancy complications, such as placental abruption and preeclampsia. Food sources of folate are liver, lentils, beans, asparagus, spinach, kidney beans, and collard greens.

Selenium, because of its antioxidant property, helps to protect the ovum and sperms from free radical injury which is a cause of miscarriages and birth defects. Selenium is also necessary for spermiogenesis.

Zinc is important in more than 300 different enzymatic reactions in the body. It helps in cell division. Low levels of zinc have been linked to miscarriage in the early stages of a pregnancy. In males, it improves the count, morphology, function, and quality of sperm and decreases male factor infertility. Zinc is an integral element in the development of spermatozoa and DNA synthesis and an important antioxidant in seminal fluid [25–27].

Zinc is damaged by cooking, and so it is important to eat foods high in zinc in their raw forms.

31.4.3 Maca

Maca *(Lepidium meyenii)* is a rootlike cruciferous vegetable from the Andes of Peru.

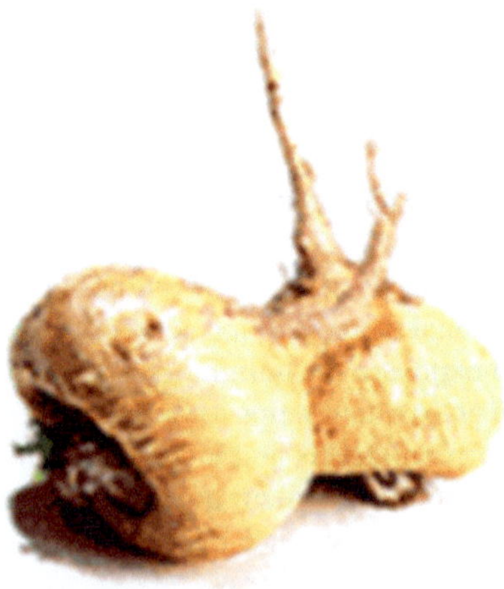

It has many phytonutrients and glucosinolates which influence fertility in both males and females. It affects the fertility of females by optimizing estrogen and progesterone levels and in males by increasing libido and sperm health [28].

31.4.4 Healthy Fats

Omega-3 fatty acids (DHA and EP) have been shown to help fertility by regulating hormones in the body, increasing cervical mucus, and promoting ovulation. Low levels of DHA lead to depression and other mental health issues [29].

Flax seeds, walnuts, and fish are important source of essential fatty acids.

31.4.5 Organic Food

Herbicides and pesticides decrease both male and female fertility. Organic vegetables and fruits have more nutritional value. Dairy which is not organic contains added hormones and antibiotics which lead to increased estrogen levels in the body. One should eat meat that is grass fed and organic as it is low in saturated fat and has high protein content.

31.4.6 Royal Jelly, Bee Pollen, and Bee Propolis for Fertility

Bees produce many substances, which have been found to have great health benefits. Apitherapy refers to the use of bee products (honey, propolis, bee pollen, and royal jelly) for enhancing fertility.

Royal jelly: Royal jelly is a substance that is secreted by worker bees' glands. It is rich in amino acids, lipids, sugars, some vitamins, fatty acids, and proteins. It also helps to balance hormones. A study has shown that royal jelly resembles estrogen and is helpful in women with low levels of this hormone [30].

Bee pollen: Bee pollen contains antioxidants, proteins, and minerals. It helps in improving immunity and fertility in both men and women [31].

Bee propolis: It is a resinous mixture of tree sap, buds, and tree leaves. It has anti-inflammatory properties and is useful in women with fibroids, endometriosis, and pelvic inflammatory disease (PID). A recent study documented improvement in infertility associated with endometriosis in women using propolis in dose of 500mg twice a day for 9 months [32].

31.5 Herbs and Reproductive Outcome

The following herbs have been found beneficial and should be started as close to the miscarriage as possible [33].

Angelica root (*Angelica archangelica*): It is a herb that increases circulation while supporting the nervous system, promoting relaxation, and reducing anxiety. It also improves immunity and general weakness.

Black cohosh root: Black cohosh has anti-inflammatory and antispasmodic action. It also promotes blood flow to the pelvic region and helps to tone the pelvic floor muscles.

Yarrow leaf/flower: It promotes circulation, relieves inflammation, and controls heavy bleeding. It is excellent for miscarriage recovery.

Vitex agnus-castus (also known as chaste tree berry): It regulates the hormonal balance by acting on hypothalamic-pituitary-ovarian axis.

Tribulus helps to cure irregular menstrual cycles and anovulation [34].

31.6 Other Non-pharmacological Methods

31.6.1 Fertility Massage

Fertility massage is a powerful, noninvasive type of natural fertility treatment which has been in use since hundreds of years. It can be used as a stand-alone treatment in the interconception period or as an adjunct with other forms of fertility treatment.

Benefits of Fertility Massage

- Increases blood circulation to pelvic organs.
- It breaks down pelvic adhesions and resolves ovarian cysts.
- Reduces dysmenorrhea and regulates menstrual cycle.

Timing: The best time for a fertility massage is during ovulatory phase (day 6–14). It should be avoided during the luteal phase as this would increase the risk of miscarriage in case implantation has occurred immediately postovulation.

Types of Fertility Massage

- Femoral fertility massage
- Acupressure fertility massage
- Reflexology massage

Femoral Fertility Massage

- Press the area between the thigh and lower abdomen with both thumbs as shown in Fig. 31.1.
- Hold down with fairly heavy pressure. The pressure should be so as to cease the blood flow for 30–40 s.

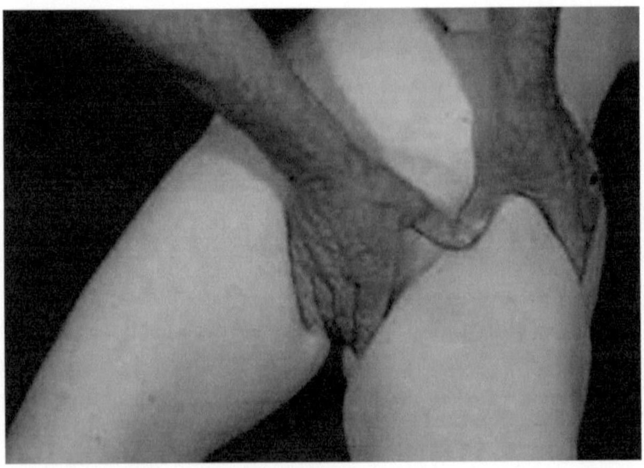

Fig. 31.1 Femoral fertility massage technique

- This pressure helps to push the blood back into the pelvic region, thereby increasing circulation in the reproductive organs.
- Release the pressure and a warm sensation runs down the lower extremities.
- Repeat the same procedure on the opposite side.
- Perform the massage twice a day, from day 6–14 of menstrual cycle.

31.7 Acupressure Fertility Massage Technique

It is an ancient Chinese technique in which pressure is applied to certain areas of the body called **acupressure points** (Fig. 31.2). It helps to increase balance and circulation and improve chances of fertility.

1. Ren 3**:** Stimulating this point helps to regulate the menses.
2. Ren 4**:** This is the site of the uterus, and stimulating this point increases chi energy to aid conception.
3. Ren 6**:** This point is also called the sea of Chi. Its stimulation increases energy and vitality to the whole body.
4. Zigong: The stimulation of this point increases blood flow to the ovaries.
5. St 30: It helps to increase the function of the ovaries, fallopian tubes, and uterus by releasing stagnation.

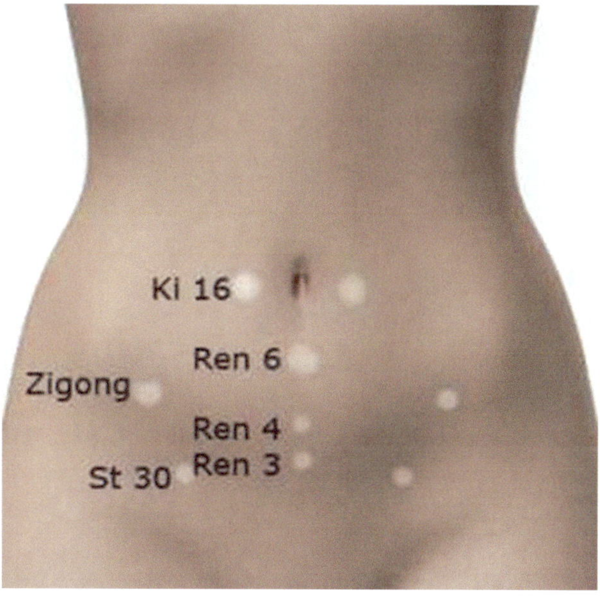

Fig. 31.2 Important acupressure points

31.8 Reflexology Fertility Massage Technique

There are certain areas on the feet that correspond to specific organs of the body. They are known as reflexology points (Fig. 31.3). When these points are stimulated or massaged with fingers, it clears blockage, thereby increasing circulation and encouraging the flow of energy to the organ.

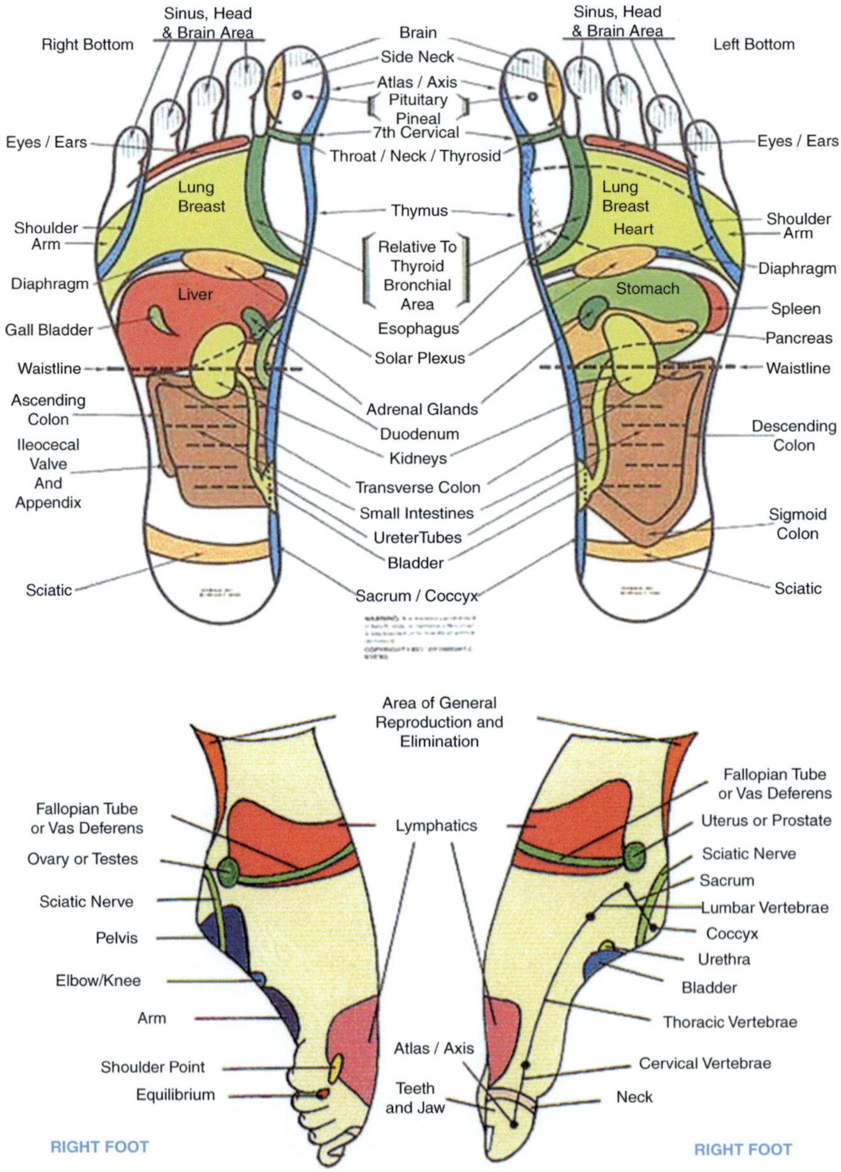

Fig. 31.3 Reflexology points

31.9 Acupuncture

Acupuncture involves insertion of ultrathin stainless steel needles into specific points on the body. Needles stimulate body meridians (channels of energy) along certain points. These points when needled regulate the way in which the body functions. It offers effective solutions for some cases of recurrent miscarriages by helping to increase blood flow to the ovaries, thereby resulting in better quality follicles and eggs. It also warms the uterus increasing blood flow and endometrial thickness. It normalizes the function of the hypothalamic-pituitary-ovarian axis and regulates body's hormonal production. It also helps males affected with sperm DNA fragmentation.

31.10 Fertility Yoga

Fertility yoga is gentle on the joints and promotes blood flow to the pelvic area while stretching and toning the body also. Meditation and pranayam along with yoga helps cognitive function and aids in balancing hormonal milieu.

31.10.1 The Bridge Pose

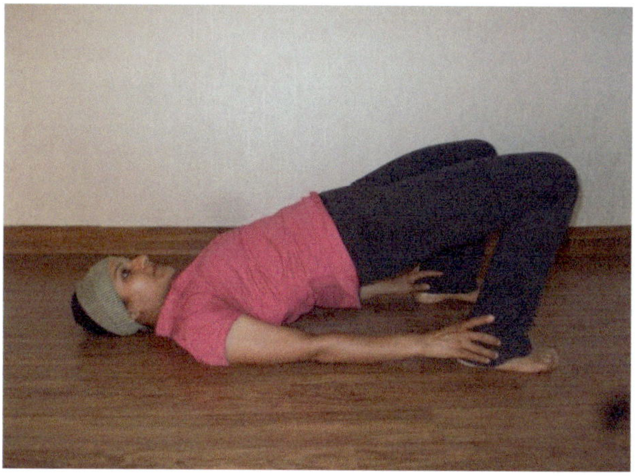

Clasp the back of the ankles with your hands and lift the pelvis. It helps energy to circulate to the uterus and ovaries and also slightly stimulates the thyroid gland. Hold this pose from 30 s to a couple of minutes; glutei muscles contract strengthening the pelvic girdle.

31.10.2 Cobra Pose

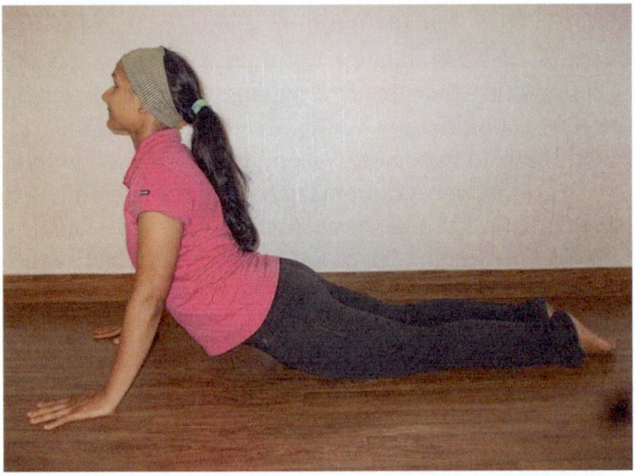

Lie prone, join both feet, and contract the glutei muscles. Lift body up, arms by the side of chest keeping wrists and shoulder at same level. This pose stimulates the hormones and brings energy to the uterus and ovaries.

31.10.3 Reclining Bound Angle Pose

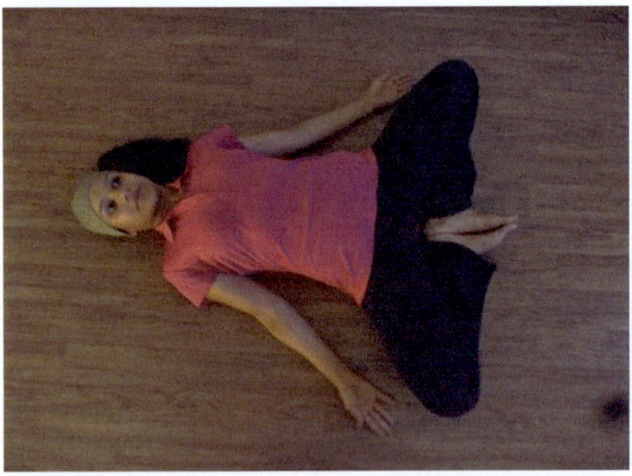

Stretch your legs in front of you. Bring your feet together, and place them flat on the floor, letting your knees fall out to the side. Lay back, open your arms, and breathe.

Key Points

- Non-pharmacological methods of management of RPL include lifestyle modifications, healthy diet, Ayurveda, various herbs, and other complementary methods like acupressure, acupuncture, and yoga.
- Antiphospholipid antibody syndrome which is linked to RPL has been reported to disappear with eradication of periodontal infection with *H. pylori.*
- Maca root contains glucosinolates which affect both men and women fertility by optimizing estrogen and progesterone levels as well as increasing libido.
- Honey, propolis, bee pollen, and royal jelly produced by bees are used for healing and enhancing fertility.
- Fertility massage is a powerful, noninvasive type of natural fertility treatment which increases blood circulation to pelvic organs, breaks down pelvic adhesions, resolves ovarian cysts, reduces dysmenorrhea, and regulates menstrual cycle.
- Fertility yoga promotes blood flow to the pelvic area and meditation, and pranayam along with yoga helps cognitive function and aids in balancing hormonal milieu.

References

1. Nybo Anderson AM, Wohlfahrt J, Christens P, Olsen J, Melbye M. Maternal age and fetal loss: population based register study. BMJ. 2000;320:1708–12.
2. Farrell S, Ide M, Wilson RF. The relationship between maternal periodontis, adverse pregnancy outcome and miscarriage in never smokers. J Clin Periodontol. 2006;33:115–20.
3. Mannem S, Chava VK. The relationship between maternal periodontitis and preterm low birth weight: a case control study. Contemp Clin Dent. 2011;2:88–93.
4. Abel EL. Maternal alcohol consumption and spontaneous abortion. Alcohol Alcohol. 1997;32:211–9.
5. Windham GC, Von Behren J, Fenster L, et al. Moderate maternal alcohol consumption and risk of spontaneous abortion. Epidemiology. 1997;8:509–14.
6. Rasch V. Cigarette, alcohol, and caffeine consumption: risk factors for spontaneous abortion. Acta Obstet Gynecol Scand. 2003;82:182–8.
7. Reprod Biomed Online. 2014;28(6):684–703. https://doi.org/10.1016/j.rbmo.2014.02.004. Epub 2014 Mar 4.
8. Weng X, Odouli R, Li DK. Maternal caffeine consumption during pregnancy and the risk of miscarriage: a prospective cohort study. Am J Obstet Gynecol. 2008;198(3):279.e1–8. [Medline].
9. Cnattingius S, Signorello LB, Anneren G, et al. Caffeine intake and the risk of first-trimester spontaneous abortion. N Engl J Med. 2000;343:1839–45.

10. Smith ML, Schust DJ. Endocrinology and recurrent pregnancy loss. Semin Reprod Med. 2011;29:482–90.
11. Rodriguez H. London school of hygiene and tropical medicine. Medical News Today. 2006.
12. Danielsson K. Homocysteine and miscarriage—what you should know. http://miscarriage.about.com/od/thrombophiliadisorders/p/homocysteine.htm
13. Glenville M. Miscarriage. (n.d). http://www.marilynglenville.com/womens-health-issues/miscarriage/–
14. Refsum H, Nurk E, Smith AD. WHO laboratory manual for the examination and processing of human semen. 5th ed. Cambridge: Cambridge University Press; 2010.
15. Erenpreiss J, Elzanaty S, Giwercman A. Sperm DNA damage in men from infertile couples. Asian J Androl. 2008;10:786–90.
16. Practice Committee of the American Society for Reproductive Medicine. The clinical utility of sperm DNA integrity testing: a guideline. Fertil Steril. 2013;99:673–7.
17. Kumar K, Deka D, Singh A, Mitra DK, Vanitha BR, Dada R. Predictive value of DNA integrity analysis in idiopathic recurrent pregnancy loss following spontaneous conception. J Assist Reprod Genet. 2012;29:861–7.
18. Aitken RJ, De luliis GN, Finnie JM, Hedges A, McLachlan RI. Analysis of the relationships between oxidative stress, DNA damage and sperm vitality in a patient population: development of diagnostic criteria. Hum Reprod. 2010;25:2415–26.
19. Takeda Y, Liu X, Sumiyoshi M, et al. Placenta expressing the greatest quantity of bisphenol A receptor ERR (gamma) among the human reproductive tissues: predominant expression of type-1 ERR gamma isoform. J Biochem. 2009;146:113–22.
20. Rogers JA, Metz L, Yong VW. Endocrine disrupting chemicals and immune responses: a focus on bisphenol A and its potential mechanisms. Mol Immunol. 2013;53:421–30.
21. http://EzineArticles.com/expert/Eric_Bakker_ND/517070 http://EzineArticles.com/?More-Plastic-Than-Plankton&id=4222200
22. Li DK, Liu L, Odouli R. Exposure to nonsteroidal anti-inflammatory drugs during pregnancy and risk of miscarriage: Population based cohort study. BMJ. 2003;327:368–72.
23. Madsen M, Jorgensen T, Jensen ML, Juhl M, Olsen J, Anderson PK, et al. Leisure time physical exercise during pregnancy and the risk of miscarriage: a study within the Danish National Birth Cohort. BJOG. 2007;114:1419–26.
24. Song GJ, Norkus EP, Lewis V. Relationship between seminal ascorbic and sperm DNA integrity in infertile men. Int J Androl. 2006;29:569–75.
25. Ebisch IM, Thomas CM, Peters WH, Braat DD, Steegers-Theunissen RP. The importance of folate, zinc and antioxidants in the pathogenesis and prevention of subfertility. Hum Reprod Update. 2007;13:163–74.
26. Zago MP, Oteiza PI. The antioxidant properties of zinc: interactions with iron and antioxidants. Free Radic Biol Med. 2001;31:266–74.
27. Littarru GP, Tiano L. Bioenergetic and antioxidant properties of coenzyme Q10: recent developments. Mol Biotechnol. 2007;37:31–7.
28. https://draxe.com/top-5-maca-root-benefits-and-nutrition/
29. Hellner M., Winter D., Von Georgi R., and Munstedt K. (2008). Apitherapy: usage and experience in German beekeepers. eCAM; 5(4)475–479. doi:https://doi.org/10.1093/ecam/nem052. downloads.hindawi.com/journals/ecam/2008/827582.pdf
30. Suzuki K-M, et al. Estrogenic activities of fatty acids and a sterol isolated from royal jelly. eCAM. 2008;5(3):295–302. https://doi.org/10.1093/ecam/nem036. http://downloads.hindawi.com/journals/ecam/2008/938757.pdf
31. en.wikipedia.org/wiki/Bee_pollen
32. Ingels D. Bee propolis may improve fertility in women with endometriosis fertility and sterility. 2003;80:S32.
33. Fetus: recurrent pregnancy loss in traditional Chinese medicine. In: Carp HJA, editors. Recurrent pregnancy loss : causes, controversies and treatment.
34. http://natural-fertility-info.com/preventing-miscarriage

Index

S. Mehta, B. Gupta (eds.), *Recurrent Pregnancy Loss*,
https://doi.org/10.1007/978-981-10-7338-0

K

L

MIX
Papier aus verantwortungsvollen Quellen
Paper from responsible sources
FSC® C105338

If you have any concerns about our products,
you can contact us on
ProductSafety@springernature.com

In case Publisher is established outside the EU,
the EU authorized representative is:
Springer Nature Customer Service Center GmbH
Europaplatz 3, 69115 Heidelberg, Germany

Printed by Libri Plureos GmbH
in Hamburg, Germany